ORGAN
PHYSIOLOGY

STRUCTURE
AND FUNCTION
OF THE
CARDIOVASCULAR
SYSTEM

Revised Reprint

With a Chapter on

ELECTRICAL ACTIVITY OF THE HEART

ROBERT F. RUSHMER, M.D.

Director, Center for Bioengineering, Professor and
Head, Division of Bioengineering, School of Medicine;
Professor of Bioengineering, College of Engineering,
University of Washington

1972

W. B. SAUNDERS COMPANY · PHILADELPHIA · LONDON · TORONTO

W. B. Saunders Company: West Washington Square
Philadelphia, Pa.   19105

12 Dyott Street
London, WC1A 1DB

833 Oxford Street
Toronto 18, Ontario

ORGAN PHYSIOLOGY — Structure and Function of the   ISBN 0-7216-7850-5
Cardiovascular System —
Revised Reprint

Print No.:   9   8   7   6   5   4   3   2   1

*This book is dedicated to
students interested in the cardiovascular system.*

PREFACE

This book (derived from CARDIOVASCULAR DYNAMICS, Third Edition) is intended for those interested from many viewpoints in the functional properties of the heart and blood vessels—from beginning students to professional cardiologists. The basic concepts of cardiovascular function and control were originally developed by means of experimental observations on excised tissues or exposed organs of animals under decidedly abnormal conditions. Since the functions of living tissues and organs are sensitive to changes induced by the process of measurement, the relevance of these concepts to the intact organism was not clear but was not commonly questioned. During the past twenty years, new techniques and technologies have been developed for continuously monitoring and quantitatively analyzing the function of internal organs in intact unanesthetized experimental animals capable of engaging in normal activity. Comprehensive descriptions of the changing function of the heart and blood vessels could be recorded during spontaneous activity, or responses to experimentally induced changes (i.e., administration of drugs, stimulation of neural structures or imposition of stresses). Fundamental discrepancies were immediately and consistently noted between the cardiovascular adaptations predicted from traditional concepts and those directly observed in these animals. On the basis of observations on intact animals, inquiries utilizing some of those techniques were directed to cardiovascular function in man. Despite the fact that quantitative measurements on human hearts and blood vessels tend to be available at relatively lower sampling rates (e.g., 1/second or 1/minute instead of 20 to 50/second), many similarities and some differences in relation to dogs and other animals could be identified. The slow sampling rates of many standard measurements on man had tended to provide a rather static picture of cardiovascular variables, but the higher frequency recordings provided more continuous indications of the fluctuations in heart size, blood pressure and blood flow and indicated the functional importance of dynamic properties of cardiovascular performance. Thus, the absolute values for pressure, dimensions or flow of blood in various components are important, but the rates of change of these variables during individual cycles or over more extended periods are just as important and perhaps more so.

In view of this history, the dynamics of the heart and blood vessels are described by drawing heavily upon rather extensive and diverse investigations in our own laboratories as they have influenced our total picture of the mechanisms involved. The observations of other investigators are included as appears essential, but it is clear that no attempt has been made to survey the fund of experimental knowledge available from the past. Instead, the structure and function of the cardiovascular system is described as specifically as possible with little discussion of alternative opinions or controversial viewpoints. It is heavily biased because of a large number of personal observations on many and diverse experimental preparations which have thoroughly colored our view of the way in which this intriguing system works. Many of the concepts are illustrated by schematic diagrams which are rendered as realistic as possible without sacrificing clarity.

ROBERT F. RUSHMER

ACKNOWLEDGMENTS

A BOOK OF THIS SORT represents a small sample of facts and concepts selectively extracted from a vast store of material on the subject. The final content of this manuscript has been greatly influenced by a series of investigations accomplished in association with a closely knit research team representing several fields of interest. The ingenuity, persistence and technical competence of this group were indispensable to the successful completion of the studies summarized in this text. The various research projects were supported in part by grants from the National Heart Institute of the National Institutes of Health, United States Public Health Service; the Washington State Heart Association and the American Heart Association.

Sandy Ritz carried the heavy secretarial load and I gratefully acknowledge her interest, cooperation and patience in the preparation of the manuscript. I gratefully acknowledge the wholehearted cooperation of the W. B. Saunders Company in the production of the book.

Most of the illustrations from the first edition were designed and executed by the author although many were refined and labeled by Miss Jessie Phillips, Miss Virginia Brooks and Mrs. Mary Jane Owens. The relatively small number of signed drawings is no indication of the extent of their contribution to the illustrations in the book. New illustrations were prepared by Mrs. Helen Halsey from rough sketches.

Several of the original illustrations in this book first appeared in articles by the author and his associates in the following journals: *American Journal of Physiology* (Fig. 7-10); *Circulation* (Figs. 2-13, 2-14, 5-2); *Circulation Research* (Figs. 3-6, 5-13); *Handbook of Physiology, Section II, Vol. I* (Figs. 3-18, 6-13, 6-14); *Physiological Reviews* (Figs. 7-4, 7-5, 7-9). I wish to express my appreciation to the publishers of these journals for permission to reproduce the illustrations.

ROBERT F. RUSHMER, M.D.

CONTENTS

CHAPTER 7

CHAPTER 8

CHAPTER 1

PROPERTIES OF THE VASCULAR SYSTEM

Living cells possess many of the attributes of microscopic chemical factories, containing many complex chemical processes producing molecular transformations to perform various specialized functions. Unicellular organisms contain all the mechanisms required to sustain life within a single membranous cell boundary. Multicellular organisms are made up of cells serving many different functions through the evolutionary process of specialization. All cells survive only so long as the logistics of metabolism are successfully met by an influx of oxygen, metabolic fuels and chemical components involved in the physiochemical processing (Fig. 1–1). Waste products, including carbon dioxide and toxic excretions, must be carried away at a rate which limits their accumulation. Some cells release energy (i.e., electrical excitation processes), others can perform external work (i.e., skeletal muscles) and virtually all cells produce heat which must be eliminated into the external environment. Our ability to perform external work often appears to be limited by the rate of delivery of the material which is used at the fastest rate in relation to its storage capacity within the body, namely oxygen. Many other tissues produce no external work

(i.e., producing movement of masses) but perform other useful functions such as the elimination of heat by the skin, digestion and absorption of foodstuffs in the gut, secretion of waste products by the kidney and elaboration of hormones by endocrine glands. In most of these tissues, the levels of activity are not limited by the rate of oxygen delivery to the tissues under normal conditions. In all tissues, the logistics of metabolism are effectively carried on by the combined effects of convection (currents of fluids near cells) and of diffusion.

Unicellular organisms such as amoebae live in large expanses of water with which they exchange these substances continuously, primarily by the process of diffusion. Diffusion is the movement of particles from regions of high concentration into regions of lower concentration. If a drop of dye is placed in a beaker of motionless water, the molecules of dye will gradually disperse until finally they are uniformly distributed throughout the water (Fig. 1–2A). This dispersion results from thermal agitation producing random movement of molecules (Brownian movement) such that at any moment more molecules are moving away from the source of dye than are moving toward it. If dye, salt, sugar and urea are

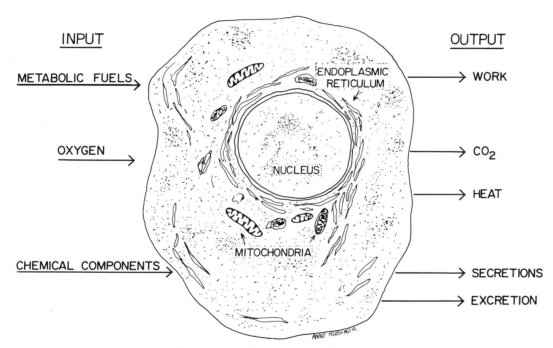

FIGURE 1–1   LOGISTICS OF METABOLISM

The nutrition of cells involves the delivery of oxygen, metabolic fuels and chemical constituents to the cells engaged in physicochemical processes to produce an output of work, CO_2 heat, secretions and excretions. The circulatory system of complex organisms must maintain an appropriate balance between the metabolic activity, the rate of delivery and the rate of removal of the chemical products from cellular activity.

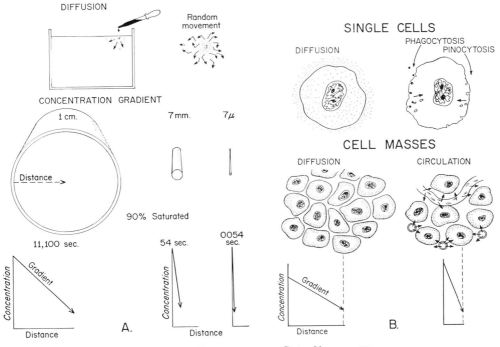

FIGURE 1–2 DIFFUSION AND CELL NUTRITION

A, The Process of Diffusion. Substances dissolved or suspended in a continuous fluid medium tend to become uniformly dispersed as the particles move from regions of higher concentration to regions of lower concentration through thermal agitation (Brownian movement). The rate of diffusion is determined by the steepness of the concentration gradient.

B, Nutrition of Cells. Many cells display active imbibition of solid particles (phagocytosis) and of droplets of fluid (pinocytosis) by envelopment or vesicle formation. Single cells may be nourished by diffusion alone. Small cell masses can also be nourished by diffusion. The concentration gradients are flattened and transport is slow. In large cell masses, steep concentration gradients are maintained by circulation of nutrient fluids or blood into the immediate vicinity of the individual cells in each tissue.

placed in four different regions of the water-filled beaker, they will all achieve uniform distribution by movement of each molecular species from the region of its high concentration into regions of its lower concentration.

By random movement, a molecule of water could theoretically pass from a man's head to his toe unassisted by circulation or flow currents, but this would require more than 100 years. The same molecule could cover a distance of 1.5 μ in approximately 0.003 second. In any particular continuous fluid phase the rate at which a substance diffuses depends primarily upon the steepness of the concentration gradient.

A cylinder of tissue 1 cm. in diameter, suddenly placed in an atmosphere of 100 per cent oxygen, would become 90 per cent saturated with oxygen after 11,100 seconds (about three hours). If the diameter of the cylinder were only 0.7 mm., the same degree of saturation would occur in 54 seconds (Fig. 1–2A). A single cell 7 μ in diameter would be saturated in .0054 second.[1] As the distance of diffusion from the surface to the center of the tissue is reduced the concentration gradient becomes very steep and diffusion occurs very rapidly. In general, a single cell, bathed in an expanse of nutrient fluid, can survive by diffusion alone (Fig. 1–2B). As the cell utilizes oxygen, its concentration drops in the protoplasm and other molecules of oxygen diffuse toward the cell from regions of higher concentration outside.

In addition, many different types of cells have the ability to engulf particles (phagocytosis) or to imbibe droplets of fluid in the form of vesicles which may move toward the center of the cell. This process of vesicle formation has long been known to occur in amoebae and has been called pinocytosis, i.e., "drinking" by cells. Infolding

of the cell membrane produces a tiny pouch which envelops a droplet of extracellular fluid (Fig. 1–2B). This process is receiving greatly increased attention since electron micrographs of many different mammalian cells show circular rings which appear to be vesicles. Indeed, this process has been proposed as a mechanism for active transport of materials across the capillary endothelium (see Chapter 4).

As cells group together to form more complex organisms, the distance of diffusion to the center of the mass increases and the shallow diffusion gradient limits the rate of transfer of various substances (Fig. 1–2B). Such organisms must either subsist on low levels of metabolism or develop a circulatory system.

In a large complex mass of cells, like the mammalian body, rapid diffusion along steep concentration gradients is achieved by providing a continuous flow of blood in the vicinity of all cells. The streams of blood must be contained within channels which retard diffusion only minimally. These requirements are satisfied by hundreds of millions of thin-walled capillaries distributed profusely throughout every portion of the body. The capillary density (number of capillaries/volume of tissue) reflects the tissue's requirements for blood flow. With the specialization of cells and tissues into complex organisms, blood flow must not only supply metabolic needs but also serve other functions such as dissipation of heat, movement, secretion, absorption and excretion (see Chapter 4).

In mammalian forms, blood with high concentrations of oxygen and nutritive substances and with low concentrations of carbon dioxide and metabolites is brought into the vicinity of each cell in the body. In skeletal muscle, for example, each capillary serves tissue with a volume only about twelve times its own. Thus, the diffusion distances are very small and the concentration gradients are extremely steep so long as the capillary blood flow is not interrupted. When capillary flow ceases, the concentration gradients immediately begin to flatten and diffusion slows as the various substances approach uniform dispersion through the fluids. If the utilization of oxygen and metabolic fuels increases, their concentrations in the cells are reduced and the steeper concentration gradients accelerate diffusion. Faster capillary flow is then required to maintain maximally steep diffusion gradients.

Blood pumped by the heart is distributed to the billions of capillaries by a diffuse arborization of the arterial tree with a single artery giving off branches which divide and subdivide to produce a complicated ramification. In the same way, blood leaving the capillaries returns to the heart by way of venous channels which have similar ramifications. The functional properties of the circulatory system reflect this architectural arrangement.

THE SYSTEMIC CIRCULATION

The patterns of circulation in various tissues have been the subject of widespread investigation in many laboratories. Until recently, the caliber, length, volume and total cross-sectional area of various components of the systemic circulation have been based on data from dead and fixed material. Wiedeman[3] described geometrical relations of the microcirculation and the branching arterial and venous channels in live animals. (Fig. 1–3). In accordance with previous concepts, the cross-sectional area increases at each branch point along the main arterial and venous trunks (Fig. 1–3A, C). The caliber of the veins is considerably greater than that of corresponding arterial channels. In the microcirculation, capillaries branch off arterioles (Fig. 1–3B) and frequently form branching networks such that the total cross section of venous capillaries and postcapillary venules is much greater than any other segment of the vascular tree (Fig. 1–3D). The volume of blood contained within the capillaries and arterioles is relatively small, particularly in comparison with postcapillary venules, venules and small veins (Fig. 1–3E). Thus, the capillaries contain a small and relatively fixed quantity of blood, the arterial system contains a larger but relatively constant quantity of blood and the veins contain a major portion of the total blood and can change their capacity to accommodate quite large variations in total and regional blood volume.

Visualization of the systemic circulation can be simplified by means of a schematic drawing in which all the capillaries are arranged in parallel (Fig. 1–4) and all arterial branches having the same caliber are arranged one above the other. Similarly, the corresponding branches of the venous system are vertically oriented. In this way it is possible to demonstrate the effects of the branching arterial and venous systems on the pressure and flow of blood in corresponding segments of the circulatory tree.

VOLUME FLOW THROUGH VARIOUS SEGMENTS OF THE CIRCULATORY SYSTEM

The anatomic complexity of the peripheral circulatory distribution tends to obscure some very basic principles which are obvious in a single tube. For example, if fluid flows into

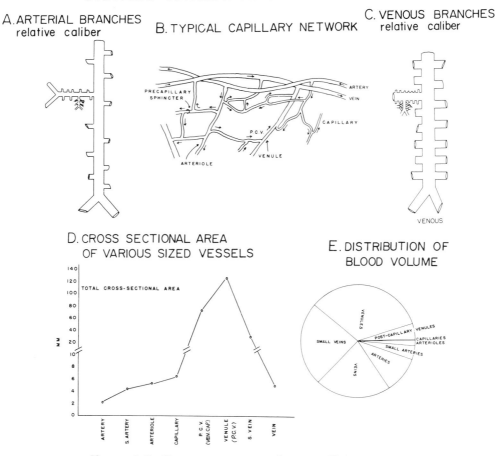

FIGURE 1–3   COMPONENTS OF THE SYSTEMIC CIRCULATION

A, The relative caliber of the aorta and its main branches are illustrated to show the increasing cross-sectional area with arborization.

B, Typical capillary networks are complex channels with flow regulated by arterioles and precapillary sphincters. (From Wiedeman, M. P., in Handbook of Physiology, Section 2: Circulation, Vol. II. W. F. Hamilton and P. Dow, eds. Washington, D. C., American Physiological Society, 1963.)

C, The relative caliber of the systemic veins is generally greater than the corresponding branches of the arterial system.

D, The cross-sectional area of the peripheral vessels increases gradually going from arteries to capillaries and then expands enormously at the postcapillary venule (more commonly known as venous capillaries) and even more at venules.

E, The total blood volume is distributed with the smallest amount in capillaries and the greatest amount on the venous side of the circulation, particularly the venules and small veins. (Presented through courtesy of Mary Wiedeman.[3])

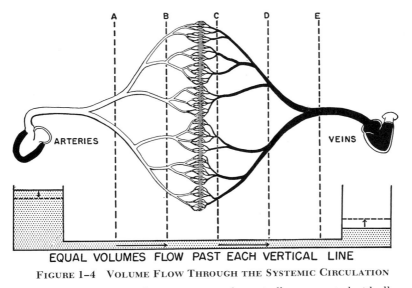

FIGURE 1–4   VOLUME FLOW THROUGH THE SYSTEMIC CIRCULATION

Arborization of the systemic circulatory system is schematically represented with all vessels of the same caliber arranged vertically. This simplified illustration emphasizes the fact that the volume of fluid flowing past each vertical line in a unit time must be equal to the quantity entering and leaving the system, just as in a single tube.

the single straight tube at the bottom of Figure 1–4 at a rate of 5 liters per minute, the same quantity of fluid must flow out of the tube. Similarly, 5 liters must flow past each of the vertical lines (A, B, C, D, E) during each minute. The only possible exception to this rule would result from a net shift of fluid from one segment to another. Such a redistribution of fluid would produce transient and relatively insignificant differences in the flow past the various regions of the tube. A schematic representation such as Figure 1–4 shows the general applicability of this rule in the systemic circulation, namely; the quantity of blood flowing past each vertical line is exactly equal to the quantity pumped into the system and the quantity leaving the system per unit time, except for slight and transient differences due to redistribution of the fluid volumes within the system. It is true that the

flow may be greater through one parallel channel than through another, but the total flow through all corresponding segments must be essentially identical. This very simple principle is neglected in many discussions of circulatory dynamics.

CROSS-SECTIONAL AREA OF THE CIRCULATORY SYSTEM
(Fig. 1-5)

When an artery or vein bifurcates, the cross-sectional area of its branches exceeds that of the parent vessel. The number of vessels formed by this branching is so great that the estimated cross-sectional area of the capillaries is approximately 625 sq. cm. in a 13 kg. dog with an aortic area of only 0.8 sq. cm.[2] This peak value from Green[2] is retained in Figure 1–5, but the maximum cross-sectional area has been shifted toward the region of the post-

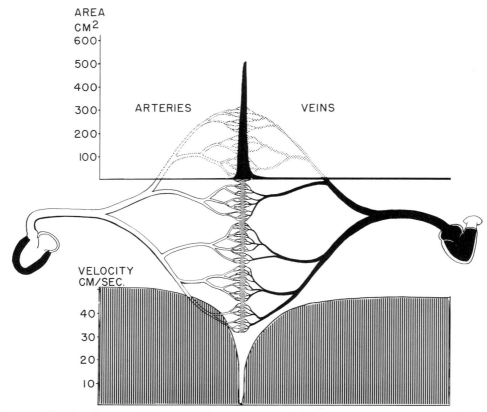

FIGURE 1–5   THE RELATION BETWEEN CROSS-SECTIONAL AREA AND THE VELOCITY OF FLOW IN THE SYSTEMIC CIRCULATION

Cross-sectional areas of various segments of the systemic circulation computed for a 13 kg. dog. Note the tremendous area in the arterioles, capillaries and venules. The velocity of blood flow is inversely proportional to the cross-sectional area so that blood flows through the capillaries at about 0.07 cm. per second (see reference 2).

capillary venule as suggested by Wiedeman's more recent data (see Fig. 1–3D). Since the volumes of blood flowing through corresponding segments of the system are equal, changes in cross-sectional area affect the velocity of blood flow.

VELOCITY OF BLOOD FLOW
(Fig. 1–5)

Just as water in a rushing stream slows down when it enters a broad pool, so the velocity of flow is reduced in regions of the circulation with large cross-sectional areas. In the aorta, blood travels at an average velocity of 40 to 50 cm. per second, and in the capillaries it moves at about 0.07 cm. per second.[2] Slow flow in the peripheral capillaries provides time for the exchange of materials across the capillary walls. After passing into the veins, the blood again accelerates as the cross-sectional area progressively decreases. However, the caliber of the veins exceeds that of corresponding arteries, so the velocity of venous blood only approaches and does not equal that of the arterial blood. It is obviously necessary to distinguish between volume flow and velocity of blood flow. The volume flow of blood through a particular tube depends upon the pressure gradient, the resistance to flow and the physical characteristics of blood.

Resistance to Blood Flow in the Circulation
(Fig. 1–6)

Fluid flows through tubes in response to a gradient in pressure. The progressive reduction in the pressure of fluid passing through a tube of constant bore represents the energy which is lost as heat due to friction, i.e., heat lost in the collisions of the moving molecules composing the fluid. The difference between the pressures at the two ends of a tube is a measure of the frictional loss of energy or of the resistance to the flow of fluid. For example, consider a laminar flow of water through the horizontal tubes in Figure 1–6. The pressure gradient is indicated by the height of the columns of water in the vertical tubes. In a tube of constant bore, the pressure drop is directly proportional to the length of the tube. Thus, if the length of the tube is doubled, the magnitude of the pressure drop is also doubled. During passage of a homogeneous fluid through the segment labeled R, the pressure drop is given as 1 cm. of water. During

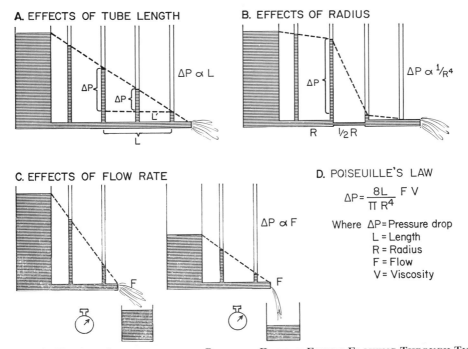

FIGURE 1–6   FACTORS INFLUENCING THE PRESSURE DROP IN FLUIDS FLOWING THROUGH TUBES (POISEUILLE'S LAW)

A, The drop in pressure (ΔP) during laminar flow of a homogeneous fluid through a rigid tube of constant caliber is directly proportional to the length of the tube.

B, Under the same conditions, the pressure drop is also inversely proportional to the reciprocal of the radius to the fourth power ($1/R^4$) and directly proportional to the volume flow (C) through the tube and to the viscosity (V) of the fluid. The relationships between these factors are included in the formula which is an expression of Poiseuille's law (D).

passage through the next segment, where the radius is only ½ R, the pressure drop is 16 cm. of water. The frictional resistance, as indicated by the pressure gradient, is proportional to $1/R^4$ (the reciprocal of the fourth power of the radius) so that reducing radius by one-half increases the pressure drop sixteenfold. The pressure drop is also directly proportional to the rate of flow. Finally, the pressure drop along a tube is directly proportional to the viscosity of the fluid. The interrelationships of these factors have been combined in a formula (Fig. 1–6) which summarizes Poiseuille's law for streamlined flow of viscous fluids through rigid tubes of constant caliber.

Poiseuille's law cannot be quantitatively applied to the circulatory system for several reasons: (a) Blood vessels are not rigid; they stretch in response to an increase in pressure. Elevated internal pressure may produce an increase in both radius and length. For this reason, the pressure and the dimensions of the tube are not independently variable. (b) Plasma is a truly viscous fluid, but whole blood is not. If plasma is perfused through an ordinary rigid tube, even the smallest differential pressure will produce some flow. On the contrary, when whole blood is perfused through the vascular system of an animal's extremity, no flow is produced until the pressure gradient from arteries to veins reaches 10 mm. Hg (even more in the presence of vasoconstriction). (c) Blood is not a homogeneous fluid since it contains large number of cellular elements which affect its flow through the vascular system.

PRESSURE GRADIENTS IN THE CIRCULATORY TREE

While Poiseuille's law is not entirely applicable to the circulatory system, the factors illustrated in Figure 1–6 apply in a qualitative sense. As the arterial blood pressure and the length of the vessels tend to remain relatively fixed and the viscosity of the blood has limited variability from moment to moment, the caliber of the vessels unquestionably plays a predominant role in determining both the pressure gradients and the flow through various segments of the circulatory system (Fig. 1–7). The blood flows through the major arterial trunks with little frictional loss, as indicated by the very gradual drop in the mean arterial pressure. As the arteries divide and sub-

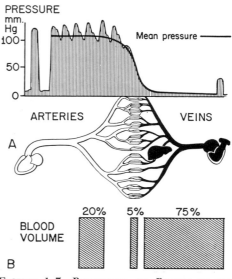

FIGURE 1–7 PRESSURES OF BLOOD IN THE SYSTEMIC CIRCULATION

A, The pressures in the arterial system are elevated and pulsatile. The mean arterial pressure declines very gradually as blood flows through the main branches of the arterial tree. In the small vessels, the pressure head diminishes rapidly and the fluctuations are damped out because of the high resistance to flow. In the major veins, the pressure gradient is again very shallow.

B, The volume of blood in the arteries is relatively fixed at about 20 per cent of the total. The veins contain about 75 per cent of the systemic blood volume but can alter their capacity over a wide range.

divide, the caliber of the vessels diminishes and the pressure gradients become correspondingly steeper. Some 80 per cent of the pressure drop along the arterial channels occurs in the terminal arteries and arterioles. Similarly, the confluence of veins is associated with a reduction in resistance as blood flows from the capillaries toward the heart. In the larger veins blood flows briskly in response to very shallow pressure gradients. The marked increase in resistance in the small vessels produces a precipitous fall in pressure which forms a functional line of demarcation between the arterial and the venous portions of the systemic circulation (Fig. 1-7).

THE RELATION BETWEEN CROSS-SECTIONAL AREA, FLOW VELOCITY AND FLOW RESISTANCE

The effects of the reduction in the caliber of a single vessel are quite different from those of a corresponding reduction in the caliber of many branching channels. The differences are presented schematically in Figure 1–8. A constricted section in a single tube (Fig. 1–8) results in a much greater resistance (pressure drop per unit length) and a much greater flow velocity. The same volume of fluid flowing through the large segment must rush through the smaller seg-

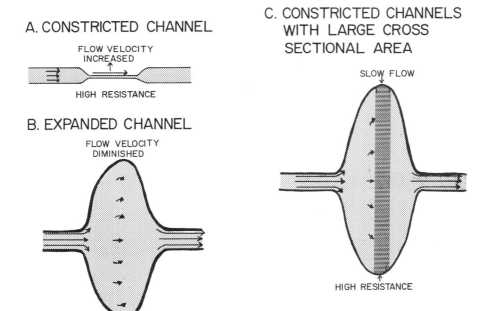

FIGURE 1–8 HYDRAULIC RESISTANCE IN BRANCHED CHANNELS OF VARYING CALIBER

A, A local constriction in a single channel produces increased flow velocity, greater resistance and steeper pressure drop.

B, In a locally expanded channel, the flow velocity, hydraulic resistance and pressure drop are all greatly diminished.

C, Liquid flowing through an expanded channel filled with many small caliber channels has low velocity, high resistance and steep pressure drop.

ment. In contrast, the flow velocity, resistance to flow and the pressure gradient per unit length are greatly reduced as liquid flows through a region of greatly increased cross-sectional area (Fig. 1–8B). Imagine the midportion of this expanded channel filled with tightly packed capillary tubes as suggested in Figure 1–8C. In this case, the flow velocity would still drop as the cross-sectional area expands, but the flow resistance and pressure drop would be greatly increased by the frictional resistance to flow of liquid through the short lengths of small caliber tubes. The same type of situation prevails in the branching arterial system and microcirculation as illustrated in Figure 1–5.

FUNCTIONS OF SYSTEMIC ARTERIES

The systemic arteries serve as a pressure reservoir by means of the elastic properties of the walls (Fig. 1–9A). The contracting left ventricle rapidly ejects blood into the aorta, which becomes distended as the arterial pressure rises. When the ventricle relaxes, the inflow ceases but the wall tension in the arteries continues to drive blood through the peripheral capillaries. The arterial pressure falls progressively until the next ventricular contraction. By this mechanism the systemic arterial pressure fluctuates above and below a mean pressure of about 90 mm. Hg and never falls to zero.

The aortic arch functions as a type of surge chamber immediately downstream from the left ventricle (Fig. 1–9A). Left ventricular ejection produces a very abrupt acceleration of blood into the arterial system which contains long columns of blood. If the arterial system were rigid, very high

pressures would develop throughout the system during contraction of the ventricles. The arterial perfusion pressure would drop to zero between ventricular contractions. The highly distensible aortic arch serves a function very much like the surge chamber often used to damp out large pressure surges produced by piston pumps as shown in Figure 1–9B. In this instance, the air is compressed during the ejection stroke and maintains pressure during the filling stroke. The function of arteries and the regulation of arterial pressure are discussed further in Chapter 5.

The pressure in an elastic tube is an expression of the tension exerted by its walls. Increased internal pressure can be attained by four mechanisms: (a) increased distention by accumulation of fluid, (b) active contraction of the walls without a change in contained volume, (c) external compression and (d) the hydrostatic effects of continuous columns of blood. If the arteries displayed purely elastic properties, the pressure-volume relations would be constant. In other words, so long as the mean arterial pressure remained the same, the mean volume of blood within the arterial system would also be constant. We know that the caliber of arteries in situ may be actively reduced by topically applied epinephrine.[4] The actual amount of significance of active constriction of the arteries is not known. In general, the arterial system is considered to have a relatively constant volume so long as the arterial pressure remains fixed.

Relatively small increments of volume change in the arteries produce large changes in pressure. For example, the arterial pulse wave at rest represents a large pressure fluctuation induced by the sudden injection of some 80 cc. of blood into the central end of the arterial system. In contrast,

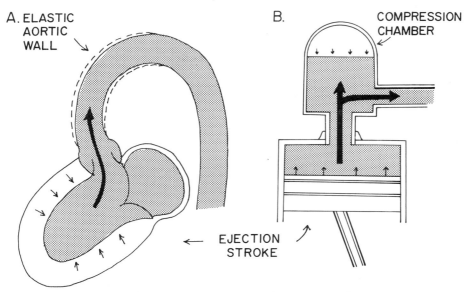

FIGURE 1–9 THE AORTIC ARCH AS A COMPRESSION CHAMBER

A, The elastic wall of the aorta distends during ejection of blood from the heart, storing pressure energy for gradual release during the interval between beats.

B, Air in a compression chamber attached to a piston pump is put under pressure during the ejection stroke and expands again during the filling stroke, damping violent fluctuations in pressure and flow.

a similar quantity of blood leaves the venous system at approximately equivalent rates during each cardiac cycle, but the venous pressure varies only a few millimeters of mercury during each cycle. This fact points up the principal differences between the relatively fixed-capacity arterial pressure reservoir and the variable-capacity, low pressure, venous volume reservoir.

THE TENSILE STRENGTH OF VASCULAR WALLS

The walls of the large arteries and veins are so thick and tough that their bursting pressure ranges in the thousands of millimeters of mercury. Interposed between the arteries and veins lie the capillaries which have exceedingly small diameters and very thin walls. Capillary walls are composed of a single layer of very thin endothelial cells. The wall thickness is of the order of a micron or less, very much smaller than the diameter of a red blood cell as illustrated in Figure 1–10. The endothelial cells are joined at their edges to form a flimsy cylindrical channel. The capillary endothelium is very easily deformed and exhibits very little tensile strength. The junctions between the edges of the endothelial cells appear in electron micrographs as being even more delicate (Fig. 1–10*B*). Thin walls and small caliber are required in capillaries for the rapid diffusion of substances between the blood and tissues. The delicate capillary walls support pressure amounting to 20 to 30 mm. Hg at heart level and more than 100 mm. Hg in the lower extremities during standing. At first sight, it is difficult to visualize how the fragile capillaries

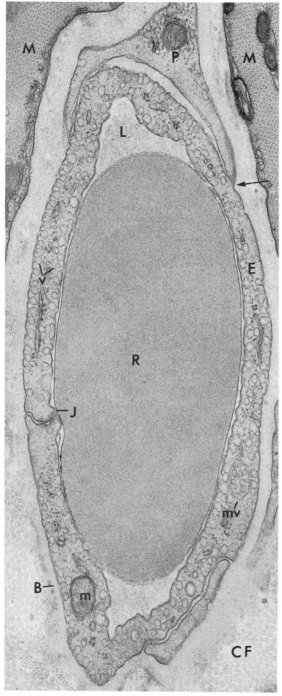

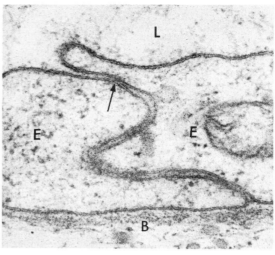

FIGURE 1–10   FINE STRUCTURE
OF CAPILLARIES

A, Capillaries are cylindrical channels formed of flat endothelial cells joined at their edges. The caliber of the capillary is about the same as the diameter of a red blood cell (R). Ring-like structures ("vesicles") are more abundant near both surfaces and have been assigned a role in transport of substances across the capillary walls.

B, The junction between adjacent endothelial cell edges appears to be tightly sealed, apparently lacking slits, pores or sieve-like structures postulated as necessary for the exchange of most constituents in the plasma. (Figs. 15–3 and 15–7 in R. S. Cotran, Fine structure of the microvasculature in relation to normal and altered permeability, in Physical Basic of Circulatory Transport, E. B. Reeve and A. C. Guyton, eds., Philadelphia: W. B. Saunders Co.).

can support such very high internal pressures. The explanation lies in the very small caliber of these vessels.

THE RELATION BETWEEN PRESSURE, WALL TENSION AND CALIBER OF VESSELS

This relationship is graphically illustrated by a partially inflated rubber balloon.[5] During inflation, the mid-portion of the balloon expands while the distal portion remains undistended (Fig. 1–11). The portion of the balloon with a large radius is very tense and resists indentation, indicating that the walls are under high tension. The pressure is equal throughout the inside of the balloon and yet in the undistended region the walls are relatively flaccid and can be easily compressed.[5] This commonplace example illustrates the law of Laplace ($T \propto p \times$

R), which states that the tension in the wall of a hollow cylinder is directly proportional to the product of the tube's radius and the pressure being supported by the wall. Burton,[6] applying this law to the vascular system, pointed out that an aorta with a radius of 1.3 cm. supports a pressure of 100 mm. Hg with a wall tension of 170,000 dynes per centimeter of length (Fig. 1–11). In contrast, capillaries with a radius of 4μ support a pressure of some 30 mm. Hg with a wall tension of only 16 dynes per centimeter of length. In other words, the pressure in the aorta is about three or four times as great as that in the capillaries while the radius is some three thousand times as great. Therefore, the wall tension in the aorta is about ten thousand times as great as that in the capillaries. In tubes of very small caliber, no great strength is required to support a high internal pressure. By the same token, the capillary walls can be very thin so that the distance of diffusion from the central portion of the capillary blood to the outside can be very short. These physical attributes of the capillaries are essential to their function.

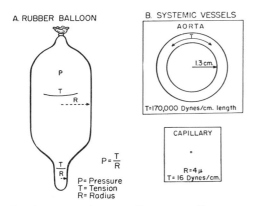

FIGURE 1–11   THE RELATION BETWEEN PRESSURE, WALL TENSION AND RADIUS IN HOLLOW ORGANS

A, In a partially expanded balloon, internal pressure is constant throughout, but the wall tension is very much greater in the distended portion than in the undistended tip because of the difference in radius. As the radius increases, the wall tension must also increase to support a given pressure.

B, Because of the tremendous differences in radius, the wall tension is approximately 10,000 times as great in the aorta as in a capillary, even though they support similar pressures.

THE STRUCTURE AND FUNCTION OF CAPILLARIES

A major portion of the pressure drop between the arteries and veins occurs at the points of controlled resistance at the entrance to the capillary channels (see Fig. 1–7). In addition, a fairly steep pressure gradient along the capillaries is required to maintain flow because of their small caliber. The velocity of blood flow is less in the capillaries than elsewhere because of their tremendous total cross-sectional area (Fig. 1-5). For the same reason, the total surface area of capillary walls is very extensive, particularly in relation to the quantity of blood within each capillary vessel and the total volume of the capillary beds (see Fig. 1–3E). All the blood in the capillaries comes very close to the extravascular tissue spaces, a condition essential for the rapid transfer of substances by diffusion.

Ions and small molecules diffuse across the capillary walls at a surprising rate. Flexner and his associates[7, 8] studied this problem with radioactive tracers and concluded that 60 per cent of the sodium in plasma was exchanged for extravascular sodium in one minute. Similarly, 64 per cent of the chloride in plasma and 140 per cent of the water were calculated to be exchanged each minute.[7] Using more quantitative techniques, Pappenheimer et al.[9] obtained evidence that the amount of water and lipid-insoluble molecules transferred is some two hundred times greater than the values calculated by Flexner and his group (see also Chapter 4). They found that the area of the capillary walls available for diffusion of a molecule the size of water is less than 0.2 per cent of the total wall surface. Ultramicroscopic holes or "pores" in the capillary wall with uniform diameters of 30 Angstrom units (A) account very well for the diffusion rates of fat-insoluble molecules ranging in size from that of sodium chloride to that of hemoglobin. The data could also be explained by a range of pore dimensions with a mean of 24 A and a standard deviation of 12 A. The total area of the "pores" is so small that they may be localized to the spaces between adjacent endothelial cells. Renkin[10] presented evidence that lipid-soluble substances may diffuse through the capillary endothelium so that capillary exchange of oxygen and carbon dioxide may utilize the entire capillary wall.

THE STRUCTURE OF CAPILLARY WALLS

The endothelial cells resemble fried eggs in shape and are only about 1μ thick except at the nucleus (Fig. 1–12). According to earlier studies these flat cells were believed to be joined at their edges by a substance called intercellular cement, which was visualized as composed of long chain molecules bridging the slit between adjacent cells. Interstices between these molecules have been considered responsible for the sieve-like properties of capillary walls and may correspond to the "pores" described previously.

The number and scale of capillaries defies the imagination. Krogh's oft quoted figures are believed to overestimate the numbers somewhat (see Majno[11]), but are still qualitatively revealing.

"It requires some mental effort to conceive how there can be room (on an area no larger than the cross section of an ordinary pin) for about 700 parallel tubes carrying blood, in addition to about 200 (skeletal) muscle fibers." Based on light microscopy, several pathways have been proposed to account for the movement of molecules and particles, large and small, to pass from the blood through the capillary wall and into the spaces between the cells in various tissues (Fig. 1–12). For example, penetration through endothelial cells has been widely accepted for small lipid-soluble molecules like oxygen and carbon dioxide and for water. Passage of other substances (including small inorganic and organic molecules and proteins) may be largely restricted by these cell membranes and occur only through the junctions between the edges of endothelial cells. The simplified schematic representation, as in Figure

STRUCTURE AND PERMEABILITY OF CAPILLARIES

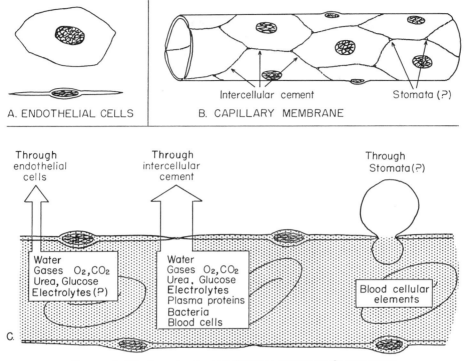

A. ENDOTHELIAL CELLS | B. CAPILLARY MEMBRANE

Intercellular cement   Stomata (?)

Through endothelial cells

Through intercellular cement

Through Stomata(?)

Water
Gases O_2, CO_2
Urea, Glucose
Electrolytes (?)

Water
Gases O_2, CO_2
Urea, Glucose
Electrolytes
Plasma proteins
Bacteria
Blood cells

Blood cellular elements

C.

FIGURE 1–12   STRUCTURE AND PERMEABILITY OF CAPILLARIES

Capillaries are formed of endothelial cells joined at their edges by "intercellular cement" to form tubes. It seems likely that water, gases, small organic molecules and possibly certain electrolytes can pass through the endothelial cells. Most of the capillary exchange probably occurs through the intercellular cement (see text). It has been postulated that blood cellular elements pass through orifices between endothelial cells, called stomata.

1–12, fails to take proper cognizance of the complexity of individual capillaries or the differences in anatomical and functional characteristics of capillaries in various tissues in the body. (See also Chapter 4 for further discussion.) The functional anatomy of capillaries has been studied intensively in recent years, particularly since electron microscopes became readily available. This body of knowledge has been ably reviewed by Majno[11] and by Contran,[12] while the functional aspects of capillary exchange have been summarized by Landis and Pappenheimer.[13]

In spite of the enormous surface area presented by the walls of millions of capillary tubes, these very thin endothelial membranes greatly retard the movement of most molecules involved in the capillary exchange processes. Water, ions and molecules in the plasma, which are relatively insoluble in lipids, are effectively retarded or blocked by the endothelial cell membranes, yet they are known to exchange rapidly between the blood and extravascular spaces. This discrepancy has been explained on the basis that the rapid capillary exchange of lipid insoluble substances must occur along the lines of junction where the edges of the endothelial cells are joined together (Fig. 1–12). For many years, the intercellular junctions were confidently regarded as the site of slits, pores or sieve-like structures through which most of the exchange took place.

This widely accepted concept was challenged when electron microscopes were employed to provide greatly increased magnification and resolution of the fine structure of capillaries. Electronmicrograms apparently failed to disclose the "pores, slits or sieves" and indicated that the lines of adhesion between the edges of endothelial cells were "anatomically tight junctions." (See Figure 1–10B.) In addition, the endothelial cells contained large numbers of circular shadows or "vesicles" which were interpreted as potential mechanisms for active transport directly through the endothelial cells by a process called "pinocytosis." According to this concept, a vacuole would form on the endothelial cell surface, enclosing a small globule of plasma or extravascular liquid, as the case may be. This vesicle would then move through the endothelial cell protoplasm to the opposite side of the cell and discharge its contents.

During the ensuing years, several pathways for transport of material were considered as illustrated in Figure 1–13A. These included (1) direct passage through endothelial cells, (2) migration of vesicles, (3) vesicles emptying from one to another, (4) passage along junctions (the dotted lines suggest diversion around tight junctions), (5) bypass of junction by diffusion through a thin layer of endothelial cells and (6) bypass of junction by vesicular transport.

This conceptual problem has now come nearly full circle with Karnovsky's[14] electron microscopic evidence that a readily identifiable peroxidase with a molecular weight of 40,000 passed directly through anatomically tight junctions and was distributed along their whole length. The passage of larger molecules (and particles) still suggests the need to postulate dispersed pores of 25 to 500 A, which might be visualized as transiently opening and closing or resealing. Alternatively the need to postulate such larger pores might be satisfied by active vesicular transport (Fig. 1–13), but this remains controversial.

In many tissues, capillaries are surrounded or enclosed by a sheath of cells or reticular fiber membranes (see also Chapter 4). This perivascular membrane forms a line of demarcation

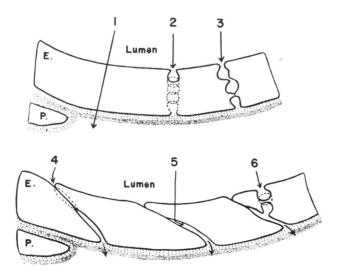

FIGURE 1–13 PREVIOUSLY POSTULATED PATHWAYS THROUGH CAPILLARY WALLS

Six possible pathways across a continuous capillary endothelium. 1. Direct pathway, mainly for gases, water and lipid-soluble substances. 2. Transport by vesicles. 3. Vesicles opening from one to another. 4. Passage along junctions, dotted lines indicate permanent sieve or intermittent opening. 5. Bypass of the junction by diffusion. 6. Bypass of the junction by vesicles. (Presented with permission of G. Majno, Ultrastructure of the vascular membrane, in Handbook of Physiology, Section 2: Circulation, Vol. 2, American Physiological Society, 1965).

between the perivascular space and the gelatinous matrix in the interstitial spaces.

The pericapillary sheath appears to give mechanical support to capillaries. Hyaluronidase applied to the frog mesentery abruptly produced microscopic petechial hemorrhages when liquefaction of the gels extended to the capilllaries, softening the supporting connective tissue sheath. It has long been recognized that increased "permeability" of capillaries may occur without increased fragility (characterized by the rupture of capillaries with the formation of petechial hemorrhages). It has been suggested that the capillary endothelium is responsible for permeability while the condition of the perivascular membrane determines the degree of capillary fragility.

Electron microscopy has demonstrated very distinctive differences in the structure of capillaries in various specialized tissues of the body. Luft and Hechter's[15] observations indicate a need for caution in basing morphologic and functional interpretations on electron micrographs of capillaries. When bovine adrenal glands were fixed one or two hours after the death of the animal, the capillary endothelium consistently exhibited fenestrations, but when adrenal glands prepared in a similar fashion were perfused with warm, oxygenated bovine blood for an hour or so, the capillaries were intact—no fenestrations could be seen. Thus, the structure of capillaries may be labile and may change under different conditions including the preparation of material for examination.

WATER BALANCE AT THE CAPILLARIES

Since water molecules move back and forth so rapidly between blood and tissues and since the pressure inside the capillaries is greater than extravascular pressure, why does water remain in the blood stream rather than pour out into the tissues? The fluid exchange across capillary walls was described by Starling[16] as follows:

In Lecture II, I called your attention to the fact that the non-diffusible constituents of the blood serum, chiefly proteins, were capable of exercising an osmotic pressure or osmotic attraction for water, which amounted to about 4 mm. Hg for every 1 per cent protein in the serum. Blood plasma with 6 to 8 per cent proteins would therefore exert an osmotic pressure of 25 to 30 mm. Hg as compared with an isotonic salt solution. The importance of these results lies in the fact that, although the osmotic pressure of the proteins of the plasma is so insignificant when contrasted with that of its saline constituents, it is of an order of magnitude comparable to that of the capillary blood pressure (see Figure 1-14); and whereas capillary pressure is the chief determining factor in the production of interstitial fluid, the osmotic difference of pressure dependent on the greater concentration of the fluid within as compared with that without the blood vessels might be sufficient to determine absorption. In fact the osmotic attraction of the serum, or plasma, for the extravascular fluid will be proportional to the forces expended in the production of the latter, so that at any given time there may be a balance between the hydrostatic pressure of the blood in the capillaries and the osmotic attraction of the blood for the surrounding fluids. With increased capillary pressure there must be increased transudation. The blood will become more concentrated until equilibrium is established at a somewhat higher point, when there is a more dilute fluid in the tissue spaces and therefore a higher absorbing force to balance the increased capillary pressure. With diminished capillary pressure there will be an osmotic absorption of salt solution from the extravascular fluid; this becomes richer in proteins, and the process will come to an end when the difference between its protein osmotic pressure and that of the intravascular plasma is equal to the diminished capillary pressure.

According to this hypothesis, the filtration or reabsorption of fluid across the capillary walls depends upon the net effect of four interdependent forces: (a) capillary pressure, (b) tissue pressure, (c) osmotic pressure of the plasma and (d) osmotic pressure of the tissue fluids. For sake of convenience, the difference between capillary pres-

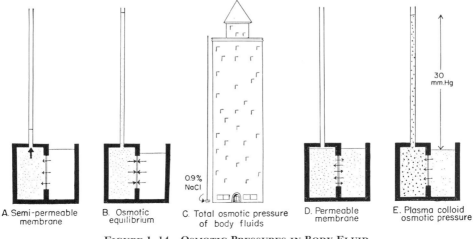

FIGURE 1–14   OSMOTIC PRESSURES IN BODY FLUID

A, When two solutions of different osmotic concentrations are separated by an appropriate semi-permeable membrane, fluid moves from the region of lower concentration through the membrane to dilute the solution with higher concentration.

B, Osmotic equilibrium is reached when the hydrostatic pressure in the vertical fluid column precisely balances the osmotic pressure exerted by the more concentrated solution.

C, The total osmotic pressure of any of the body fluids is about 7.9 atmospheres when equilibrated with pure water. This pressure is equivalent to the vertical column of 0.9 per cent saline solution extending to the top of a 20-story building.

D, If solutions of different osmotic concentration are separated by permeable membranes, no osmotic pressure is present at equilibrium because both the water and solutes diffuse to produce equal osmotic concentrations throughout the fluid phase. For this reason the tremendous potential osmotic pressure of body fluid (*C*) serves merely to maintain osmotic equilibrium throughout the fluid compartments of the body.

E, Since the capillary walls are highly permeable to solutes other than plasma proteins, the osmotic pressure of the plasma is determined by the difference in concentration of the proteins and amounts to only about 25 to 30 mm. Hg.

sure and tissue pressure will be called *effective capillary pressure* or *filtration pressure*. The difference between plasma and tissue osmotic pressure will be termed *effective plasma osmotic pressure*. The maximal effective plasma osmotic pressure ranges around 30 mm. Hg in regions where the capillaries are virtually impermeable to proteins. The average effective capillary pressure is in this range at heart level. Starling's hypothesis calls for a fairly complete balance of filtration and reabsorption in relatively impermeable capillaries at heart level when the mean capillary pressure approximates effective colloid osmotic pressure (Fig. 1–15). Under these con-

ditions, no filtrate or lymph would be formed.

VARIATIONS IN CAPILLARY PRESSURE

Most of the confirmatory evidence for Starling's hypothesis has been derived from experiments with capillaries at or near heart levels in small animals.[17] Clearly, filtration is most likely to predominate in regions where marked elevation in capillary pressure is not balanced by a corresponding increase in extravascular pressure.

Since fluid flows from regions of high pressure to regions of lower pressure, the pressure in peripheral veins

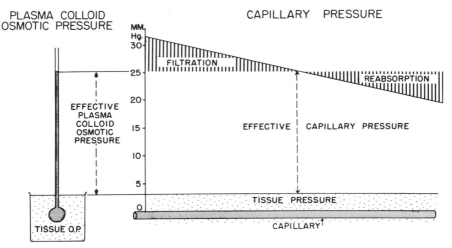

FIGURE 1–15   FACTORS DETERMINING FLUID EXCHANGE IN CAPILLARIES

The effective colloid osmotic pressure of the plasma is determined by the difference in protein concentration in tissues and in the plasma. The effective capillary pressure is the difference between capillary pressure and tissue pressure. The pressure gradient in capillaries under a specific set of conditions may produce filtration at the arteriolar end of the capillary and reabsorption in the venular end of the capillary with no net fluid exchange. Such complete fluid balance is the exception rather than the rule.

establishes the minimal capillary pressure in each capillary network. Similarly, the filling pressure of the right ventricle establishes the lower end of the shallow gradient in venous pressure (Fig. 1–7). Thus, the capillary pressure is affected by changes in either local venous pressure or the diastolic pressure in the right ventricle.

Some factors which affect capillary fluid balance are illustrated schematically in Figure 1–16. When a man stands up, the long hydrostatic columns of blood tend to produce great increases in capillary pressure without corresponding increases in effective osmotic pressure of the blood. This problem will be considered in Chapter 6.

CAPILLARY PERMEABILITY IN DIFFERENT REGIONS

The effective plasma osmotic pressure is markedly reduced in capillaries with greater permeability to protein.

Judged from the protein concentration of lymph from different regions, capillary permeability is not uniform throughout the body (Fig. 1–16). For example, lymph actively flowing from skin and connective tissues generally contains less than 1 per cent protein. Lymph from heart, lungs, intestines and kidney usually contains protein in concentrations between 3 and 4 per cent. Liver lymph carries as much as 6 per cent protein when the plasma concentration is only about 7 per cent, suggesting an effective colloid osmotic pressure of about 4 mm. Hg in the liver sinusoids. In tissues where protein escapes from capillaries in concentrations of 3 per cent or more, lymph flows continuously. However, lymph is not universally accepted as an example of tissue fluid.

THE LYMPHATIC SYSTEM

The filtrates from plasma which pass into the tissue spaces are either

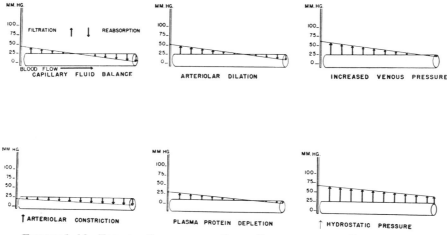

FIGURE 1–16   FACTORS INFLUENCING FLUID BALANCE AT THE CAPILLARIES

Filtration and reabsorption of fluid are balanced only when the effective plasma osmotic pressure precisely equals the mean effective capillary pressure. Dilatation of arterioles causes a steeper capillary pressure gradient with little change in venous pressure. Increased venous pressure and hydrostatic pressure in dependent parts elevates the pressures along the whole length of the capillary. Plasma protein depletion and increased capillary permeability reduce the tendency for reabsorption and foster excess filtration. Net reabsorption of fluid is aided by arteriolar constriction or by elevating the capillaries above heart level. (From Sodeman, W. A.: Pathologic Physiology: Mechanisms of Disease. Philadelphia, W. B. Saunders Co., 1956.)

reabsorbed into the blood or returned to the circulation by the lymphatic system. The lymphatic system is fundamentally a drainage system phylogenetically developed to return to the circulating blood fluids which have escaped from capillaries.[18] Although lymph flow appears to be rather sluggish, the amount of lymph returned to the blood stream in a day is roughly equivalent to the total plasma volume.

Lymphatic collecting vessels tend to travel in close anatomic relation to the veins and have a similar function, i.e., the return of blood elements from the tissues to the venous reservoirs near the heart (Fig. 1–17). The lymphatic and venous systems both have superficial and deep distributions. On the surface of the body, the superficial lymphatic collecting vessels usually accompany the superficial veins just beneath the skin. They also lie just beneath the mucous membrane throughout the whole length of the di-

gestive, respiratory and genito-urinary tracts. These networks of collecting lymphatics drain lymphatic capillaries abundantly distributed in the submucosa and in the dermis of the skin, forming a continuous network throughout all the internal and external linings of the body except the cornea of the eye.

The *deep* lymphatic vessels intertwine and anastomose around the veins which accompany the deep arteries in their regional distribution to the organs of the body (Fig. 1–17). Arteries, veins and deep lymphatics tend to share the same sheaths and are distributed to the same tissues and organs.

The lymphatic system has two transport functions: (*a*) the return of capillary filtrate to the circulation and (*b*) the removal of foreign particles and exudates from tissue spaces and serous cavities. Since the lymphatic capillary networks are distributed through the interstitial spaces along with the blood

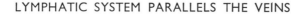

LYMPHATIC SYSTEM PARALLELS THE VEINS

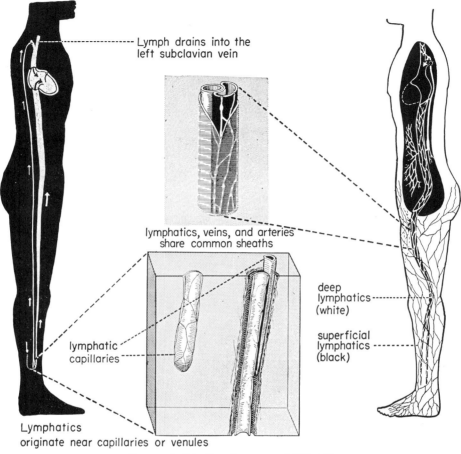

Lymph drains into the
left subclavian vein

lymphatics, veins, and arteries
share common sheaths

lymphatic
capillaries

deep
lymphatics
(white)

superficial
lymphatics
(black)

Lymphatics
originate near capillaries or venules

FIGURE 1–17   THE LYMPHATIC SYSTEM

The lymphatic system is essentially a "paravenous system" since the lymphatic capillaries lie in close association with the capillaries and veins of the blood vascular system; the collecting lymphatics tend to accompany veins and arteries and drain into the central veins. Like the veins, the lymphatic system consists of both deep and superficial distributions of vessels and carries constituents of the blood back to the region of the heart.

capillaries, the terminal vessels of the two systems must lie very near each other (Fig. 1–17). Most commonly, the lymphatic capillaries are believed to end blindly in interstitial spaces at varying distances from the capillaries of the blood vascular system. There is also evidence that lymphatic capillaries may develop along the perivascular spaces where growth appears to be less impeded. Lymphatic vessels which terminate within the pericapillary spaces are ideally located for the transportation of filtrate from the capillary beds. Lymphatics lying free within the interstitial spaces may remove foreign particles and inflammatory exudates. Under certain conditions, apertures have been observed in lymphatic capillaries surrounded by inflammatory exudate.[19] When the tissues are clear of free fluid the lymphatic capillaries have continuous unbroken endothelial membranes.

There are many gaps in our knowledge of lymphatic function. The forces driving a fluid laden with protein and cellular elements through the continuous wall of a lymphatic capillary have not been clearly elucidated. This problem is most acute in the skin of a dependent extremity where vascular pressures are very high and the tissue pressures very low. The exact mechanisms elevating lymph from dependent extremities to the level of the subclavian vein are not universally agreed upon, although a number of possibilities exist. The lymphatic collecting vessels are intimately associated with the veins and are subject to the same muscular and abdominothoracic pumping actions (see Chapter 6). Confined within the same sheath as arteries and veins, the lymphatics would tend to be compressed by changes in the caliber of these vessels. Even the arterial pulse may act as an accessory pump, displacing lymph upward with each wave of distention. Irisawa[20] showed that both leg movements and weight bearing elevate lymphatic pressure propelling the lymph toward the heart. Finally, there is some evidence that certain lymphatics have independent contractility which could propel lymph by a peristaltic type of action. The lymphatic pressure in the thoracic duct must exceed the pressure in the subclavian veins into which it empties.

THE VENOUS SYSTEM

The veins not only act as conduits to channel blood from the capillaries to the heart, but they also adjust their total capacity to accommodate variations in total blood volume. The pressure at the point of outflow from a system of tubes establishes the lower end of the pressure gradient which promotes flow through the tubes. The point of outflow from the systemic veins is the right ventricle during each diastole. If the pressure in the right atrium fell below the pressure outside the wall of this vessel, the filling pressure of the right ventricle would be zero. Actually, the pressure within the right atrium and ventricle remains within a narrow range at very low levels in spite of changes in the total blood volume or the distribution of blood in the circulation. For example, the average normal adult can walk into a blood bank, give up 500 cc. of blood and, after a few minutes, walk out again.

The maintenance of a fairly constant right atrial and right ventricular pressure under varying conditions requires adjustments in the capacity of various portions of the venous system. Measurements on *isolated* segments of veins reveal smaller pressure increments with increasing volume than occur in arteries. The greater venous distensibility represents only part of the adaptability of the venous system. The venous system is of primary importance in its capacitance function since it contains 65 to 75 per cent of the total blood volume. In peripheral vascular beds, most of the blood is contained in the venules and small veins (see Fig. 1–3E) where relatively small changes in caliber of large numbers of small veins can greatly change the quantity of blood they contain. The variable capacity of the venous system is also vested in specialized venous reservoirs and in alterations in the caliber of venous channels through venoconstriction.

It has long been recognized that the spleen acts as a depot from which blood may be expressed in times of stress. This function is not well developed in the human spleen since it contains only some 200 to 250 cc. The subpapillary plexus of the skin has a potential role as a blood depot, but this function is intimately related to dissipation of heat. In other words, this blood is rarely released into the general circulation at the expense of temperature regulation. The pulmonary veins are generally believed to have a role in cushioning transient differences in the output of the right and left ventricles. Although measuring the capacity of internal organs is very difficult, there is some evidence that the capacity of the venous channels may also be controlled by "venomotor" activity. Variations in venous "tone" would contribute to adjustment in the capacity of the circulation in response to alteration in blood volume.

VENOUS RESISTANCE AND CAPACITANCE EFFECTS

The resistance to blood flow through the venules and veins is much less than that encountered in the precapillary resistance vessels (arterioles and precapillary sphincters). This fact is clearly shown in the steep pressure drop just upstream from the capillaries as illustrated schematically in Figure 1–8. However, the resistance to blood flow through postcapillary venules and small veins is not negligible because of their strategic position just downstream from the capillaries. For example, constriction of venules would elevate capillary pressure and promote increased filtration of fluid from the capillary blood. Conversely, venodilation accompanied by precapillary constriction could result in increased resorption of extravascular fluid into capillary blood, dehydrating the tissue and expanding the plasma volume. This kind of phenomenon is most obvious in the glomeruli of the kidney where a meshwork of capillaries is located between precapillary and postcapillary sphincters with extremely well developed control over the filtra-

tion rate. Folkow and Mellander[21] have stressed the importance of the changing ratio of precapillary and postcapillary resistance in other peripheral vascular beds. In skeletal muscle this factor plays an important role in the partititioning of fluid between the intravascular and extravascular spaces. Furthermore, contraction of skeletal muscles compresses the veins between the muscle bundles, expressing blood from the veins, propelling it toward the heart and reducing venous and capillary pressures in dependent extremities. The muscle pumping action on venous flow is discussed in greater detail in responses to arising (see Chapter 6). The capacity of the veins in the legs may be reflexly diminished by vasomotor reflexes when man stands. If so, this is a portion of the compensatory response to the erect stance.

Shepard[22] summarized evidence indicating that the output of the heart increased as the total peripheral resistance diminished (vasodilation) and the wall tension of the venous capacity vessels increased (venoconstriction). Among these conditions were exercise, hyperventilation, strong emotions, cold showers, severe anemia and the cardiovascular hormones epinephrine and isoproterenol. The stiffness and blood content of the peripheral venous channels is primarily controlled by autonomic reflexes involving pathways to the base of the brain and above, including the cerebral cortex as a part of complex neural control patterns as will be discussed in greater detail in many subsequent portions of this book, particularly Chapter 4.

PULMONARY CIRCULATION

The systemic and pulmonary vascular beds are connected in series to

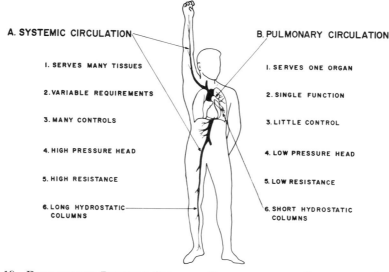

A. SYSTEMIC CIRCULATION

1. SERVES MANY TISSUES

2. VARIABLE REQUIREMENTS

3. MANY CONTROLS

4. HIGH PRESSURE HEAD

5. HIGH RESISTANCE

6. LONG HYDROSTATIC COLUMNS

B. PULMONARY CIRCULATION

1. SERVES ONE ORGAN

2. SINGLE FUNCTION

3. LITTLE CONTROL

4. LOW PRESSURE HEAD

5. LOW RESISTANCE

6. SHORT HYDROSTATIC COLUMNS

FIGURE 1–18 DIFFERENCES BETWEEN SYSTEMIC CIRCULATION AND PULMONARY CIRCULATION

  The systemic circulation differs from the pulmonary circulation in a number of distinctive characteristics. These differences may be related to the differences in the functions, organization and environment of the two vascular beds.

form a continuous circuit. Although these two vascular systems are superficially similar, the following important differences between them are summarized in Figure 1–18. The systemic circulation is a high-resistance circuit with a large difference in pressure between the arteries and veins, while the pulmonary circuit normally offers very slight resistance to flow. The pulmonary vessels supply only one type of tissue (alveolar membranes), so the requirements for vasomotor control are not as great as those in the systemic circulation. The volume of blood in the pulmonary system is neither so great nor so variable as that in the systemic circulation. Since the lungs immediately enclose the heart, hydrostatic columns are fairly short even from the most distant portions of the pulmonary parenchyma. The pulmonary circulation is confined within the thoracic cage, so extravascular conditions are fairly uniform throughout.

ANATOMY OF THE PULMONARY CIRCULATION

  The ramifications of the pulmonary arterial system closely parallel the arborization of the bronchial system. The mainstem bronchi give off lateral branches which divide and subdivide like the branches of a tree. At the tip of each terminal branch is a bronchiole which divides into two respiratory bronchioles. In turn, these divide into two branches, each of which gives off alveolar ducts. The alveolar ducts are connected through a variable number of atria to a tuft of alveolar sacs (air cells). A wax model of part of the bronchial tree of an infant, reconstructed by Boyden and Tompsett[23] is reproduced in Figure 1–19 to illustrate the complexity of the terminal airways and alveoli even at that early age. Gaseous interchange between the air and blood may occur in all divisions beyond the bronchioles.

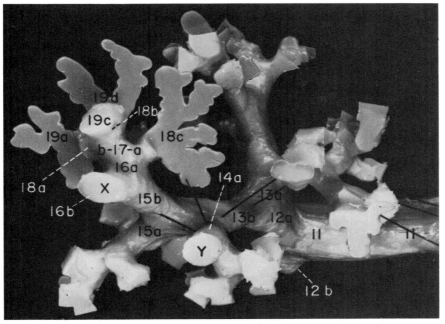

FIGURE 1–19   TERMINAL BRONCHIOLES AND ALVEOLI

A wax model of terminal respiratory airways of an infant. Ramus 16a, a respiratory bronchiole of the first order, gives rise to six terminal clusters of alveolar sacs. (Reproduced by the courtesy of Dr. Allen Boyden.[23])

Structurally, the main pulmonary arteries closely resemble the aorta. The walls of the main arteries and their branches remain essentially the same down to the intrapulmonary branches with outside diameters of about 1 mm., except that the amount of smooth muscle in the wall progressively increases in the smaller branches.[24] Muscular arteries ranging in diameter from 1 to 0.1 mm. have a prominent media of circularly arranged smooth muscle between the internal and external elastic laminae. The walls of arterial branches less than 0.1 mm. in diameter consist essentially of poorly supported endothelial tubes which abruptly break up into a profusely anastomotic capillary network. Thus, the pulmonary circulation does not contain any vessels corresponding to the muscular arterioles in the systemic circulation. The alveolar capillaries are the principal structural elements in the walls of the respiratory membranes (see Fig. 1–24A). The capillary network is so dense that in many alveoli the space between capillaries is less than their diameter.[25]

RESISTANCE TO BLOOD FLOW THROUGH THE PULMONARY CIRCUIT

For several reasons the normal intravascular pressures do not fall abruptly in the small vessels of the lung (Fig. 1–20): (a) There are no high-resistance muscular arterioles in the terminal ramifications of the vascular tree. (b) The pulmonary capillaries are extremely voluminous, diffusely anastomotic and of relatively large caliber. (c) The pulmonary vessels are passively distended in response to increased pulmonary blood flow. (d) There is a large reserve capacity in the lung which is not fully utilized except

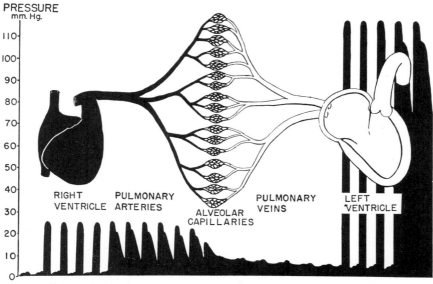

FIGURE 1–20   PRESSURES IN THE PULMONARY VASCULAR SYSTEM

Since the pulmonary arterial system offers slight resistance to blood flow, the mean pressure difference between pulmonary artery and left atrium amounts to only 4 to 6 mm. Hg. This low-pressure head drives the same volume of blood through the pulmonary circuit as flows through the systemic circulation with a gradient of some 90 mm. Hg.

under conditions of stress. For example, an entire lung with all its capillary bed can be removed without increasing the pulmonary arterial pressure. (e) Finally, all vessels in the pulmonary vascular tree have a somewhat larger caliber than corresponding vessels in the systemic circulation. The net effect is a total pulmonary resistance to flow only about one eighth of that in the systemic circulation.

During systole, the right ventricular pressure rises to about 22 mm. Hg. The pulmonary arterial pressures average about 22/8 mm. Hg with a mean arterial pressure of about 13 mm. Hg.[26] The pressure at the point of outflow from the pulmonary circuit (the left ventricular diastolic pressure) is about 7 mm. Hg (Fig. 1–20). Thus, a pressure gradient of only about 6 mm. Hg will force through the pulmonary circuit the same quantity of blood propelled through the systemic circuit by a gradient of 90 mm. Hg. Furthermore,

the pulmonary arterial pressure may remain unchanged or diminish slightly when the cardiac output increases threefold. One case has been described in which a pressure gradient of 4 mm. Hg propelled 15 liters of blood per minute through the pulmonary circuit.[27] The small pressure gradient between the pulmonary artery and the left atrium is the basis for the statement that the pulmonary circuit is a low resistance system.

FUNCTIONS OF THE PULMONARY CIRCULATION

The pulmonary circuit simultaneously performs three functions: (a) gaseous exchange of oxygen and carbon dioxide between the alveolar air and blood, (b) storage of blood in a variable volume reservoir and (c) blockade of foreign particles, thrombi and other types of emboli circulating in the systemic venous blood.

Gas Exchange: The Principal Function of the Lungs. Blood passing through the alveolar capillaries of the lungs is effectively spread into a layer about 10μ thick and 100 sq. m. in area. The alveolar air is separated from the hemoglobin in the blood by the alveolar epithelium, a thin basal membrane, the capillary endothelium, a layer of plasma and the red cell membrane. These barriers appear formidable when highly magnified in an electron microgram (Fig. 1–21), but these thin layers represent very slight obstacles to the rapid exchanges of alveolar gases with the blood. The oxygen tension is lower and the carbon dioxide tension is greater in blood entering the alveolar capillaries than in the alveolar air. Blood traverses the alveolar capillaries in about 1 second. Propelled by their diffusion gradients, oxygen and carbon dioxide are exchanged so rapidly that blood leaving the alveolar capillaries is normally in virtual equilibrium with the alveolar air (Fig. 1–22A). The action of carbonic anhydrase in the erythrocytes and rapid dissociation of carbon dioxide from reduced hemoglobin as it is converted to oxyhemoglobin facilitate exchange of carbon dioxide. The gaseous exchange remains this rapid only when the diffusion distances are extremely small. Thus, very thin layers of fluid accumulating between the al-

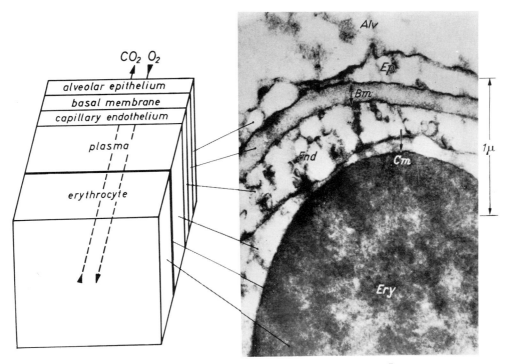

FIGURE 1–21   BARRIERS TO DIFFUSION OF GASES IN THE LUNGS

Interposed between the alveolar air and the hemoglobin in the blood are the alveolar epithelium, a basal membrane, the alveolar capillary endothelium, plasma, the red cell membrane and protoplasm. Despite these barriers, equilibrium is very rapidly established in blood flowing through the pulmonary capillaries despite their very short length. (From G. Thews, Gaseous diffusion in the lungs and tissues, in Physical Bases of Circulatory Transport: Regulation and Exchange, E. B. Reeve and A. C. Guyton, eds. Philadelphia. W. B. Saunders Co., 1967.)

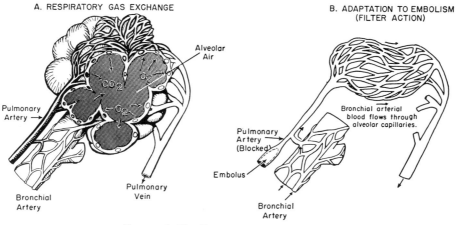

FIGURE 1–22   FUNCTIONS OF THE LUNG

A, Gas exchange, the principal function of the lungs, occurs because of the higher concentration of oxygen and lower concentration of carbon dioxide in the alveolar air than in the venous blood arriving at the pulmonary capillaries.

B, Embolic obstruction of pulmonary arteries does not produce necrosis of pulmonary parenchyma because bronchial arterial blood is diverted through dilated channels into the alveolar capillaries. Because of this dual blood supply, the lungs can serve as filters for emboli without self-destruction.

veolar air and the blood can seriously retard respiratory exchange.

Oxygen and carbon dioxide cannot be exchanged when the blood flows through collapsed alveoli because it does not come in close proximity to alveolar air. Thus, blood passing through non-aerated alveoli would retain the character of venous blood. However, resistance to flow increases markedly in atelectatic lung tissue, automatically shunting blood from non-aerated portions into the inflated regions of the lung.

Reservoir Function of the Lungs. Since the pulmonary vessels constitute a low-pressure, distensible system, any slight increase in outflow pressure at the left ventricle or relative increase in input from the right ventricle can cause considerable quantities of blood to accumulate within the lungs. Presumably, engorgement of the lungs will cause elevated pressure throughout the pulmonary circuit because the pressure gradient is so shallow. However, it seems likely that considerable distention may occur with little eleva-

tion in pressure. For example, there is evidence that substantial quantities of blood are displaced into the heart and lungs after reclining. Sjöstrand[28] reported that an average of more than 600 ml. of blood was shifted from the lower extremities to the rest of the body when standing subjects reclined. He concluded that more than half of this volume was accommodated in the lungs.

As much as 25 per cent of the blood in the thorax (heart and lungs) may be shifted to the legs. This reserve volume in the pulmonary circuit appears to be distributed diffusely through the lungs, where it is held "on tap" until drawn from in order to effect the rapid readjustment of the circulation required for larger cardiac output. Reserve blood in the lungs has been compared with water dammed up behind a sluice gate where it compensates for occasional variations in supply and output. On this basis, the lungs have an important reservoir function. This distensible vascular network may also serve to cushion transient differences in right and left ventricular output, e.g., at the onset of violent exercise.

Filter Action of the Lungs. If foreign bodies, thrombi, air bubbles or fat particles enter the systemic arterial system, they generally occlude a terminal artery within some organ. This reduces or eliminates circulation to the tissues supplied by that arterial branch, and the tissue cells frequently die. If it occurs in a vital organ such as the brain or heart, this is a serious event. Fortunately, most of the emboli enter the blood stream on the venous side of the circulation and lodge in the lungs. By virtue of a double circulation, the pulmonary vascular tree is particularly adapted to filtering out these circulating vascular plugs without self-destruction.

In parallel with the pulmonary arterial system, the bronchial arteries transmit oxygenated blood throughout the walls of the bronchial tree as far peripherally as the bronchioles.[25] Anastomotic connections between pulmonary and bronchial arteries are not believed to occur normally. However, anastomoses of small caliber exist in the walls of the bronchioles and alveolar ducts, where they share common capillary beds (Fig. 1–22*B*). The venous drainage from the bronchial arterial system is by way of the pulmonary vein except in the first two or three divisions of the bronchial tree. Obstruction or occlusion of a branch of the pulmonary artery does not affect the blood supply to the bronchial system. Dilatation of channels in the common capillary networks provides a mechanism for diverting oxygenated blood through the alveolar membranes when pulmonary arterial flow is arrested or reduced (Fig. 1–22*B*). Thus, lung tissue is rarely destroyed by obstruction of the pulmonary blood supply. The diffuse anastomotic connections between adjacent alveoli provide additional protection against occlusion of small peripheral branches of the pulmonary arterial system. The affected lung tissue survives while the embolus is resorbed or recanalized, after which the tissue resumes its activity. There is every reason to believe that this sequence of events occurs repeatedly during any person's lifetime without producing symptoms unless the embolus is very large or is located in a critical position.

SUMMARY

The systemic circulation consists of three functional divisions, the arterial pressure reservoir, the venous volume reservoir and the capillary networks. The precipitous drop of pressure due to high resistance to flow through the arterioles, capillaries and venules forms the functional region of demarcation between the arterial and venous systems. So long as the pressure difference between arteries and veins remains constant, the blood flow through the capillaries is determined by the resistance to flow through the minute vessels. The quantity of blood flowing per unit time through the arteries, capillaries and veins must be identical except for insignificant differences in flow involved in shifting blood from one region to another. The central arterial and venous pressures tend to remain fixed within relatively narrow ranges regardless of the total amount of blood flowing through the system per unit time (cardiac output). The average volume of blood in the arterial system tends to remain fairly constant so long as the mean arterial blood pressure is unchanged. In contrast, the central venous pressure tends to remain relatively constant in spite of variations in the total quantity and distribution of blood through adjustments in the capacity of venous reservoirs. Cardiovascular response to disease cannot be fully understood without consideration of the mechanisms by which the normal circulatory system adjusts to various conditions including changes in body posture, changes in regional blood flow and cardiac output.

REFERENCES

1. HILL, A. V. The diffusion of oxygen and lactic acid through tissues. *Proc. Roy. Soc.,* B104:39-96, 1928.
2. GREEN, H. D. Circulation: physical principles. Pp. 208-232 in *Medical Physics,* Vol. 1, O. Glasser, Ed. Chicago, Year Book Publishers, 1944.
3. WEIDEMAN, MARY P. Architecture of the terminal vascular bed. Chapter 18 in *Physical Bases of Circulatory Transport: Regulation and Exchange,* E. B. Reeve and A. C. Guyton, Eds. Philadelphia, W. B. Saunders Co., 1967.
4. HEYMANS, C., and VAN DEN HEUVAL-HEYMANS, G. New aspects of blood pressure regulation. *Circulation,* 4:581-586, 1951.
5. WOLF, A. V. Demonstrations concerning pressure-tension relations in various organs. *Science,* 115:243-244, 1952.
6. BURTON, A. C. On the physical equilibrium of small blood vessels. *Amer. J. Physiol.,* 164:319-329, 1951.
7. COWIE, D. B., FLEXNER, L. B., and WILDE, W. S. Capillary permeability, rate of transcapillary exchange of chloride in the guinea pig as determined with radiochloride. *Amer. J. Physiol.,* 158:231-236, 1949.
8. FLEXNER, L. B., COWIE, D. B., and VOSBURGH, G. J. Studies on capillary permeability with tracer substances. *Cold Spr. Harb. Symp. Quant. Biol.,* 13:88-98, 1948.
9. PAPPENHEIMER, J. R., RENKIN, E. M., and BORRERO, L. M. Filtration, diffusion and molecular sieving through peripheral capillary membranes. A contribution to the pore theory of capillary permeability. *Amer. J. Physiol.,* 167:13-46, 1951.
10. RENKIN, E. M. Capillary permeability to lipid-soluble molecules. *Amer. J. Physiol.,* 168:538-545, 1952.
11. MAJNO, G. Ultrastructure of the vascular membrane. Chapter 64 in *Handbook of Physiology, Section 2: Circulation,* Vol. 3, W. F. Hamilton and P. Dow, Eds. Washington, D.C., American Physiological Society, 1965.
12. COTRAN, R. S. The fine structure of microvasculature in relation to normal and abnormal permeability. Chapter 15 in *Physical Bases of Circulatory Transport:*

Regulation and Exchange, E. B. Reeve and A. C. Guyton, Eds. Philadelphia, W. B. Saunders Co., 1967.
13. LANDIS, E. M., and PAPPENHEIMER, J. R. Exchange of substances through the capillary walls. Chapter 29 in *Handbook of Physiology, Section 2: Circulation,* Vol. 2, W. F. Hamilton and P. Dow, Eds. Washington, D.C., American Physiological Society, 1963.
14. KARNOVSKY, M. J. Ultrastructural basis of capillary permeability studied with peroxidase as a tracer. *J. Cell Biol.,* 35:213-236, 1967.
15. LUFT, J., and HECHTER, O. An electron microscopic correlation of structure with function in the isolated perfused cow adrenal, preliminary observations. *J. Biophys. Biochem. Cytol.,* 3:615-620, 1957.
16. STARLING, E. H. *The Fluids of the Body.* Chicago, W. T. Keener & Co. 1909, 186 pp.
17. LANDIS, E. M. Capillary permeability and factors affecting composition of capillary filtrate. *Ann. N. Y. Acad. Sci.,* 46:713-731, 1946.
18. MAYERSON, H. S. The physiologic importance of lymph. Chapter 30 in *Handbook of Physiology, Section 2: Circulation,* Vol. 2, W. F. Hamilton and P. Dow, Eds. Washington, D.C., American Physiological Society, 1963.
19. CLARK, E. R., and CLARK, E. L. Further observations on living lymphatic vessels in the transparent chamber in the rabbit's ear—their relation to the tissue spaces. *Amer. J. Anat.,* 52:273-305, 1933.
20. IRISAWA, A., and RUSHMER, R. F. Relationship between lymphatic and venous pressure in leg of dog. *Amer. J. Physiol.,* 196:495-498, 1959.
21. FOLKOW, B., MELLANDER, S., and SWEDEN, G. Veins and venous tone. *Amer. Heart J.,* 68:397-408, 1964.
22. SHEPHERD, J. T. Role of veins in the circulation. *Circulation,* 33:484-491, 1966.
23. BOYDEN, E. A., and TOMPSETT, D. H. The changing patterns in the developing lungs of infants. *Acta anat.,* 61:164-192, 1965.
24. BRENNER, O. Pathology of the vessels of the pulmonary circulation. *Arch. Int. Med.,* 56:211-237, 1935.
25. MILLER, W. S. *The Lung,* 2nd ed. Springfield, Illinois, Charles C Thomas, 1947, 222 pp.
26. COURNAND, A. Some aspects of the pulmonary circulation in normal man and in chronic cardiopulmonary diseases. *Circulation,* 2:641-657, 1952.
27. HICKAM, J. B. Atrial septal defect. A study of intracardiac shunts, ventricular outputs, and pulmonary pressure gradients. *Amer. Heart J.,* 38:801-812, 1949.
28. SJÖSTRAND, T.: Volume and distribution of blood and their significance in regulating the circulation. *Physiol. Rev.,* 33:202-228, 1953.

CHAPTER 2

FUNCTIONAL ANATOMY OF CARDIAC CONTRACTION

Blood is propelled along the branched vascular channels by the energy represented by pressure gradients, shallow in the arteries and veins and very steep at the sites of controlled resistance. As blood flows through the various series and parallel channels, pressure energy is dissipated in the form of heat due to friction. The energy lost during the circulation of the blood is restored by the contracting heart.

The two fundamental requirements of the cardiovascular system are (a) circulation of blood without interruption and (b) adjustment of blood flow in response to varying demands of the tissues. If the circulation is interrupted, even momentarily, survival of the individual is jeopardized because nervous tissue in the brain can suffer lasting damage from transient deprivation of oxygen. Thus, the heart must continue to beat repetitively and without a sustained interruption for a lifetime. Furthermore, the heart must adapt its output to balance the changing total flow through the billions of capillaries in the body.

The energy released during ventricular systole represents the combined output of the various bundles of myocardial fibers. The contribution of each bundle depends not only on its contractile power, but also on its anatomic orientation within the cardiac walls. This chapter is devoted to describing the functional anatomy of cardiac contraction as a background which is essential for an understanding of cardiac adaptability and control.

THE DEVELOPMENT OF THE NORMAL HEART

During embryologic development, the various tissues and organs rapidly pass through stages representing the evolutionary development of the species. For this reason, the extensive investigation of embryology in the chick is generally applicable to human embryos, but there is one important difference: the chick embyro is attached to the surface of an abundant yolk.

The heart develops from a pair of primordial tubes derived from clusters of endothelial cells which proliferate, become organized into strands of cells and acquire a lumen. These primitive tubes meet in the midline

33

and fuse into a single elongated chamber which will ultimately develop into the ventricles. From the simple cardiac tube, the endocardial primordia proliferate toward the head to form the aortic arch system. The caudal extensions of the primordial tubes become the omphalomesenteric veins. As the formation of gut proceeds caudally, fusion of the primordial tubes continues, forming the primitive atrium and finally the sinus venosus.

CONVOLUTION OF THE CARDIAC TUBE

The primitive cardiac tube grows longer more rapidly than either the investing pericardium or the surrounding somatic structures. It is anchored above by the arterial trunks and below by developing venous channels. Since the tube is fixed at both ends, its rapid elongation causes flexion, initially toward the right side of the embryo. As elongation continues, the cardiac tube becomes more tortuous (Fig. 2–1A). At the same time, constrictions develop which indicate the ultimate division of this single convoluted tube into atria and ventricles. As the ventricular region progressively expands and grows longer, it swings back toward the midline to cover the atrial region, which remains relatively fixed in position. In this process, the primitive atrium and arterial trunks, which were originally on opposite ends of the cardiac tube, are brought into apposition. Thus, the inflow tract and outflow tract are adjacent and all four valve rings ultimately merge into a single fibrous skeleton (see Fig 2–7). The developing atria expand laterally to form two extensive sacculations, the primitive right and left atria. These sacculations ultimately become the right and left auricles, while the main atrial chambers develop by progressive incorporation of the venous channels into the posterior wall (Fig. 2–1A, bottom).

THE INITIAL CARDIAC CONTRACTION

According to Patten,[1] the first signs of contraction of the heart in chick embryos appear while it is represented by only the ventricular portion of the cardiac tube (Fig. 2–1). Localized slow contractions usually are noted first on the right margin near the root of the primitive arterial trunks. However, the site and spread of these earliest undulations vary considerably. The initial contractions in the embryonic rat heart occur a few hours before the elaboration of fibrillae or cross striations.[2] About an hour after the first fibrillar contraction appears, the entire primitive ventricle contracts regularly and synchronously, but slowly. The nature of the contraction changes a few hours later as the atrium is formed. At this time, contractions originate in the atrial region and sweep over the ventricle like a peristaltic wave. The atrium assumes the role of pacemaker because its inherent rate of impulse formation is higher than that of the ventricle. The sinus venosus has an even faster inherent rhythm and assumes control as soon as it is formed. The sinus venosus ultimately forms the sinoatrial node, the normal pacemaker of the fully developed heart.

By the time the atrium and sinus venosus are formed, this primitive tubular heart is actively pumping blood through the developing circulatory system. During the peristaltic type of cardiac contraction, retrograde flow of blood is prevented by developing mounds of endocardial tissue which project into the lumen at the junction of the primitive atria and ventricles.[3] During each contraction

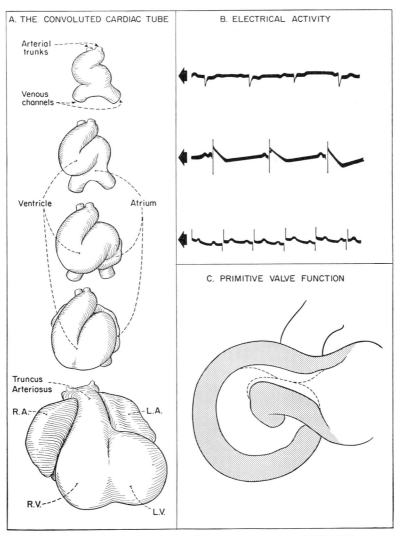

FIGURE 2–1 EMBRYOLOGIC DEVELOPMENT OF THE HEART

A, The initial stage in the development of the heart is the formation of a single cardiac tube which will ultimately evolve into the ventricular portion of the heart. At this very early stage, contractions occur repetitively at a slow rate. Being anchored above by the developing arterial trunks and below by extensive venous channels, the cardiac tube, growing rapidly in length, is bent into a loop to the right of the midline. By progressive fusion of the cardiac primordia, the primitive atrium is formed and remains relatively fixed in position as the cardiac loop grows longer and swings back to the midline to cover the expanding atrial chambers. In this process the ventricle assumes a position anterior and caudal to the atria.

B, Electrical activity can be recorded from the heart of the chick embryo at the very early stages of development, indicated by the first three drawings in part *A*. As the cardiac tube becomes convoluted, the electrocardiographic patterns produced by this electrical activity begin to resemble the patterns observed in fully developed hearts. (After Hoff *et al*.[4])

C, Contraction of the cardiac tube is peristaltic in character, beginning in the atrial region and progressing toward the truncus arteriosus. During contraction at the atrioventricular junction, the endocardial surfaces come into apposition to prevent retrograde flow of blood. A similar valve action may be observed at the root of the truncus arteriosus. (After Patten *et al*.[3])

these endocardial cushions meet each other, completely blocking the channel (Fig. 2–1C). Thus, simple but effective atrioventricular valves are formed at this very early stage of development. Similar endocardial cushions develop in the outflow tract near the ventricular conus. This region ultimately becomes the conus of the right ventricle.

THE DEVELOPMENT OF THE ELECTROCARDIOGRAM

According to Hoff et al.,[4] electrical activity can be consistently recorded from chick embryos at the stage of development illustrated in Figure 2–1A. A few hours later a sharp downward deflection appears, which is interpreted as equivalent to a QRS complex. In the next three or four hours the atrium has become differentiated and the sinus venosus is formed. At about this time, downward deflections (P waves) can be recorded just preceding the QRS. As the primitive cardiac tube becomes convoluted, the electrocardiogram assumes a configuration similar to that of the adult (Fig. 2–1B). The fetal electrocardiogram in the human cannot be recorded by external electrodes on the maternal abdomen until about the twelfth week of gestation.

PARTITIONING OF THE ATRIOVENTRICULAR CANAL

At six weeks of age, the major components of the human heart can be readily identified. A shallow, interventricular groove forms a line of demarcation between the future right and left ventricles.

In spite of the apparent separation of the atria from the ventricles at the atrioventricular junction (Fig. 2–2A,

arrow), the heart actually consists of a common atrioventricular canal which empties into a single arterial trunk. A four-chambered heart is developed from this convoluted, dilated tube by the formation of three partitions separating the atria, the ventricles and the two main arteries.

The first step in the separation of the atrial and ventricular chambers begins with the growth of endocardial cushions from the dorsal and ventral portions of the atrioventricular groove. These masses of endocardial tissue later fuse to form a column which splits the stream of blood flowing from atrium to ventricle (Fig. 2–2C). At the same time a muscular septum develops from the interventricular groove toward the base of the heart, separating the right and left ventricles.

In the atrium, a crescentic ridge (septum primum) appears on the dorsocephalic part of the atrium and rapidly grows down toward the ventricle. As this septum grows across the common atrial chamber, the aperture between the right and left atria (foramen primum) is progressively constricted (Fig. 2–2D). However, before the foramen primum is completely closed, a new opening (foramen secundum) appears high on septum primum (Fig. 2–2E). The timely development of the foramen secundum prevents interruption in the shunting of blood from the right atrium into the left.

Another septum (secundum) develops just to the right of the septum primum and extends like a curtain down over the aperture in the septum primum (Fig. 2–2F). The septum secundum grows beside the septum primum to become a second atrial partition which is complete except for a persistent aperture adjacent to the foramen secundum. The thickened

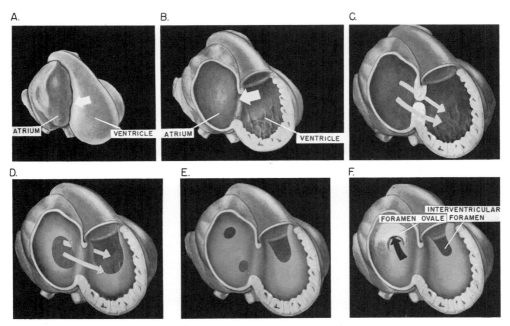

FIGURE 2–2 PARTITIONING OF THE HEART

A, When the cardiac tube illustrated in Figure 2–1*A* is observed in a lateral view, the atrium and ventricles appear to be divided by a deep atrioventricular invagination.

B, Actually, this groove is merely a constriction at the atrioventricular junction. The embryonic heart at this stage is still a simple tube which has become convoluted and expanded into primitive chambers. A four-chambered heart with corresponding arterial trunks is formed by the elaboration of three septa dividing the atria, ventricles and truncus arteriosus.

C, First, the atrioventricular channel is divided at its waist by proliferating endocardial cushions which fuse into a column.

D, Septa dividing the atrium and ventricle grow simultaneously toward the atrioventricular grooves. If either of these partitions fails to form, the fully developed heart has only a single atrium or a single ventricle.

E, An aperture in the developing atrial septum persists near its junction with the endocardial cushions (the foramen primum). Before foramen primum is closed, a new aperture appears high on the interventricular septum (foramen secundum). These two embryonic apertures are the most common sites of interatrial septal defects.

F, The foramen secundum is covered by the developing septum secundum which grows down over the aperture. Its advancing edge becomes thickened to produce the foramen ovale, which acts as a unidirectional flutter valve. Closure of the interventricular foramen awaits the development of a complex spiral septum dividing the truncus arteriosus and conus region of the primtive ventricle (see Fig. 2–3).

edge of this aperture forms the margin of the foramen ovale. The thin septum primum acts as a unidirectional flutter valve, permitting blood to flow only from the right atrium into the left. The functional significance of this unidirectional valve in relation to circulatory adjustments after birth will not be considered in this book. Closure of the interventricular foramen awaits the partitioning of the conus and truncus arteriosus.

THE SPIRAL AORTIC PULMONARY SEPTUM

The truncus arteriosus resembles a cylinder (Fig. 2–3*A*), extending from the conus region just above the partially divided ventricular chambers to its bifurcation into the aorta and pulmonary arteries. A pair of ridges appearing at the bifurcation and on opposite sides of the truncus arteriosus pursue a spiral course toward the ventricles (Fig. 2–3*B*). These ridges

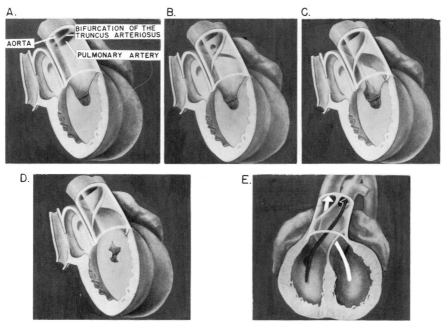

FIGURE 2–3   PARTITIONING OF THE ARTERIAL TRUNKS

A, The truncus arteriosus is illustrated as a transparent cylinder with the heart viewed in the right anterior oblique position.

B, A pair of spiral ridges develop in the internal surface of the truncus arteriosus, beginning at the bifurcation of the truncus arteriosus into the fourth and sixth aortic arches. Retaining their positions on opposite sides of the cylinder, the ridges pursue a spiral course toward the ventricles.

C, The ridges grow into the lumen and fuse to produce a spiral septum which extends into the conus region of the ventricles where they swing into line with the upper margin of the interventricular septum.

D, The interventricular foramen is normally obliterated by masses of endocardial tissue growing from the ventricular septum, the endocardial cushions and the spiral aortic pulmonary septum. This mass of endocardial tissue thins out to form the membranous portion of the interventricular septum just below the origin of the aorta and pulmonary artery. This is the most common site of interventricular septal defects.

E, The significance of the spiral aortic septum is more readily appreciated in a frontal view of the heart. The aortic pulmonary septum executes a spiral of about 180 degrees and swings into line with the superior margin of the interventricular septum. This process accounts for the manner in which the aortic and pulmonary trunks are entwined in the fully developed heart. Blood from the left ventricle enters the aorta, which passes to the right behind the pulmonary artery. The pulmonary artery passes in front of the aorta and turns posteriorly on the left side of the mediastinum.

grow toward the axis of the cylinder and fuse to form a continuous spiral septum which twists 180 degrees and swings into line with the advancing edge of the interventricular septum (Fig. 2–3*C*). The spiral form of the aortic pulmonary septum accounts for the manner in which the pulmonary artery and aorta intertwine in the fully developed heart (Fig. 2–3*E*).

The remaining interventricular foramen is closed by developing endocardial tissue from the atrioventricular cushions, the interventricular septum and the spiral aortic pulmonary septum (Fig. 2–3*D*). The connective tissue which occludes the interventricular foramen gradually thins out to form the membranous portion of the interventricular septum.

THE FORMATION OF CARDIAC VALVES

The semilunar valves begin to form during the division of the truncus arteriosus into the aorta and pulmonary artery (Fig. 2–4A). At the junction of the ventricular conus and the truncus arteriosus, the spiral ridges on opposite sides of the channel develop localized pads of embryonic connective tissue (Fig. 2–4B). As the spiral ridges grow across the lumen, these endocardial cushions form two projections into each vessel and a third pad of tissue grows into each vessel from a point opposite the line of fusion of the spiral septum (Fig. 2–4B). In this way, three pads of connective tissue project into the lumens of the vessels and are gradually excavated and molded into valve cusps forming semilunar valves (Fig. 2–4C). The formation of the atrioventricular valves cannot be visualized so easily. Thick flaps of tissue proliferate from the region of the atrioventricular junction down into the ventricular chamber. The exact mechanism by which these crude flaps are converted into beautifully formed valve cusps, intricately guyed by chordae tendineae arising from the appropriate papillary muscles, is not clear.

THE DUCTUS ARTERIOSUS

Both the pulmonary arteries and the ductus arteriosus are remnants of the sixth pair of aortic arches. Like all the other pairs of aortic arches, the sixth connects the ventral and the dorsal aorta and corresponds to the gill arches in fishes. Branching vessels arise from both the right and left limbs of the sixth aortic arch to supply the developing lungs. As the pulmonary branches from the right aortic arch develop, communication with the

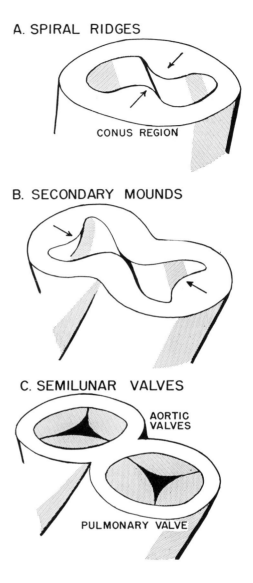

A. SPIRAL RIDGES

CONUS REGION

B. SECONDARY MOUNDS

C. SEMILUNAR VALVES

AORTIC VALVES

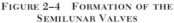

PULMONARY VALVE

FIGURE 2–4   FORMATION OF THE SEMILUNAR VALVES

A, The semilunar valves develop during the separation of the truncus arteriosus by the spiral aortic pulmonary septum (see Fig. 2–3).

B, Pads of endocardial tissue develop at the sites of the valves. These pads originate from the spiral aortic pulmonary septum and as secondary mounds on opposite sides of the channel.

C, When partitioning of the truncus arteriosus is complete, three pads of endocardial tissue appear in the aorta and in the pulmonary artery. These pads are shaped and thinned out to produce the semilunar aortic and pulmonary valves.

dorsal aorta regresses and ultimately disappears. The remnant of the sixth aortic arch between the pulmonary artery and the left aortic arch persists as the ductus arteriosus. During fetal life, blood ejected by the right ventricle can bypass the pulmonary circuit and enter the descending aorta. The functional significance of this short circuit is more clearly visualized in relation to the fetal circulation as a whole.

CONCEPTS OF MUSCULAR CONTRACTION

The walls of the heart are composed of bundles and sheets of myocardial fibers intertwined in a very complex fashion. Electron micrographs show that myofibrils are made up of still smaller filaments, each about 50 to 100 Å in diameter (Fig. 2–5). Huxley[5] has clearly demonstrated that there are two types of myofilaments, one being almost twice as thick as the other. These thick and thin filaments are linked together by an intricate system of cross bridges which project from the thick fibers at fairly regular intervals. He proposed a sliding model concept of muscular contraction, summarized schematically in Figure 2–5. This concept rapidly achieved wide acceptance because it was consistent with much other evidence and supported by crisp, detailed electron micrographs.[6] The two types of myofilaments have been identified in association with the cross bands of muscle. The thin filaments extend in both directions from the Z band. The dark A band is occupied by the thick filaments, which are partially overlapped by the thin filaments. The central light area (H zone) of the A band represents the region occupied only by the thicker filaments. Over a wide range of muscle lengths, the A bands remain of constant length during both contraction and stretching. The I bands shorten in relation to the shortening of the muscle. As the width of the I band diminishes, the H zone shrinks as these two sets of filaments slide past each other. Actually, the tips of filaments may meet and deform at extreme degrees of shortening, and the expected new sets of bands appear at the points of contact.

Ample evidence indicates that the thin filaments are indeed actin and the thick filaments are myosin. The nature of the cross bridges is not known, but they have been assigned an important role in a theory proposed by Huxley.[6] According to this scheme, the cross bridges oscillate and are able to form attachments at specific sites on the thin actin filaments and draw them a short distance.

THE RELATION OF MYOCARDIUM TO OTHER TYPES OF MUSCLE

Since the contractile mechanisms are similar in the various kinds of muscle, the principle differences in their function arise from differences in the mechanisms for excitation and control. Because myocardium superficially resembles skeletal muscle in its cross striation, in color and in the speed, vigor and duration of its contraction, the common tendency is to assume that cardiac muscle is only slightly different from skeletal muscle. On the contrary, myocardium more closely resembles visceral smooth muscle with respect to its functional characteristics and control (Fig. 2–6). Bozler[7,8] has classified smooth muscle into two main divisions, (a) multiunit smooth muscle and (b) visceral smooth muscle. Multiunit smooth muscle, in the peripheral vascular

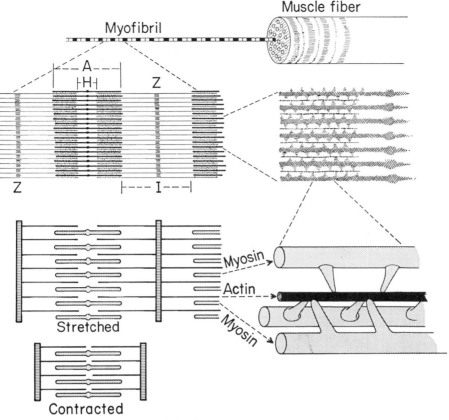

FIGURE 2–5 MUSCULAR CONTRACTION

The myofibrils are composed of overlapping thick myosin filaments and thin actin filaments. The amount of overlap is diminished during stretching and increased during contraction. Many cross bridges are observed at regular intervals between the actin and myosin filaments. These cross bridges have been visualized as forming linkages at specific sites on the actin fibers and drawing them onward during contraction. (After Huxley.[6])

system and the bladder, is directly innervated by motor nerves originating in the autonomic nervous system and resembles skeletal muscle in many aspects of its excitation and control.

In contrast, visceral smooth muscle, in the ureter, uterus and gastrointestinal tract, is not directly innervated by motor nerves (Fig. 2–6). Waves of excitation originate in the muscle fibers and are conducted throughout the contiguous cells. Although protoplasmic continuity between adjacent cells cannot be demonstrated, a mass of visceral smooth muscle functions like a syncytium, so that excitation originating at one site may spread to all other portions. In the ureter, pacemaker activity is well developed at a point near the hilus of the kidney. Waves of excitation originate at this point at fairly regular intervals and proceed in an orderly fashion down the length of the tube. Thus, the electrical activity of visceral smooth muscle is similar to that of the myocardium but very different from that of skeletal muscle (Fig. 2–6). Visceral smooth muscle is

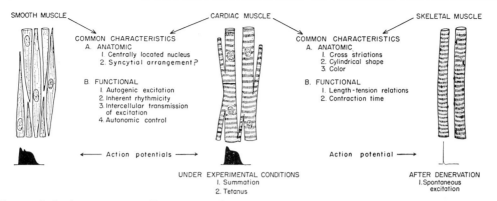

FIGURE 2–6   ANATOMIC AND FUNCTIONAL SIMILARITY BETWEEN DIFFERENT TYPES OF MUSCLE

Properties common to visceral smooth muscle and myocardium are listed between schematic drawings of these fibers. Functional characteristics shared by myocardium and skeletal muscle are similarly indicated between drawings. These different types of fibers are distinguished by their controlling mechanisms, the fundamental contractile process being very similar in each type. As far as control is concerned, myocardium is more closely related to visceral smooth muscle than to skeletal muscle. Schematic representations of action potentials from three types of muscle are indicated at the bottom of respective drawings. Smooth muscle has a rapid depolarization which is sustained for an extended period and may have multiple superimposed spikes (after Bozler[7,8]). Myocardium tends to remain depolarized for a period approximately equal to the duration of contraction. In contrast, skeletal muscle rapidly recovers its polarization after excitation and responds to repetitive stimulation to produce sustained contractions. Under experimental conditions summation and tetanus can be produced in myocardial fibers, even though such a response is usually considered typical of skeletal muscle. Denervated skeletal muscle exhibits spontaneous autogenic excitation (fibrillation), which is the typical form of excitation in myocardium and visceral smooth muscle.

controlled by the autonomic nervous system principally through the release of hormonal substances rather than through direct motor innervation. Thus, visceral smooth muscle is closely related to myocardium so far as its excitation and control are concerned. If the completeness of contraction or relaxation can vary in smooth muscle, there is no *a priori* reason for discarding this possibility in the myocardium.

The similarity of the basic contractile mechanisms is emphasized by the fact that apparent differences among the various types of muscle can be largely eliminated under specific conditions. For example, tetanus can be produced in papillary muscle from a mammalian heart maintained at 27° C. and electrically stimulated at a rapid rate.[9] A skeletal muscle deprived of its motor nerve supply exhibits

fibrillation due to myogenic impulses which spread along the individual fibers to produce asynchronous contractions. This phenomenon can be directly observed on the surface of the tongue after degeneration of its motor nerves.

ANATOMIC COMPONENTS OF THE HEART

Four rings of dense connective tissue are joined to form a single fibrous "skeleton" of the heart. The atria, ventricles, valves and arterial trunks are all firmly attached to this skeleton (Fig. 2–7). The two atria resemble a thin-walled, shallow cup of myocardium divided by a partition down the center. Each atrium has an atrial appendage, the functional significance of which is completely un-

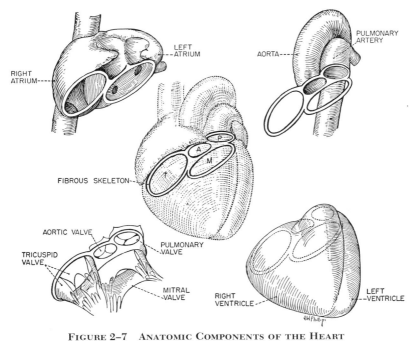

FIGURE 2–7   ANATOMIC COMPONENTS OF THE HEART

The fibrous skeleton of the heart consists of four valve rings joined together. To these dense connective tissue annuli fibrosi are fastened the two major arterial trunks and all four cardiac chambers. The atria and arterial trunks are attached to the superior surface of this fibrous skeleton and the ventricles and atrioventricular valve leaflets are fastened to its inferior aspect.

known. The margins of the atrial shell are fastened to the superior surface of the mitral and tricuspid valve rings.

The aorta and the pulmonary artery originate at the superior surface of the corresponding semilunar valve rings. Thus, the atrial chambers and the arterial trunks are anchored to the superior surface of the fibrous skeleton. The inflow and outflow channels of each ventricle lie side by side. The atrioventricular (A-V) valves are fastened to the inferior surface of the mitral and tricuspid valve rings, with the fibrous connective tissue at the root of each valve leaflet merging with that of the corresponding valvular ring. Chordae tendineae, extending from the inferior margins of each leaflet of the A-V valves, are fastened directly to the internal surface of the

ventricular walls and to papillary muscles projecting from the endocardial surface of the ventricular chambers.

The right and left ventricles are fastened to the entire circumference of the fibrous skeleton of the heart. The upper margin of the interventricular septum is attached along the line of fusion between the mitral and tricuspid valve rings. The membranous portion of the septum is fused at the junction of the pulmonary and aortic valve rings.

THE ANATOMY OF THE VENTRICULAR WALLS

The ventricles serve as the major source of energy for the circulation of blood and are composed of sheets of myocardial fibers encircling the ventricular chambers in a complex fashion[10, 11] reminiscent of the windings of a turban. The various muscular layers in the ventricles are so tightly bound together that they are very difficult to dissect into individual components. According to Robb and Robb,[11] the ventricular walls are composed of four different muscles: the superficial sinospiral and bulbospiral muscles and the deep sinospiral and bulbospiral muscles (Fig. 2–8). This traditional view of ventricular anatomy was

based on a special technique of dissection by a kind of unrolling process of hearts which had been prepared by prolonged soaking in strong chemicals to release binding between layers. This method was challenged by Grant,[12] and the concept tested by Streeter and Bassett[13] who measured the angles subtended by the myocardial fibers measured at 1 mm. intervals from endocardium to epicardium in pigs' hearts. The successive layers of myocardium displayed a progressive change in orientation like an open Japanese fan, without abrupt changes in fiber orientation (Fig. 2–9). The same kind of pattern was described for the interventricular septum and the anterior, posterior and free walls of the left ventricle, except at the root of papillary muscles. These measurements do not reveal discrete layers or sheets of myocardium in the ventricular walls.

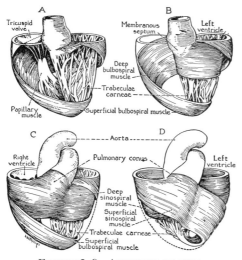

FIGURE 2–8   ANATOMY OF THE
VENTRICULAR WALLS

A, The superficial bulbospiral muscle bundles arise principally from the mitral ring and form the external investment for portions of the left and right ventricles as they spiral toward the apex. Emerging from the vortex on the inside of the chambers, these muscle bundles spiral back toward the valve rings either as trabeculae carneae or as papillary muscles which are joined to the valves through chordae tendineae.

B, The deep bulbospiral muscle fibers encircle the basilar portions of the left ventricle.

C, The deep sinospiral muscle encircles both the right and the left ventricular chambers.

D, The superficial spinospiral muscle is a counterpart of the superficial bulbospiral muscle. The anatomic distinction between the superficial sinospiral and bulbospiral muscles is arbitrary and functionally unimportant. (After Robb and Robb.[11])

Comparing myocardial orientation in the distended and contracted state, Streeter *et al.*[14] observed that, despite an increase in wall thickness as the chamber was compressed, the fiber orientation was not apparently rearranged, except at the apical portion of the lateral wall. These observations indicate that minimal tension should develop between successive layers of myocardium during contraction, contrary to my views expressed in previous publications[17, 18] and in the previous edition of this book. It would now appear that the concept of tension or force stored in the form of "interfascicular tension" between myocardial layers during systole and released during diastole should be reevaluated, perhaps abandoned.

THE FUNCTIONAL ANATOMY OF HEART VALVES

The heart valves are so simple and effective that the best available man-

FIGURE 2–9   ORIENTATION OF THE
MYOCARDIAL FIBERS

The orientation of myocardial
fibers in the left ventricular wall of a
pig's heart displays a progressive
angular displacement when examined
at 1 mm intervals. Abrupt changes in
fiber orientation representing discrete
layers (as in Fig. 2–8) were not found.
(From Streeter.[13])

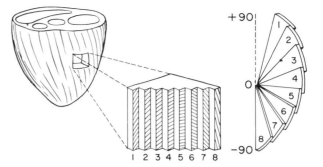

made substitutes are gross caricatures
by comparison. Not only do they open
and close rapidly and seal completely
against high pressures, but their
delicate-appearing cusps may endure
the ravages of repetitive closure for
more than 80 years.

Semilunar Valves.   The aortic and
pulmonary valves are similar, each
consisting of three symmetrical valve
cusps. Two cusps of equal size could
close tightly but would not open completely without considerable elastic
stretch. Three cusps can theoretically
open to the full dimensions of the valve
ring and yet produce a perfect seal
when closed. Behind the aortic valve
cusps are three outpouchings, the
sinuses of Valsalva, which help prevent obstruction of the coronary ostia.
If a valve leaflet came in contact with
the coronary orifice, shutting off the
flow of blood from the aorta, coronary
pressure would fall rapidly as blood
left the coronary arterial system, and
the valve cusp would be sealed against
the coronary ostium by a high differential pressure. This unfortunate accident is presumably prevented by the
presence of adequate space behind
the open valve cusps.

Atrioventricular Valves.   The tricuspid and mitral valves are larger and
much more complicated than the semilunar valves. The anatomic distinction
between the mitral valve and the tricuspid valve is largely artificial since
both valves consist fundamentally of

two large opposing cusps and small
intermediary cusps at each end. However, the chordae tendineae of the
tricuspid valve usually insert on three
fairly distinct groups of papillary
muscles, while only two principal
papillary muscles serve the mitral
valve. The anatomy of the papillary
muscles is subject to considerable
individual variability, some being
deeply notched, grooved or separated into multiple heads. Since the
structure and function of the mitral
and tricuspid valves are similar,
only the former will be described
in detail.

THE MITRAL VALVE.   The mitral
valve is interposed between the low-
pressure left atrium and high-pressure
left ventricle. The two valve cusps are
unequal in size. The large anterome-
dial (aortic) cusp hangs down like a
curtain between the mitral and aortic
orifices, while the shorter postero-
lateral cusp originates from the lateral
portions of the mitral ring. The combined surface area of the two valve
cusps is nearly twice as great as the
area of the mitral orifice which they
must occlude. The mitral valve orifice
is considerably smaller than the mitral
ring because the valve cusps are joined
at the commissures so the upper portion of the mitral valve resembles a
funnel.

The chordae tendineae correspond
to multiple guy lines extending from
the papillary muscles into the struc-

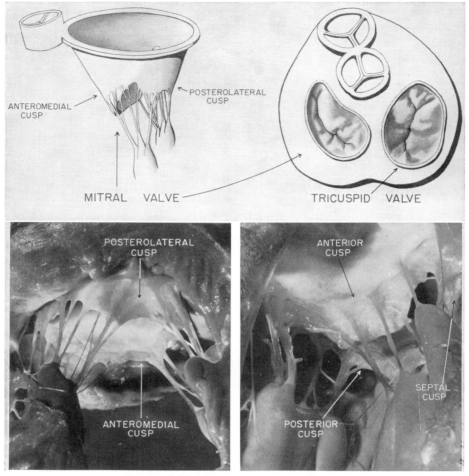

FIGURE 2–10　ATRIOVENTRICULAR VALVES

A, The mitral valve is shaped like a funnel when open and is closed by the approximation of two broad, membranous cusps. The chordae tendineae originate from the tips of two sets of papillary muscles and prevent eversion of the valve cusps into the left atrium during ventricular systole. The major chordae merge into the edge of the short leaf, but may insert several millimeters back from the edge of the larger aortic leaf.

B, The mitral and tricuspid valves are similar in both structure and function. They both consist primarily of two broad, opposing valve cusps with smaller intermediate cusps situated at each end. The tricuspid valve has a somewhat larger intermediate cusp and a total of three separate papillary muscles. (After Spalteholz, W.: Hand Atlas of Human Anatomy. Philadelphia, J. B. Lippincott Co., 1933.)

C, In a normal heart specimen, the walls of the left ventricle were excised to illustrate the postero- lateral aspect of the mitral valves, chordae tendineae and papillary muscles. Transillumination reveals that fibers of the chordae tendineae extend long distances within the valve cusps.

D, The three papillary muscles and corresponding valve cusps of the tricuspid valve were photo- graphed as viewed from within the right ventricular cavity.

ture of the valve cusps (see Fig. 2–10). It is important to recognize that the chordae tendineae from adjacent re- gions of the two valve cusps insert upon the same or adjacent papillary muscles (Fig. 2–10). Thus, tension ex-

erted through the chordae tends to draw the two valve cusps together. If the papillary muscles begin their con- traction early in ventricular systole, traction on the valve cusps should facilitate apposition of the valves.

COORDINATION OF THE HEART BEAT

To produce efficient pumping, the complex mass of myocardial fibers must contract more or less simultaneously. The effectiveness of the ventricles is lost if the individual myocardial bundles contract in a random fashion, e.g., in ventricular fibrillation. Coordinated contraction of the complex pattern of myocardial bundles stems from the functional continuity of the myocardial fibers; excitation beginning at one site spreads to all other contiguous areas. Excitation of the thick ventricular walls is facilitated by a rapidly conducting system of Purkinje fibers. The conduction system is responsible for periodic initiation of excitation (pacemaker activity), a delay between atrial and ventricular contraction (A-V nodal delay) and the rapid spread of excitation to all portions of the ventricular walls so that their contraction is sufficiently simultaneous to produce effective pumping action. When the conduction system is operating normally, this stereotyped sequence of events is repeated during each successive cardiac cycle.

THE CONDUCTION SYSTEM OF THE HEART

The sino-atrial (S-A) node is a small mass of specialized myocardial tissues embedded in the atrial wall near the entrance of the superior vena cava (Fig. 2–11). This node consists of an accumulation of modified myocardial cells. Shaped like an Indian war club, it has a fringe of delicate fibers merging with surrounding myocardial fibers. The S-A node is the normal pacemaker, spontaneously originating the spreading waves of excitation at a more rapid rate than any other part of the heart. A large number of fibers from the parasympathetic and sympathetic nervous systems terminate in the vicinity of the S-A node. Discharge of the vagal fibers releases acetylcholine, which tends to slow the rate of impulse formation, and the sympathetic fibers release epinephrine-like substances, which act to accelerate the frequency of impulse formation. If it were iso-

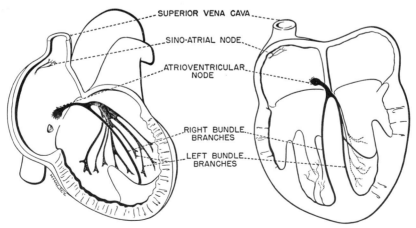

FIGURE 2–11   CONDUCTION SYSTEM OF THE HEART

The sino-atrial node is the normal pacemaker of the heart. No specialized conduction system has been described in the atria. The A-V node, common bundle and bundle branches conduct the wave of excitation from the atrium to the ventricular myocardium.

lated from all neural and hormonal control, the S-A node would probably generate impulses at a rate in excess of 100 per minute. Since the vagal influence generally predominates, the "normal" heart rate ranges between 60 and 100 impulses per minute. The S-A node retains its position as pacemaker for the entire heart so long as it generates impulses at a faster rate than any other region of the myocardial syncytium and so long as the spreading wave of excitation is rapidly conducted from the atria into the ventricles.

THE SEQUENCE OF EXCITATION

Apparently no conduction system serves the atria, so a wave of excitation originating in the S-A node spreads in all directions like the concentric wave produced by dropping a pebble into a pool of water. It travels at a rate of about 1 meter per second and reaches the most distant portions of the atrium in about 0.08 second. As it approaches the interatrial septum, the wave of excitation reaches another mass of specialized conducting tissue, the atrioventricular (A-V) node.

The A-V node is located on the right side of the interatrial septum close to the entrance of the coronary sinus (Fig. 2–12). When the wave of excitation reaches the A-V node, it does not proceed directly to the ventricles but is delayed there for intervals ranging around 0.08 to 0.12 second. It has been suggested that this delay is due to slow conduction along delicate fibers connecting the atrial myocardium with A-V nodal tissue. During the A-V nodal delay, atrial contraction is largely completed. The A-V node is the bulbous end of a bundle of Purkinje fibers—the bundle of His—which passes forward along the right side of the interatrial septum before plunging downward across the A-V junction to the upper margin of the muscular interventricular septum. There the bundle divides into two branches—the right and left bundles—which descend on opposite sides of the interventricular septum. The bundle branches ramify into a network of Purkinje fibers which are distributed over the inner surface of the ventricular chambers.

After leaving the A-V node, the wave of excitation passes rapidly (4 to 5 meters per second) along the Pur-

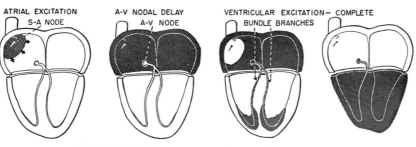

FIGURE 2–12   SEQUENCE OF CARDIAC EXCITATION

Excitation of the heart is normally initiated by an impulse which is generated by the S-A node and which spreads rapidly in all directions through the atrial musculature. After a slight delay at the A-V node, impulses are conducted by the Purkinje system into the ventricles where a wave of excitation spreads from the endocardial surfaces through the ventricular musculature.

kinje fibers of the common bundle and the bundle branches.[15] The endocardial surfaces of the ventricular chambers are excited early, and the endocardial layers (trabeculae carneae and papillary muscles) are first to contract. Thus, the wave of excitation probably penetrates the ventricular walls from the endocardial to the epicardial surface. The rapid spread of excitation through the ventricles produces more or less simultaneous contraction of the ventricular musculature.

THE SEQUENCE OF EVENTS DURING THE CARDIAC CYCLE

So long as the heart receives excitation along the normal pathways and the heart rate remains constant, each successive cardiac cycle tends to follow the same pattern of contraction and relaxation. A clear picture of the mechanical events of the cardiac cycle is required for logical interpretation of many physiologic events, e.g., timing of heart murmurs and analysis of electrocardiograms or arterial and venous pulse contours.

THE CARDIAC CYCLE: CINEFLUOROGRAPHIC ANGIOCARDIOGRAPHY

X-rays penetrating the body of a dog illuminate a fluorescent screen, producing an image of the cardiac silhouette. Motion pictures of these images record changes in the size and shape of the heart. If a radiopaque substance such as Diodrast is rapidly injected into the jugular vein, the course of the opacified blood can be followed through the heart and great vessels.[16] The changes in size and configuration of the individual cardiac chambers can be visualized as a two-dimensional projection or silhouette.

For purposes of orientation, the anatomic relations of the great vessels and cardiac chambers in the heart of the dog are indicated in Figure 2–13 as viewed from the right side. Note that the right ventricle does not extend to the apex of the heart in the dog. Further, the configuration of the ventricular chambers is not the same in dogs and in man. Although the fundamental principles of cardiac contraction in dogs probably resemble those in humans, caution must be exercised in applying the discussion which follows to cardiac function in man.

The typical sequence of events which occurs during filling and contraction of the right atrium and right ventricle of a dog is illustrated in Figure 2–14. Diodrast flowed along the superior vena cava during the eight frames in column A and entered the right atrium in the third frame of column B (B-3). In frame B-5, the tricuspid valves everted into the right atrium and blood gushed into the right ventricle (B-6). The variations in density of the right ventricular shadow in frames B-7 and B-8 represent the mixing of the incoming blood with the residual blood remaining in the ventricle after the preceding systole. The next contraction began in frames C-5 and C-6, as indicated by the protrusion of the right atrial appendage associated with atrial systole. In frame C-6, the right ventricle began to contract and in the next three frames was reduced to a small triangular area with its base at the tricuspid valves. Between frames C-8 and D-1 (1/15 second), the right ventricle was filled and apparently remained unchanged in size until the succeeding contraction (D-8). During the remainder of this cycle, Diodrast passed through the right atrium and flowed into the inferior vena cava down to the level of the diaphragm against the oncoming

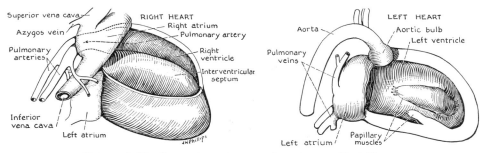

FIGURE 2–13   ROENTGENOGRAPHIC ANATOMY OF DOG HEART

The anatomic relations of the cardiac chambers and arterial trunks in the dog as viewed from the right side for comparison with angiocardiograms presented in subsequent figures. The right atrium lies above the left atrium on the posterior aspect of the heart. The interventricular septum presents a convex surface to the right ventricular cavity. Thus, the right ventricular cavity has a crescentic transverse section and partially encircles the left ventricular cavity.

stream of blood. The opacified blood in the inferior vena cava returned to the heart during the next filling period. The right ventricle did not distend noticeably during the latter part of diastole even when there was sufficient pressure to force Diodrast against the stream of blood into the inferior vena cava. Diastolic filling appears to be largely complete very early in the diastolic interval.

Filling of the Right Ventricle. Diastolic filling of the right ventricle can be studied by injecting Lipiodol into a systemic vein. Lipiodol is a radiopaque, viscous oil which is very cohesive and tends to flow along with the stream of blood as a long ribbon or as multiple globules, depending upon how it is injected. The course of one Lipiodol streamer ascending the inferior vena cava is indicated by serial tracings in Figure 2–15. The movement was relatively slow during systole. At the beginning of the rapid filling in early diastole the Lipiodol streamer accelerated rapidly, passing along the inferior vena cava, through the atrium and into the right ventricle. Thus, the blood which fills the right ventricle comes not only from the atrium but also from a considerable distance down the inferior vena cava.

Blood streams from the superior and inferior venae cavae converge at the right atrium. Streamers of Lipiodol and Diodrast moving down the superior vena cava frequently exhibit a spiral flow as they enter the ventricle (Fig. 2–15). This is attributed to a swirling motion of the blood produced by the confluence of the two streams. These currents tend to mix the venous blood within the right ventricle.

Contraction of the Right Ventricle. Cinefluorographic films indicate that a longitudinal section of the right ventricular chamber is roughly triangular. It is bounded by a convex septal wall and the concave free wall, which enclose a crescent-shaped slit between them (Fig. 2–13). The action of the right ventricle resembles that of the old-fashioned bellows used to kindle fires. Since the sides of the bellows are large compared to the space between them, their very slight movement toward each other causes displacement of a large volume from within. In the right ventricular cavity, a relatively narrow space is confined between two broad surfaces so that the surface area of the chamber is very great in relation to the volume.[17, 18]

Blood is ejected from the right ventricle by three separate mechanisms occurring more or less simultaneously (Fig. 2–16): (*a*) Contraction

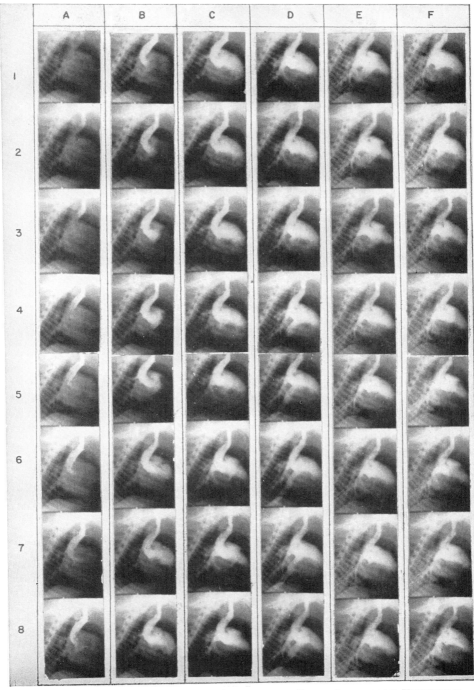

FIGURE 2–14   CHANGES IN SIZE AND SHAPE OF THE RIGHT ATRIUM AND VENTRICLE

Successive frames from a cinefluorographic film exposed at 15 frames per second illustrate the filling and contraction of the right atrium and right ventricle during 3.2 seconds following the injection of contrast medium. Examine each column in succession from above downward to observe the sequence of events.

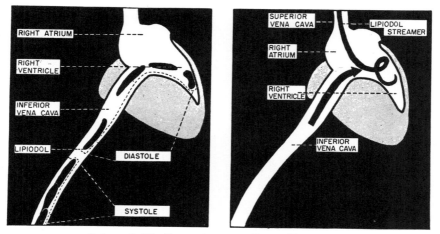

FIGURE 2–15   FILLING OF THE RIGHT VENTRICLE

Lipiodol streamers, floating freely in the blood, move relatively slowly during one phase of the cardiac cycle, then suddenly accelerate and move without hesitation into the right ventricular cavity, presumably during the rapid filling phase of ventricular diastole (see text). Similar streamers of Lipiodol descending along the superior vena cava frequently display a swirling motion which may be due to the convergence of the two currents of blood flowing into the atrium.

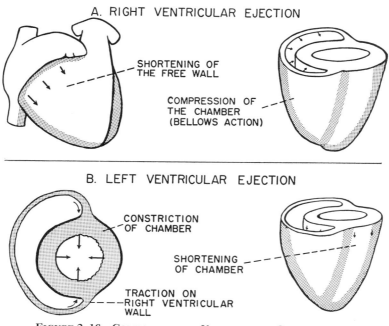

FIGURE 2–16   COMPONENTS OF VENTRICULAR CONTRACTION

A, Blood is ejected from the right ventricle by shortening of the free wall with downward displacement of the tricuspid valve ring and movement of the free wall toward the interventricular septum by myocardial shortening. Compression of the right ventricular cavity may be supplemented by traction exerted on the free wall by left ventricular contraction.

B, Left ventricular ejection is accomplished primarily by a reduction in the diameter of the chamber with some additional shortening of the longitudinal axis.

of the spiral muscles draws the tricuspid valve ring toward the apex of the heart and shortens the longitudinal axis of the chamber. This shortening is the most obvious movement but is much less effective than the bellows action in ejecting blood. (*b*) The free wall of the right ventricle moves toward the convex surface of the interventricular septum. This movement is very slight but extremely effective in ejecting blood. (*c*) Contraction of the deep circular fibers enclosing the left ventricular cavity must produce a greater curvature of the interventricular septum (Fig. 2–16), although the midportion (central axis) of this septum remains remarkably fixed in both position and length. Since the free wall of the right ventricle is attached to the left ventricle along the interventricular groove, traction on this wall will also contribute to the bellows action on the right ventricular cavity. This effect is so slight that it cannot be readily demonstrated on cinefluorographic films. It has been clearly shown, however, that the free wall of the right ventricle can be almost completely destroyed by cauterization in dogs[19] or by coronary occlusion in man[20] without obvious effects on the circulatory efficiency.

Clearly, the configuration of the right ventricle is ideally suited to the ejection of large volumes of blood with minimal amounts of myocardial shortening. On the other hand, this architectural design is not conducive to the development of high intraventricular pressure.[17] If the normal right ventricle were suddenly required to provide the intraventricular pressures normally developed in the left ventricle, the right ventricular myocardium would have to develop tension many times as great as that in the left ventricle. Thus, we see that the right ventricle is specifically adapted to the task of pumping large or widely varying volumes of blood against a very

low outflow pressure. Since the pulmonary vascular tree normally offers slight resistance to flow, the right ventricle normally ejects blood at relatively low pressure into the pulmonary artery. A sudden increase in pulmonary arterial pressure (massive pulmonary embolism) frequently leads to sudden death because the right ventricular myocardium cannot sustain the higher pressures needed to provide adequate flow through the lungs.

Contraction of the Left Ventricle. Contraction of the left ventricle involves both a reduction in the diameter of the cylindrical portion and a shortening along the longitudinal axis of the chamber. Contraction of the circumferential muscle bundles acts to reduce the diameter of the chamber (see Fig. 2–16). This action accounts for most of the power and volume of the ejection, since the volume contained decreases with the square of the radius in a cylinder. Shortening of the longitudinal axis is less prominent and less effective in ejecting blood because the volume displacement is directly proportional to the change in length.

Shortening of the chamber involves movement of the mitral valve ring toward the apex of the heart. During diastole, the A-V junction rapidly ascends toward the left atrium. Since the interventricular septum shortens very little, the distance between the root of the aorta and the apex of the heart changes very little.

In contrast to the right ventricle, the left ventricular cavity has a small surface area in relation to the contained volume by virtue of its cylindrical contour. The thick cuff of deep myocardial bundles is ideally situated to develop a very high internal pressure during contraction. Thus, the left ventricle is architecturally designed as a high-pressure pump, which is consistent with its role of supplying energy for the flow of blood through the high-pressure, high-resistance, systemic circulation. The normal left ventricle has less adaptability than the right ventricle in ejecting large volumes of blood. When the left ventricle is exposed to an excessive volume load for extended periods of time, e.g., in aortic insufficiency, the chambers often become tremendously dilated so that the surface area per unit volume is increased. In other words, the left ventricle assumes some of the characteristics of the right ventricle when large volumes must be ejected during each stroke.

Clearly, the anatomic and architectural features of the ventricular chambers reflect the type of work which each must perform. By the same token, the functional characteristics of the circulatory trees which they serve establish the nature of the load or the working conditions for each ventricular chamber.

Continuous measurements of the various ventricular dimensions provide an opportunity to synthesize a description of the changes in the volume.

Techniques for Recording Cardiac Performance in Intact Dogs. Although it has not been possible to measure directly the absolute ventricular volume in intact animals, new techniques have been devised[21, 22] for continuously recording the circumference, diameter and length of the left ventricular chamber. The left ventricular pressure and the flow of blood through the aorta have also been measured in intact dogs, and records of all these parameters of ventricular function have been obtained during a wide range of activities for periods of days or weeks. These methods are described here briefly because they are recent developments which are not generally familiar; much of the data

discussed in the remainder of this section have been obtained by these means.

Left ventricular diameter has been measured by variable inductance gauges installed within that chamber and connected to a recorder by wires on the outside. The gauge comprises a coil, anchored at one end to the free wall of the left ventricle, and a stylus, anchored to the midportion of the interventricular wall and free to move within the coil. The position of the stylus within the coil can be recorded to a fraction of a millimeter by recording changes in inductance of the coil (see Fig. 2–17A).

Left ventricular length can also be determined with a variable inductance gauge. For this measurement the gauge is installed between the root of the aorta and the apex of the chamber (Fig. 2–17C).

Left ventricular circumference has been measured by a variable resistance gauge (a mercury-filled rubber tube) encircling the chamber; a wire from one end of the gauge passes into the right ventricular cavity to follow the contour of the interventricular septum. The absolute circumference of the gauge is determined from roentgenograms exposed perpendicular to the long axis of the ventricle (see Fig. 2–17C).

SONOCARDIOMETERY.[21, 22] Alternatively, a ventricular dimension may be measured in the intact dog with the sonocardiometer. With this instrument, the distance across the ventricular cavity is determined as the transit time of bursts of ultrasonic vibrations passing between barium titanate crystals installed on its walls. These sound waves travel through blood and the ventricular walls at 1.5 mm./msec., so that this transit time can be continuously recorded and calibrated as ventricular diameter.

The internal diameters and in-

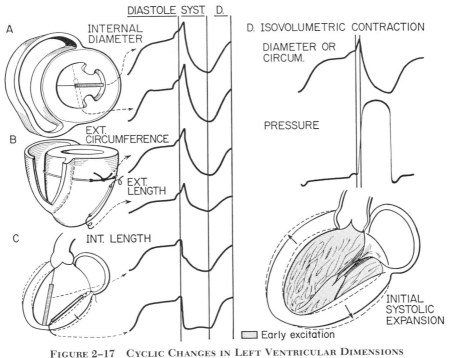

FIGURE 2-17 CYCLIC CHANGES IN LEFT VENTRICULAR DIMENSIONS

A, During ventricular diastole, all dimensions increase, rapidly at first and more gradually during the latter part of the filling interval. Atrial contraction adds a slight additional increment of blood. At the onset of ventricular systole, the internal diameters (A), external circumference and length (B) abruptly increase because the internal length (C) shortens during this interval which is called the isovolumetric contraction (D). The external length increases during this interval when the internal length is abruptly diminishing because of the outward bending of the thick-walled ventricle.

ternal length of the left ventricle have been measured by variable inductance coils (Fig. 2-17A,C). The external circumference and the length of the left and right ventricles have been measured by variable resistance gauges (delicate rubber tubes filled with mercury). These records illustrate the following characteristics of the filling and emptying of the ventricles. At the beginning of the diastolic interval, all dimensions of the ventricular chamber increase rapidly. This phase of rapid diastolic filling is very brief and merges abruptly or gradually into the phase of slow filling which persists until atrial contraction ensues. When the ventricles are maximally distended, the dimensions reach a plateau

at the end of the rapid filling phase and do not increase further during the remainder of diastole. Such an interval of unchanging ventricular volume is termed *the period of diastasis*. The diastolic interval normally ends with the onset of atrial contraction, which begins as the wave of excitation spreads over the atrium. Contraction of the atrial musculature reduces the capacity of the atrial chambers and displaces blood forward into the ventricles or backward into the great veins, depending on which course offers the least resistance.

The Isovolumic Phase of Ventricular Systole. As the wave of excitation extends rapidly along the Purkinje system (Fig. 2-12) and spreads over the endocardial surface of the ventricles, the trabeculae carneae and the papillary muscles are excited and begin to contract. The shortening papillary muscles exert traction on the chordae tendineae, drawing the atrioventricular valves into apposition, and the rising ventricular pressure seals them tight. The contracting papillary muscles draw the antrioventricular valve edges toward the apex,[23, 24] and the shortening endocardial layers draw the atrioventricular valve rings toward the apex of the heart. Since all four valves are closed, the contracting muscles elevate the pressure within the ventricle but do not change the volume they contain. Thus, the interval during which ventricular pressure rises to a level sufficient to open the semilunar valves has been called the period of isovolumic contraction. At the onset of systole, the length of the ventricles is abruptly shortened as the atrioventricular diaphragm rapidly descends. The other dimensions (diameter, circumference and external length) of the ventricle simultaneously expand. The sudden lengthening of the circumferentially oriented constrictor muscles in the ventricle, just before they contract, may increase the effectiveness of their contraction.

Ventricular Systole. As the full thickness of the ventricular wall becomes excited, pressure in the ventricles exceeds corresponding arterial pressure and blood is very rapidly ejected from the ventricles. The rapidity of ventricular emptying is indicated by the reduction in the ventricular dimensions, rapid during early systole and slowing during the last part of systole. The various dimensional changes illustrated in Figure 2–17 are applicable to ventricular systole when the heart is normally well filled at the end of diastole. If the ventricular chambers are not well filled during diastole, the circumference is reduced at the onset of systole and systolic ejection is accomplished primarily by shortening of the longitudinal ventricular axis. This type of ejection occurs when cardiac size is below the normal range as a result of extremely fast heart rates, positive radial acceleration or exposure of the heart for experimental purposes.

THE MECHANICAL EFFECTS OF CARDIAC CONTRACTION

The cyclic changes in the various dimensions of the ventricles combine to produce alternating expansion and contraction of total ventricular volume. Such changes in volume have been recorded by inserting the exposed hearts of animals into rigid chambers called cardiometers. (See Fig. 2–18.)

Myocardial contraction produces a sequence of changes in the pressure and volume of blood in the ventricles which is traditionally described in terms of the atrial, ventricular and arterial pressures and of the variations in the combined volume of both ventricles measured by a cardiometer as illustrated schematically in Figure 2–18.

During the later portion of diastole, the ventricular pressure equals the atrial pressure because the two chambers are connected through the wide A-V orifices and little or no blood is flowing between them. The wave of excitation spreading over the atrium is followed by atrial contraction. The contraction slightly increases both intra-atrial and intraventricular pressures because it suddenly compresses this portion of the venous volume reservoir. As the atrium contracts, blood may be displaced into the ventricular chambers or back into the large venous

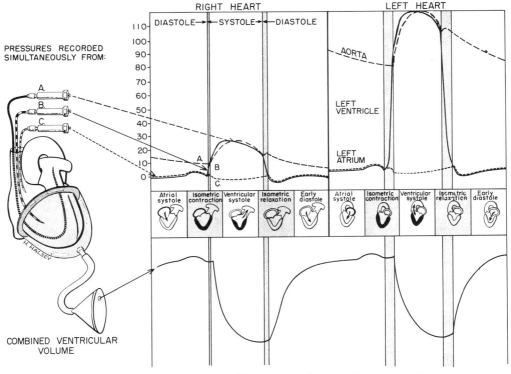

FIGURE 2–18 MECHANICAL EFFECTS OF CARDIAC CONTRACTION

Simultaneous changes in atrial, ventricular and arterial pressures in the right and left ventricles are illustrated schematically along with fluctuations in combined ventricular volume to indicate the sequence of events during a single cardiac cycle. Note that ventricular pressure exceeds corresponding arterial pressure only during the first portion of systole (see text). The great difference in pressure developed by the two ventricles is consistent with the differences in their architecture (see Fig. 2–16).

channels, depending upon which course offers the least resistance. The quantity of blood which enters the ventricle in response to atrial contraction is quite variable.

Excitation of the ventricles begins as atrial contraction is being completed, and ventricular contraction begins about 0.075 second later.[25] Ventricular pressure rises to exceed arterial pressure during the period of isometric contraction, which lasts about 0.013 second in the right ventricle[26] and about 0.06 second in the left ventricle (Fig. 2–18).

During this period the ventricular volume is unchanged except for the movement of blood required to close and displace the valves. This period of isovolumic contraction is characterized by a slight reduction in recorded ventricular volume and a slight increase in atrial pressure due to ballooning of the A-V valves. The atria relax and begin to refill during ventricular systole. Isovolumic contraction of the ventricle ends when ventricular pressure exceeds the arterial pressure and is followed by rapid ejection of blood into the arterial system. Thus, the arterial pressure is elevated while the ventricular volume is abruptly diminished.

During the initial portion of systolic ejection, the ventricular pressures rise well above the pressure in the arterial channels into which they discharge. This transient, steep pressure gradient (somewhat exaggerated in Fig. 2–18) produces rapid acceleration of outflowing blood to produce a peak flow rate early in systole. During the later portion of systole, pressure in the ventricles actually drops slightly below the pressure in the corresponding artery, even though the ventricular volume continues to diminish, indicating persistent outflow of blood. These changes in pressure gradient and volume changes in the ventricles find important functional significance in the performance of the heart in terms of blood flow rates.

The intraventricular and arterial pressures tend to level off and descend as the rate of ejection from the ventricles drops below the rate at which blood leaves the arterial system through the capillaries. The onset of ventricular relaxation is associated with a rapid drop in ventricular pressures below arterial pressure. The semilunar valves become approximated by a retrograde surge of blood in the root of the aorta, which produces the dicrotic notch in the arterial pressure wave. During isovolumic relaxation, ventricular pressure rapidly drops below atrial pressure. The A-V valves swing open before a gush of blood from the atrium. The ventricles rapidly refill with blood from the thoracic veins and atria, as indicated by the abrupt upswing in the ventricular volume curve. The slope of the volume curve indicates that early filling of the ventricles is more rapid than the ejection of blood by ventricular contraction. Ventricular filling is largely complete very soon after the onset of ventricular relaxation and, if the diastolic interval is sufficiently long, ventricular volume reaches a plateau during which no more blood enters from the atrium—the period of

diastasis. The length of the diastolic interval is determined largely by the time required for the pacemaker to discharge the new wave of excitation which initiates another cardiac cycle.

BLOOD FLOW: METHODS OF MEASUREMENT

The rate of ventricular ejection can be estimated from the systolic downslope on cardiometer records. Obviously, the rate of change of ventricular volume is related to the flow velocity and volume flow rates of blood leaving the ventricles. A clear picture of ventricular ejection cannot be obtained from measurements of changing dimensions and pressures. Detailed information regarding the blood flow out of each ventricle and at various key arteries and veins is absolutely essential for a comprehensive understanding of cardiovascular function and control. A wide variety of flow measuring devices have been employed in physiological and clinical studies. Extensive discussion of methodology is not appropriate in this type of discussion. However, some representatives examples of flow detecting devices are presented schematically in Figure 2–19 as representative examples, divided into five rather arbitrary categories.

Some Volume Sensors. If fluid flow is defined as the change of volume or displacement of a volume per unit time, (dV/dt), a most direct approach would utilize sensors responding to changes in volume, such as the cardiometer illustrated in Figure 2–18. Each of the methods illustrated in the left hand column of Figure 2–19 has been employed in physiological investigations, and many other techniques in the same category have been described in other publications.[27–29] A volumetric container and a timer

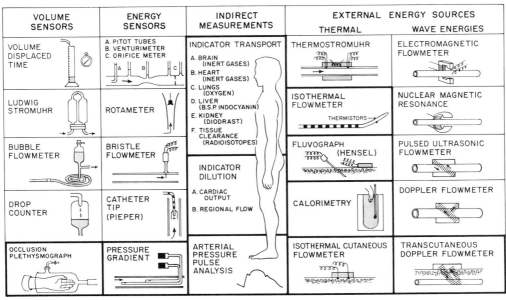

VOLUME SENSORS	ENERGY SENSORS	INDIRECT MEASUREMENTS	EXTERNAL ENERGY SOURCES	
			THERMAL	WAVE ENERGIES
VOLUME DISPLACED TIME	A. PITOT TUBES B. VENTURIMETER C. ORIFICE METER	INDICATOR TRANSPORT A. BRAIN (INERT GASES) B. HEART (INERT GASES) C. LUNGS (OXYGEN) D. LIVER (B.S.P. INDOCYANIN) E. KIDNEY (DIODRAST) F. TISSUE CLEARANCE (RADIOISOTOPES)	THERMOSTROMUHR	ELECTROMAGNETIC FLOWMETER
LUDWIG STROMUHR	ROTAMETER		ISOTHERMAL FLOWMETER THERMISTORS	NUCLEAR MAGNETIC RESONANCE
BUBBLE FLOWMETER	BRISTLE FLOWMETER	INDICATOR DILUTION A. CARDIAC OUTPUT B. REGIONAL FLOW	FLUVOGRAPH (HENSEL)	PULSED ULTRASONIC FLOWMETER
DROP COUNTER	CATHETER TIP (PIEPER)		CALORIMETRY	DOPPLER FLOWMETER
OCCLUSION PLETHYSMOGRAPH	PRESSURE GRADIENT	ARTERIAL PRESSURE PULSE ANALYSIS	ISOTHERMAL CUTANEOUS FLOWMETER	TRANSCUTANEOUS DOPPLER FLOWMETER

FIGURE 2–19   BLOOD FLOW DETECTING AND MEASURING DEVICES

Various types of flow detecting and measuring devices are illustrated schematically to indicate the diversity of methods that have been used in the past. The indirect techniques have found common use in clinical diagnosis and are described in greater detail in Chapter 3, Section 2.

serve as a standard for calibrating flowmeters just as a mercury column is a common standard for calibrating pressure gauges. The Ludwig strohmuhr, bubble flowmeter and drop counter and plethysmograph all monitor changes in volume which can be calibrated in terms of flow rates of blood. To directly measure volumetric blood flow requires gaining access to the entire volume of blood flowing through a blood vessel, which generally requires undesirably preliminary steps such as cannulation or exposure under surgical conditions. A notable exception is the venous occlusion plethysmograph by which arterial inflow is collected within the veins and measured by a volume sensor; it is applicable only to accessible peripheral vascular beds.

Some Energy Sensors. The energy content of moving blood may be used to activate sensors such as Pitot tubes, venturimeters, orifice meters, rotameters and bristle flowmeters as illustrated schematically in Figure 2–19. These have been described in considerable detail elsewhere.[27–29] The catheter tip flowmeter of Pieper[30] responds to the momentum of flowing blood impinging upon a very small plate exposed to the blood streaming along a channel. The flow rate along an artery can be continuously computed from the pressure gradient measured at two sites at known distances along a vascular channel by means of double lumen catheters and carefully matched pressure transducers in accordance with a technique described by Fry and his associates.[31] All of these techniques have provided information of value in controlled experiments on experimental animals. Pieper's catheter has been employed to provide information about dynamic changes in flow rates in intact healthy animals, and the pressure gradient technique has been employed in both animals and man.

Some Indirect Measurements. Most of our available information about blood flow in man has come from various techniques by which blood flow is estimated by measurement of the concentration of substances in blood or tissue.[32] In this connection, the term indirect is used to imply that the recorded variable is distinctly dissimilar to the target variable, a distinction which is sometimes quite arbitrary Clearly, the estimation of blood flow by measuring the changing concentrations of dyes or radioisotopes or dissolved gases conforms to this definition. The quantity of blood required to transport the oxygen taken into the lungs per minute can be calculated by means of the Fick formula.[33] This and other techniques applicable to man are described in Section 2 of Chapter 3. Blood flows computed from oxygen transport or indicator dilution are very useful but share two common deficiencies: flow rates can be estimated only at low sampling rates so that rapid changes cannot be followed and the sampling requires withdrawal of samples which can be obtained only by inserting needles or catheters through the skin into the blood vessels. Estimation of blood flow from a continuous record of central aortic pressure has theoretical and practical limitations.[34]

External Energy Sensors. The rate at which heat is carried away from a heat source is an indirect method of estimating flow which has been widely used in both engineering and basic medical science. The hotwire anemometer is practically a standard for fluid dynamics of gases, but its application to liquid poses serious problems. The thermostromuhr of Rein had a distinguished place in physiological research but rapidly faded into obscurity after a critical evaluation by Shipley, Gregg and Warn.[35] Since heat can be so easily generated and controlled by electronic circuitry, and since temperatures can be precisely measured by thermocouples or thermistors, many thermal flowmeters have been proposed for application to the body surface or to internal structures.[36-38] However, these devices all have a common source of uncertainty due to the fact that heat flows so readily between continuous media of all sorts. In other words, it is very difficult to confine induced thermal energy to the blood or to a single tissue.

Electromagnetic and ultrasonic wave energies have produced a growing selection of new types of flow detecting devices applicable to physiological experiments on healthy animals and man.[39] They are capable of responding rapidly to dynamic responses. Since they have contributed greatly to our knowledge in the past decade, these techniques are described in somewhat greater detail.

Two main types of flow detecting devices have been developed to the point that the transducers could be chronically implanted on the outside of arteries or veins during aseptic surgery so that cardiovascular responses could be studied during spontaneous and experimentally induced changes in activity for days, weeks or months after recovery.

Electromagnetic Flowmeters. If a strip of metal moved through the magnetic field between the poles of a magnet at right angles to the lines of force, a voltage or potential difference is generated in the metal strip in accordance with Faraday's induction law (Fig. 2–19). The induced voltage could be registered using electrodes in contact with the metal strip. An ionic solution, such as blood plasma, is also an electrical conductor. If blood flows between the poles of a magnet, a potential difference can be registered between electrodes making electrical contact with the fluid. To avoid polarization of electrodes and artifacts from extraneous electrical currents (i.e., electrocardiogram), fluctuating magnetic fields have been used by energizing the magnet with fluctuating currents (sine wave, square wave, trapezoidal and so forth). Since 1936 Kolin's early application of the Faraday principle[40] has been followed by extensive development, notably by Denison and Spencer[41] and many others, including industrial concerns. As a result, electromagnetic flowmeters with good stability, rapid response and reliable calibrations are available commercially. The principles and characteristics of these devices are covered in greater detail in other publications.[42, 43]

Pulsed-Ultrasonic Flow Sensor. A flow detecting device has been developed in the laboratory utilizing bursts of ultrasound and based on the simple principle that sound travels faster in fluid when moving with the stream than against the stream.[44] In other words, sound will take longer to travel upstream between two points than to travel downstream between the same two points. If the separation of the two points and the velocity of the sound in the still medium are known, then the velocity of the medium may be calculated or recorded based on the difference in the transit times upstream and downstream.

Two ultrasonic transmitting crystals are mounted diagonally at opposite ends of a plastic cylinder which is bivalved and fitted on the outside of an artery. Bursts of ultrasound (i.e., 5 megacycles/second) are transmitted diagonally across the stream of blood, alternately upstream and downstream. The transit time of these paired bursts are compared, amplified and recorded to represent the velocity of blood flow, averaged across the channel.

Ultrasonic Doppler Shift Blood Flow Detection. Everyone is familiar with the Doppler shift in frequency which causes the change in pitch in a railroad whistle as it passes a stationary observer. If a continuous beam of ultrasound is transmitted diagonally into a column of blood, a small fraction of the sound energy backscatters from particles in the blood to reach a receiver on the opposite side of the channel.[45] If the blood is stationary, the ultrasonic frequency at the receiver is the same as the transmitter frequency. If the blood is moving, however, a Doppler shift in frequency occurs such that the ultrasound reaching the receiver differs from the transmitted frequency by the amount dependent in part upon the velocity with which the backscattering particles are moving. By mixing the transmitted frequency with the backscattered frequency, a beat frequency is generated which is audible (0 to 10,000 c.p.s.) under normal blood flow conditions and can be recorded to indicate dynamic changes in blood flow velocity in arteries or veins. In its simplest form, this device does not distinguish forward from backward flow. The ultrasonic flowmeters are less accurate than the electromagnetic flowmeters on both theoretical and practical grounds. However, these and other flow detecting devices have potential value in various applications to basic medical science or clinical diagnosis.[46]

DYNAMIC PROPERTIES OF LEFT VENTRICULAR EJECTION

The availability of sensors which can be chronically implanted in animals has provided opportunities to study changes in pressures, dimensions and flows in strategic locations in the cardiovascular system during spontaneous and induced responses in intact healthy animals after recovery from the surgery (Fig. 2–20A). Since the sampling rates of these techniques are very rapid, they can accurately follow rapid changes in aortic flow, left ventricular diameter and arterial pressure (Fig. 2–20B). The recorded wave forms contain a great deal more

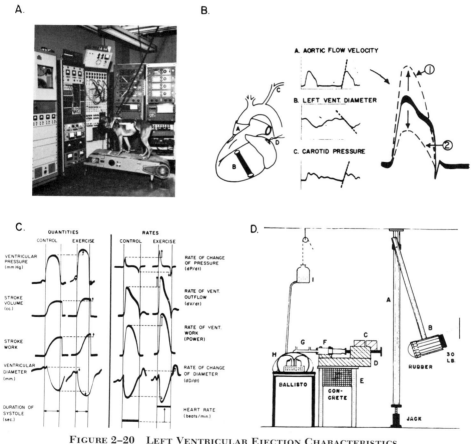

FIGURE 2–20   LEFT VENTRICULAR EJECTION CHARACTERISTICS

A, Chronically indwelling flow sensors, catheters and dimensional gauges provide an opportunity to study spontaneous cardiovascular responses in healthy dogs fully recovered from the surgery.

B, Typical wave forms of aortic flow rates, ventricle diameter and systemic arterial pressure all reveal very steep slopes during the initial stages of ventricular ejection when blood is being rapidly propelled out of the left ventricle.

C, Many characteristics of ventricular performance can be derived from direct measurements of pressure dimensions and flow.

D, To simulate the rapid acceleration of blood accomplished by the normal left ventricle in cadavers required blows by a 30 pound mass on a 8 foot lever arm striking a piston to drive blood into the aorta. (After Starr *et al.*[48])

information than is apparent from merely measuring either the mean values or the magnitudes at the peaks and valleys of the deflections. For example, the upslope of the aortic flow velocity recording is very steep, indicating that ventricular myocardium not only develops very high pressures very quickly, but also accelerates the blood very rapidly to high peak flow velocity very early during the ejection period. The downslope on the left ventricular diameter record confirms reduction in chamber diameter as the ventricle rapidly ejects blood into the aorta. As blood rapidly enters the root of the aorta, the pressure abruptly rises, inducing a pulse wave which spreads rapidly through the arterial tree. From direct recordings of aortic flow rate and left ventricular pressure and diameter, additional information can be derived using simple analogue computers and ratemeters as illustrated in Figures 2–20 and 2–22. The most significant features of left ventricular ejection are very steep slopes on the records of ventricular pressure, ventricular outflow rate (aortic flow) and ventricular diameter during the initial phases of left ventricular systole. These steep slopes indicate exceedingly rapid rates of increase in ventricular pressure and ventricular ejection velocity.

One might imagine that the muscular ventricular walls squeeze down on the contained blood much as one would milk a cow or squeeze a lemon in a clenched fist. According to Spencer and Greiss,[47] blood accelerates in the aorta exceedingly rapidly (averaging 4650 cm./sec.^{2}) to the peak velocity early in systole. To produce such rapid acceleration of blood, the ventricle must develop forces some five times the force of gravity.

Thus, the contracting myocardium propels outflowing blood with a sudden impulse like a piston struck with a mallet. For example, everyone is aware of the fact that every heart beat causes the whole body to recoil slightly, a phenomenon which can be directly observed while standing quietly on a sensitive scale. This phenomenon has been utilized in the development of a "ballistocardiograph" for studying cardiac function (see Fig. 3–25). When Starr and his associates[48] attempted to reproduce in a cadaver a recoil sufficient to simulate the normal ballistocardiographic record, they found that no available pumps could discharge blood into the aorta with sufficient acceleration to equal that of the normal heart. They finally found it necessary to use a 30 pound mass on an eight foot lever arm, striking a piston and driving blood into the cadaver's aorta (Fig. 2–20D) to produce ballistocardiographic deflections of an amplitude approaching that of normal men of equivalent size. The functional importance of these dynamic characteristics will be discussed in more detail in Chapter 3.

RIGHT VENTRICULAR EJECTION

The pattern of ejection from the normal right ventricle differs from that described for the left ventricle. The velocity of ejection increases more gradually and reaches its peak near mid systole. Flow from the ventricle also decelerates more gradually, and ejection persists longer. The retrograde flow usually associated with the closure of the semilunar valves at the end of systole occurs later. The average acceleration is lower (i.e., 2480 cm/sec.^{2}), and the pressure reversal occurs later.

These differences in the ejection patterns of the two ventricles may be attributed to their architecture and

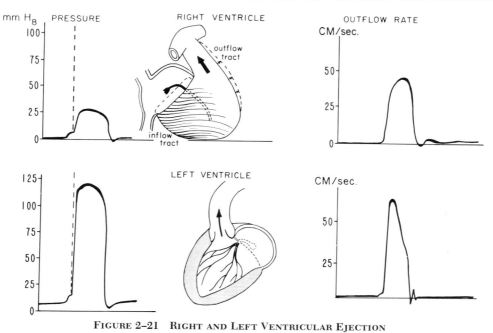

FIGURE 2–21   RIGHT AND LEFT VENTRICULAR EJECTION

In contrast with the left ventricle, right ventricular ejection produces a much more gradual pressure rise to a lower peak ventricular pressure and more gradual fall in pressure at the end of systole. Similarly, right ventricular outflow begins earlier, accelerates more gradually to a lower peak velocity occuring near mid-systole and decelerates more gradually than left ventricular outflow.

function. The rapid acceleration of blood and early peak flow velocity from the left ventricle suggest a powerful and effective mechanism for pumping against a high pressure. The thick walls of myocardium must contract very nearly synchronously to generate such a powerful impulse. In contrast, the right ventricular chamber can be likened to a crevice between two broad surfaces which exert a bellows type of action in ejecting blood. Further, a substantial body of evidence indicates that the inflow tract of the right ventricle contracts early and displaces the blood into the outflow tract. The conus region contracts last. Since the pressure in the pulmonary artery is very low at the onset of right ventricular systole, ejection begins as soon as right ventricular pressure rises only 8 to 10 mm. Hg. These factors

appear to account, at least in part, for the early onset of pulmonary flow, the gradual increase in outflow velocity from the right ventricle and the longer duration of ejection.

This description of right ventricular ejection patterns has been based on records obtained from indwelling gauges in healthy dogs with minimal intrathoracic pathology. In a few dogs with atelectasis and hydrothorax persisting after the surgical implantation of the gauges, the right ventricular ejection pattern closely resembled the normal left ventricular ejection pattern. A high peak flow velocity developed very early in systole, implying a greatly increased right ventricular impulse. Apparently, the right ventricle responds to an increase in outflow pressure by assuming the ejection properties of the left ventricle. This finding is not entirely surprising in view of the fact that during chronic pulmonary hypertension the right ventricle changes into a thick-walled chamber, very much like the left ventricle in form. Thus, the right ventricle is capable of conversion into a high-impulse pump like the normal left ventricle.

LEFT VENTRICULAR PERFORMANCE IN QUANTITATIVE PHYSICAL TERMS

A description of ventricular function solely in terms of absolute values of pressures, dimensions and flows is incomplete because a great deal of valuable information is contained within the waveforms, produced by recording systems capable of faithfully reproducing rapid changes. A more comprehensive description of cardiac function can be obtained[49] by extracting additional derived information using relatively simple analogue computers. For example, the signals from a pulsed ultrasonic flow sensor implanted on the aorta, along with ventricular pressure and diameter recordings, can be stored on magnetic tape and subsequently analyzed to provide 11 important variables as illustrated in Figure 2–22.

The pulsed ultrasonic flow sensor (or an electromagnetic flowmeter) inscribes a characteristic flow velocity wave indicating the rate at which blood is flowing from the left ventricle through the root of the aorta. This flow signal can be recorded directly without modification as at the top of the right hand column (Fig. 2–22). At the end of the experiment, known flows may be passed through the flow section in place on the aorta to provide a calibration for the system in terms of instantaneous volume flow rates (ml./ sec.). The aortic flow signals can also be processed by a simple integrator

that adds up to the flow occurring during each successive cardiac cycle to provide a deflection proportional to stroke volume. This process is equivalent to measuring the area under the original flow curve and calibrating it in terms of volume flow per stroke. Similarly, the aortic flow signal can be integrated by a circuit that adds up the flow over a set period of time (i.e., each 2.5 seconds). The height of each successive series of steps indicates the volume flow per unit time and can be calibrated as cardiac output (ml./min. or liters/min.). The slope of aortic flow wave form indicates the rate of change of velocity or acceleration of the blood. During the initial steep upslope on the flow record, a sharp spike is inscribed in the acceleration record indicating that the steepest slope and maximal increase in velocity occurs very early in systole.

The acceleration record, which was obtained by differentiating the flow waveform, indicates the rate at which the flow was increasing or decreasing. Since the flowmeter samples the average flow velocity across the vascular lumen, a reliable value for the peak linear velocity cannot be derived unless the profile of the flow velocity is known. The estimated peak acceleration is very high, e.g., 3000 cm./sec.^{2} during exercise on these records. Values reported by Noble (see Ref. 63, Chapter 3) are even higher (5000 to 10,000 cm./sec.^{2}). During the latter portions of systole, the acceleration record drops below the baseline, indicating the progressive slowing of ventricular outflow after the early peak flow velocity is attained.

The left ventricular pressure can be recorded directly from an indwelling catheter extending from the left ventricle to a high fidelity pressure gauge either just outside the heart or outside the body. The form of the ven-

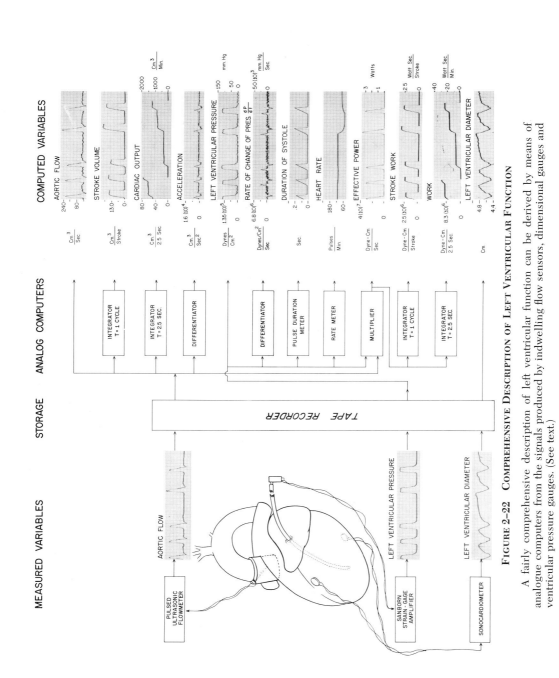

FIGURE 2–22 COMPREHENSIVE DESCRIPTION OF LEFT VENTRICULAR FUNCTION

A fairly comprehensive description of left ventricular function can be derived by means of analogue computers from the signals produced by indwelling flow sensors, dimensional gauges and ventricular pressure gauges. (See text.)

tricular pressure pulse is generally familiar, although attention is usually directed to the peak amplitude rather than to the details of the waveform. Tracings of the systolic pressure frequently exhibit a rounded dome shape, but the pressure may peak early in systole when ventricular ejection is exceptionally rapid and peripheral resistance is less than normal. The steep upslope and downslope of the ventricular record represents the rapid rate of rise and fall of pressure in the ventricle. This rate of change of pressure can be directly inscribed by passing the signal through a differentiating circuit to provide deflections, an upward spike followed by a downward spike, representing the slopes on the ventricular pressure record. The amplitudes of these spikes reflect the maximum rates of rise or fall (slope) of the ventricular pressure pulses. These amplitudes are very labile, indicating that the rate at which the ventricular pressure changes is readily altered under such conditions as spontaneous changes in heart rate, exercise, sympathetic stimulation and administration of catecholamines. The rate of change of pressure must be influenced by the degree of synchronization in the activation of the myocardial bundles and in the rate at which tension develops in these fibers.

The duration of ventricular systole in seconds can be indicated by the height of a ramp which begins as the ventricular pressure rises above some low level and is terminated when the pressure returns to the low level. The heart rate can be indicated in terms of the reciprocal of the interval between each pair of successive beats. The recorded heart rate refers to the heart rate represented by the duration of the preceding cycle (Fig. 2–22).

In a mechanical pump, the duration of the stroke is determined by the r.p.m. of the crankshaft. Similarly, there is an inverse relationship between the duration of systole and the heart rate. This relationship tends to be preserved under many different conditions, although the reasons are not so apparent in the heart as they are in a mechanical pump.

Effective power indicates the rate at which the ventricle was performing work and was derived by continuously multiplying the aortic flow rate by the ventricular pressure. This deflection continuously indicates the rate of effective energy conversion by the contracting ventricle calibrated in terms of dyne-cm./sec. or watts. Effective power is not a measure of the total rate of energy liberation because the viscous losses within the myocardium are not measured. Instead, the power record is interpreted as a measure of the rate at which energy is transferred from the left heart to the peripheral vasculature. Since peak outflow occurs early in systole when the pressure is achieving its maximum levels, power is also attaining its peak at this time. The stroke work record, derived by the integration of the power record for each successive cycle, is a measure of the total energy transferred to the peripheral vasculature during the cardiac cycle. Again, this process is similar to a manual measurement of the area under the waveform on the effective power record. Work per unit time (i.e., 2.5 seconds) can be recorded as a series of steps very much as the cardiac output was recorded in the third record from the top.

Finally, the changing ventricular diameter can be recorded directly to indicate the changing dimensions of the chamber. A much more appropriate dimension for completeness would be the changing volume of the left ventricle but we are not able to make this measurement at sampling rates approaching those of the other recorded variables in Figure 2–22.

REFERENCES

1. PATTEN, B. M. The first heart beats and the beginning of the embryonic circulation. *Amer. Scien.*, 39:225–243, 1951.
2. GOSS, C. M. First contractions of the heart without cytological differentiation. *Anat. Rec.*, 76:19–27, 1940.
3. PATTEN, B. M., KRAMER, T. C., and BARRY, A. Valvular action in the embryonic chick heart by localized apposition of endocardial masses. *Anat. Rec.*, 102:299–311, 1948.
4. HOFF, E. C., KRAMER, T. C., DuBOIS, D., and PATTEN, B. M. The development of the electrocardiogram of the embryonic heart. *Amer. Heart J.*, 17:470–488, 1939.
5. HUXLEY, H. E. The double array of filaments in cross-striated muscle. *J. Biophys. Biochem. Cystol.*, 3:631–648, 1957.
6. HUXLEY, H. E. The contraction of muscle. *Sci. Amer.*, 199:66–82, 1958.
7. BOZLER, E. An analysis of the properties of smooth muscle. *Cold Spr. Harb. Symp.*, 4:260–266, 1936.
8. BOZLER, E. Action potentials and conduction of excitation in muscle. *Biol. Symp.*, 3:95–110, 1941.
9. DiPALMA, J. R., and MASCATELLO, A. V. Excitability and refractory period of isolated heart muscle of the cat. *Amer. J. Physiol.*, 164:589–600, 1951.
10. MALL, F. P. On the muscular architecture of the ventricles of the human heart. *Amer. J. Anat.*, 11:211–266, 1911.
11. ROBB, J. S., and ROBB, R. C. The normal heart. *Amer. Heart J.*, 23:455–467, 1942.
12. GRANT, R. P. Notes on muscular architecture of the left ventricle. *Circulation*, 32:301–308, 1965.
13. STREETER, D. D., JR., and BASSETT, D. L. An engineering analysis of myocardial fiber orientation in pig's left ventricle in systole. *Anat. Rec.*, 155:503–512, 1966.
14. STREETER, D. D., JR., SPOTNITZ, H. M., PATEL, D. J., ROSS, J., JR., and SONNENBLICK, E. H. Fiber orientation in the canine left ventricle during diastole and systole. *Circulat. Res.*, 24:339–347, 1969.
15. CURTIS, H. J., and TRAVIS, D. M. Conduction in Purkinje tissue of the ox heart. *Amer. J. Physiol.*, 165:173–178, 1951.
16. RUSHMER, R. F., and CRYSTAL, D. K. Changes in configuration of the ventricular chambers during the cardiac cycle. *Circulation*, 4:211–218, 1951.
17. RUSHMER, R. F., and THAL, N. The mechanics of ventricular contraction: a cinefluorographic study. *Circulation*, 4:219–228, 1951.
18. RUSHMER, R. F., and THAL, N. Factors influencing stroke volume: a cinefluorographic study of angiocardiography. *Amer. J. Physiol.*, 168:509–521, 1952.
19. KAGAN, A. Dynamic responses of the right

ventricle following extensive damage by cauterization. *Circulation*, 5:816–823, 1952.
20. ZAUS, E. A., and KEARNS, W. M., JR. Massive infarction of the right ventricle and atrium. *Circulation*, 6:593–598, 1952.
21. BAKER, D., ELLIS, R. M., FRANKLIN, D. L., and RUSHMER, R. F. Some engineering aspects of modern cardiovascular research. *Proc. Inst. Radio Engrs.*, 47:1917–1924, 1959.
22. RUSHMER, R. F., FRANKLIN, D. L., and ELLIS, R. M. Left ventricular dimensions recorded by sonocardiometry. *Circulat. Res.*, 4:684–688, 1956.
23. RUSHMER, R. F. Initial phase of ventricular systole: Asynchronous contraction. *Amer. J. Physiol.*, 184:188–194, 1956.
24. RUSHMER, R. F., FINLAYSON, B. L., and NASH, A. A. Movements of the mitral valve. *Circulat. Res.*, 4:337–342, 1956.
25. WIGGERS, C. J., and KATZ, L. N. The contour of the ventricular volume curves under different conditions. *Amer. J. Physiol.*, 58:439–475, 1921–22.
26. COBLENTZ, B., HARVEY, R. M., FERRER, M. I., COURNAND, A., and RICHARD, D. W., JR. The relationship between electrical and mechanical events in the cardiac cycle of man. *Brit. Heart J.*, 11:1–22, 1949.
27. BRUNER, H. D. Peripheral blood flow measurement. P. 222 in *Methods in Medical Research*, Sect. 3, Vol. 8, W. S. Root, Ed. Chicago, Year Book Publishers, 1960.
28. BURTON, A. C. A critical survey of methods available for the measurement of human peripheral blood flow. *Ciba Found. Symp. Peripheral Circulation in Man*, 1954.
29. GREEN, H. D. Circulation blood flow measurement. P. 66 in *Methods in Medical Research*, Sect. 2, Vol. 1, V. R. Potter, Ed. Chicago, Year Book Publishers, 1948.
30. PIEPER, H. P. Catheter-tip blood flowmeter for measurement of pulmonary arterial blood flow in closed-chest dogs. *Rev. Sci. Instrum.*, 34:908–910, 1963.
31. GREENFIELD, J. C., JR., and FRY, D. L. Measurement errors in estimating aortic blood velocity by pressure gradient. *J. Appl. Physiol.*, 17:1013–1019, 1962.
32. KETY, S. S. Theory and applications of the exchange of inert gas at the lungs and tissues. *Pharmacol. Rev.*, 3:1–41, 1951.
33. VISSCHER, M. B., and JOHNSON, J. A. The Fick principle: Analysis of a potential error in its conventional application. *J. Appl. Physiol.*, 5:635–638, 1953.
34. VAN CITTERS, R. L., and BARNETT, G. O. Computation of blood flow velocity from the pressure pulse compared with direct measurement by the ultrasonic flowmeter. *Proc. San Diego Symp. Biomed. Engrs.*, pp. 79–86, 1963.
35. SHIPLEY, R. E., GREGG, D. E., and WARN, J. T. Operative mechanism of some errors

in the application of the thermostromuhr method to the measurement of blood flow. *Amer. J. Physiol.*, 136:263–274, 1942.

36. HENSEL, H. Messkopf zur Durchblutungs-registrierung an Oberflächen. *Arch. Ges. Physiol.*, 268:604–606, 1959.

37. HARDING, D. C., BAKER, D. W., and RUSH-MER, R. F. Isothermal cutaneous blood flowmeter. *Proc. Ann. Conf. Engr. Med. Biol., 17th*, 6:77, 1964.

38. KATSURA, S., WEISS, R., BAKER, D. W., and RUSHMER, R. F. Isothermal blood flow velocity probe. *IRE Trans. Med. Electron.*, ME6:283–285, 1959.

39. WATSON, N. W., and RUSHMER, R. F. Ultra-sonic blood flowmeter transducers. *Proc. San Diego Symp. Biomed. Engrs.*, pp. 87–91, 1963.

40. KOLIN, A. An electromagnetic flowmeter: Principles of the method and its applica-tion to blood flow measurements. *Proc. Soc. Exp. Biol. Med.*, 35:53–56, 1936.

41. DENISON, A. B., and SPENCER, M. P. Mag-netic flowmeters. P. 178 in *Medical Phy-sics*, Vol. 3. Chicago, Year Book Publish-ers, 1960.

42. SPENCER, M. P., and DENISON, A. B. Square-wave electromagnetic flowmeter for surgi-cal experimental application. Pp. 321–341 in *Methods in Medical Research*, Vol. 8. Chicago, Year Book Publishers, 1960.

43. WETTERER, E. Flowmeters: Their theory, construction and operation. Pp. 1294–1324 in *Handbook of Physiology, Section 2: Circulation*, Vol. 2, W. F. Hamilton and P. Dow, Eds. Washington, D. C., American Physiological Society, 1963.

44. FRANKLIN, D. L., BAKER, D. W., ELLIS, R. M., and RUSHMER, R. F. A pulsed ultra-sonic flowmeter. *IRE Trans. Med. Elec-tron.*, ME6:204–206, 1959.

45. FRANKLIN, D. L., SCHLEGEL, W., and RUSH-MER, R. F. Blood flow measured by Dop-pler frequency shift of back-scattered ultrasound. *Science*, 134:564–565, 1961.

46. RUSHMER, R. F., BAKER, D. W., and STE-GALL, H. F. Transcutaneous Doppler flow detection as a nondestructive tech-nique. *J. Appl. Physiol.*, 21:554–566, 1966.

47. SPENCER, M. P., and GREISS, F. S. Dynamics of ventricular ejection. *Circulat. Res.*, 10:274–279, 1962.

48. STARR, I., SCHNABEL, T. G., JR., and MAY-OCK, R. L. Studies made by simulating systole at necropsy. II. Experiments on the relation of cardiac and peripheral factors to the genesis of the pulse wave and ballistrocardigram. *Circulation*, 8:44–61, 1953.

49. FRANKLIN, D. L., VAN CITTERS, R. L., and RUSHMER, R. F. Left ventricular function described in physical terms. *Circulat. Res.*, 11:702–711, 1962.

CHAPTER 3

THE CARDIAC OUTPUT

I. FACTORS AFFECTING CARDIAC OUTPUT

An understanding of the principles governing cardiovascular responses in the normal person is a prerequisite for interpreting changes induced by disease. The five basic mechanisms by which cardiac output can be adjusted are indicated in Figure 3–1. The cardiac output is determined by the product of the heart rate and stroke volume. Stroke volume is the diastolic volume of the ventricle minus the volume of blood in the ventricle at the end of systole. Diastolic filling is determined by the effective filling pressure and the resistance to distension offered by the ventricular wall. The degree of systolic ejection depends upon the degree of shortening which the ventricular myocardium can attain while working against the arterial pressure. The changes in contractile properties of the myocardium are manifest in many different ways, affecting the rate, amount and duration of tension development, shortening and relaxation. All or parts of these changes in ventricular performance have been included rather indiscriminately under the general term "contractility." Cardiac control clearly involves all five major factors: (1) heart rate, (2) ventricular filling or distending pressure, (3) ventricular "distensibility," (4) contractile proper-

ties of the myocardium and (5) arterial pressure. A comprehensive discussion would include the contributing factors to each and the interactions of all the mechanisms, a most complex and perplexing problem.

The following discussion will be devoted to a consideration of the control of the heart rate and some of the

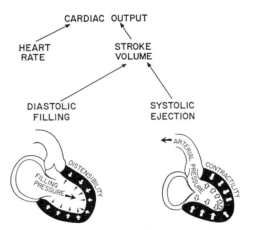

FIGURE 3–1 FACTORS AFFECTING STROKE VOLUME

The cardiac output is influenced by at least five different factors which include changes in heart rate and by four mechanisms which influence the stroke volume, namely (a) filling pressure, (b) ventricular distensibility, (c) arterial pressure and (s) contractility. Distensibility and contractility are terms which may in fact cover a number of additional independent factors.

70

factors affecting contraction and distention of the cardiac chambers. Some mechanical and architectural features of the ventricles will receive attention because they also may affect the function of the heart as a pump.

CONTROL OF HEART RATE

Normally the heart rate is determined by the frequency with which the sinoatrial (S-A) node generates the impulses which spread over the atrium and ultimately activate the heart in the sequence illustrated in Figure 2–12. Given suitable conditions, any myocardial fiber is capable of generating a conducted impulse, but the S-A node retains its role as a pacemaker of the heart (1) so long as it generates impulses more rapidly than any other part of the heart and (2) so long as the conduction system continues to function normally. During the embryonic development of the heart, the ventricle forms first; initially it contracts very slowly and irregularly (see Fig. 2–1). As the atrium develops, its faster inherent rate of impulse formation becomes manifest. The atrium takes over the pacemaker role, and the embryonic heart rate quickens. The sinus venosus, the last portion of the heart to appear, has the highest rate of impulse formation and takes over the role of pacemaker. The S-A node is a vestigial remnant of the sinus venosus and is the pacemaker of the fully developed heart.

THE NATURE OF PACEMAKER ACTIVITY

The heart is only one example of a structure with an autogenic pacemaker. The ureter displays contraction waves that originate at a point near the pelvis of the kidney and descend at regular intervals toward the urinary bladder.

The point where these conducted waves of excitation originate is also called a *pacemaker*, capable of spontaneously generating conducted impulses at regular intervals. The electrical potentials associated with this wave of excitation can be readily recorded. During the interval between the action potentials representing waves of excitation, the recorded potentials along the ureter remain steady at a low level. At the site of the pacemaker, however, the cellular potentials rise progressively until they reach the threshold of excitability which sets off a conducted impulse (Fig. 3–2A). This gradual rise in potential between action potentials is called a *prepotential* and apparently represents a spontaneous phasic swing in the potential on the membranes of cells which establishes the rate at which contraction waves descend the ureter.[1] If the ureter is transected below the normal pacemaker, a new pacemaker site becomes established in the lower segment. This new pacemaker displays a prepotential but generates impulses at a slower rate than the normal site. The inherent rate of pacemaker activity is progressively slower at greater and greater distances below the pelvis of the kidney.

The correspondence between the pacemakers of the ureter and of the heart is obvious. The specialized myocardial fibers in the S-A node generate spontaneous swings in membrane potential, recorded as prepotentials within those myocardial cells which serve as pacemakers. When the membrane potential reaches the critical threshold level, a conducted impulse spreads in all directions over the atrial musculature. No prepotentials are visible in recordings from within other atrial myocardial cells; the resting membrane potentials remain steady between each period of excitation.

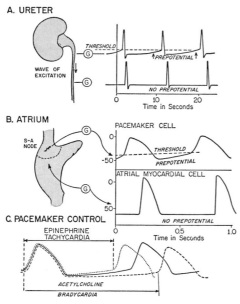

A. URETER

WAVE OF
EXCITATION

THRESHOLD

PREPOTENTIAL

NO PREPOTENTIAL

0   10   20
Time in Seconds

B. ATRIUM

S-A
NODE

PACEMAKER CELL

0-
-50-

THRESHOLD
PREPOTENTIAL

ATRIAL MYOCARDIAL CELL

0-

50-

C. PACEMAKER CONTROL

NO PREPOTENTIAL

0   0.5   1.0
Time in Seconds

EPINEPHRINE
TACHYCARDIA

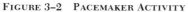

ACETYLCHOLINE
BRADYCARDIA

FIGURE 3–2   PACEMAKER ACTIVITY

A, Waves of excitation periodically pass down the ureter from a "pacemaker" site at which the membrane potentials of the cells spontaneously change (prepotentials) until threshold is reached to produce a propagated impulse spreading from cell to cell down the ureter.

B, Pacemaker cells in the sinus node normally exhibit spontaneous changes in membrane potentials (prepotentials) which lead to waves of excitation spreading centripetally from this site over the atrium.

C, Changes in heart rate induced by epinephrine or acetylcholine, acting at the pacemaker site, result from changes in the rate of membrane depolarization (slope of the prepotential) with very little alteration in the level of the threshold of excitability.

The heart rate is normally adjusted through a change in the discharge rate of the S-A node. If the slope of the prepotential is altered, the interval required to reach the threshold level would change. West *et al.*[2] inserted very fine ultramicroelectrodes into individual S-A nodal cells which were apparently acting as pacemaker. When epinephrine was applied to the site, the rate of discharge was accelerated and prepotential slope became much steeper (Fig. 3–2C). In contrast, administration of

acetylcholine produced slowing of the heart rate, associated with a much more gradual prepotential slope and a smaller action potential. Although changes in discharge rate could theoretically be achieved by alterations in threshold, this mechanism apparently is not as significant as the prepotential slope (Fig. 3–2C). Acetylcholine is the transmitter substance released from the parasympathetic nerves to the heart and norepinephrine is generally regarded as the transmitter substance released by sympathetic nerves distributed to the heart. Thus, the influences of these substances applied directly to pacemaker sites are believed to mimic the action of the sympathetic and parasympathetic nerves in the control of heart rate.

AUTONOMIC CONTROL OF HEART RATE

In 1899, Hunt[3] concluded that the accelerator (sympathetic) nerves of the heart are almost always in tonic activity. The action potentials arriving at the region of sinus node are believed to trigger the release of an epinephrine-like substance at the nerve endings. At the base of the brain, in the medulla oblongata, is the region where electrical stimulation produces large effects on both the heart rate and peripheral vascular resistance.[4] The term *cardio-regulatory center* for such poorly localized sites is somewhat misleading, but is common usage. From the "medullary centers," nerve fibers descend to the intermediolateral columns of the spinal cord (see Chapter 4). The fibers course out to the sympathetic trunk through T_1, T_2, T_3, T_4 and sometimes T_5 and pass up to the stellate ganglion and to the heart through the cardiac nerves (Fig. 3–4). Although the accelerator nerves cannot be dissociated from the other sympathetic nerves to the heart, the sympathetic accelerator fibers appear to be more prominent on the right than on the left.[5]

The motor nucleus of the vagus nerve lies not far from the medullary sites where electrical stimulation produces tachycardia. However, the vagal nerve endings distributed to the S-A node produce a profound slowing of the heart by the mechanism illustrated in Figure 3–2C.

The actions of acetylcholine and the sympathetic transmitter substance are mutually antagonistic. For example, if the vagus nerve is stimulated, the heart rate promptly slows.[6] If sympathetic accelerator fibers are simultaneously stimulated at an appropriate frequency, the heart rate can be brought back to the control levels (Fig. 3–3A). Then if the vagal stimulation is discontinued so that the sympathetic stimulation is unopposed, the heart rate promptly accelerates. An acceleration of the heart rate alone is not a very effective mechanism for increasing cardiac output without additional mechanisms to maintain or to increase the stroke volume (Fig. 3–3B).

The heart rate can be precisely adjusted by balancing the retarding effects of vagal discharge against the accelerating effects of sympathetic stimulation. This is a form of reciprocal innervation at the effector organ, the S-A node. In addition, reciprocal innervation is also prominent in the central control over heart rate (i.e., at the medullary center). For example, the neural connections are so organized that activation of the motor nucleus of the vagus is associated with simultaneous inhibition of the medullary accelerator centers. The medullary centers of cardiac and peripheral vascular control are important in the control of blood pressure.[7] However, these control centers are influenced

by nerves converging from a wide variety of sites and sources (Fig. 3–4).

ORIGINS OF AFFERENT NERVES CONVERGING ON THE CARDIOREGULATORY CENTERS

The vagus and sympathetic nerves conduct impulses which result from a more or less continuous bombardment of the cardioaccelerator and cardioinhibitor centers by afferent nerves from all over the body. The cardioregulatory centers are influenced by afferent fibers corresponding to those which play upon the vasomotor centers (see Chapter 4).

Impulses from the cerebral cortex impinge upon the cardioaccelerator and cardioinhibitor centers, as evidenced by many common experiences. Excitement, anxiety, fear and depression[8, 9] affect the heart rate without any direct relation to metabolic activity. Cardioacceleration occurs in anticipation of physical exertion before there is any significant increase in metabolism. An occasional individual can voluntarily alter his heart rate.[10] Clearly, the influence of higher centers on cardiovascular regulation cannot be ignored.

Stretch receptors in the carotid sinus and aortic arch exert a powerful influence on the cardioregulatory centers. A change in arterial blood pressure is reflected in a corresponding change in the frequency of impulses from the baroceptors which in turn influences the cardioregulatory centers and the heart rate. In general a drop in arterial blood pressure induces an acceleration of the heart and vice versa.

Digital pressure on a hypersensitive carotid sinus promptly produces bradycardia, reduced peripheral resistance, a severe drop in arterial

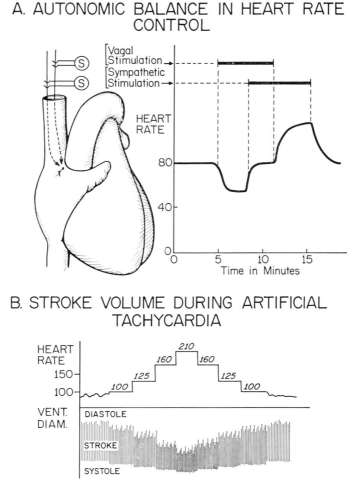

A. AUTONOMIC BALANCE IN HEART RATE CONTROL

B. STROKE VOLUME DURING ARTIFICIAL TACHYCARDIA

FIGURE 3–3   HEART RATE

A, Impulses descending the vagus nerve to the sinus node tend to produce slowing of the heart which can be precisely countered by activity of the sympathetic nerves to this site. Thus, the heart rate is regulated in terms of the balance between the sympathetic and vagal effects on the pacemaker.

B, An artificially induced tachycardia produces a progressive reduction in ventricular dimensions and in stroke deflection indicating that tachycardia alone is not an efficient mechanism for increasing cardiac output unless other mechanisms act to maintain or increase stroke volume.

blood pressure and syncope.[11] Insertion of a needle into the brachial artery of subjects in the erect position frequently produces a very similar response.[12] Such syncopal reactions, termed *vago-vagal reactions*, may be produced by many conditions.[13, 14] Since sensory fibers from virtually all parts of the body influence heart rate and peripheral resistance, only a few

of the more prominent examples can be mentioned.

Stimulation of internal organs may produce drastic cardiac inhibition. For example, stimulation of nerve endings in the upper portion of the respiratory tract may produce intense vagal depression of the heart rate. Thus, anesthetists must be extremely careful during intubation of the trachea be-

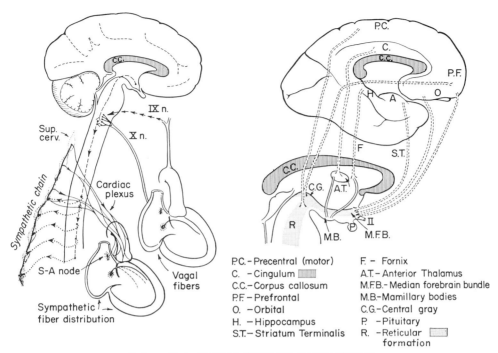

P.C. – Precentral (motor)
C. – Cingulum
C.C. – Corpus callosum
P.F. – Prefrontal
O. – Orbital
H. – Hippocampus
S.T. – Striatum Terminalis

F. – Fornix
A.T. – Anterior Thalamus
M.F.B. – Median forebrain bundle
M.B. – Mamillary bodies
C.G. – Central gray
P. – Pituitary
R. – Reticular formation

FIGURE 3–4 NEURAL CONTROL OF THE HEART

A, The vagus nerve endings are concentrated in the region of the sinus node and atrioventricular node and are more diffusely distributed over the atrium. They do not extend to the ventricular myocardium. Sympathetic fibers from $T_1 - T_5$ are distributed to all parts of the atrium and ventricles. Impulses traveling along the vagus and sympathetic nerves to the heart come from the medulla or the diencephalon.

B, Neural pathways from many parts of the brain converge on the diencephalic region to influence autonomic outflow to the heart and other visceral structures.

cause increased vagal activity may lead to cardiac standstill and death. Inhalation of irritant gases may intensely affect the heart rate. Phasic changes in heart rate (sinus arrhythmia) occur during normal respiratory cycles.

The gastrointestinal tract is supplied with afferent nerve fibers which travel along the vagus to the medulla. Nausea and vomiting are commonly associated with slowing of the heart whether they are due to digital stimulation of the pharynx or to ingestion of toxic substances. Visceral pain fibers are widely distributed and have a powerful slowing effect on heart rate. Painful stimulation of skeletal muscles may produce a similar autonomic

response. Pressure on the eyeball may produce a profound slowing of the heart through the "oculocardiac reflex." In general, visceral afferent nerves, originating in nearly all tissues and organs except the skin, produce bradycardia. In contrast, somatic pain from the skin generally produces tachycardia along with some increase in arterial blood pressure. Additional details concerning the origins of nerve impulses which influence both heart rate and contractile properties of the heart are presented in Figure 3–4.

If a stepwise increase in heart rate is produced by stimulating electrodes installed upon the right atrium near the S-A node, a progressive reduction in the diastolic dimensions—and in stroke volume—is seen (Fig. 3–3B). An increase in heart rate accompanied by a diminution in stroke volume is not an efficient mechanism for increasing total cardiac output. Thus, it is important to consider the factors which influence the quantity of blood ejected during each systole (the stroke volume).

CONTROL OF STROKE VOLUME

Most mechanical or piston pumps with which we are familiar have a constant displacement and eject precisely the same quantity of liquid during each successive stroke. The output of such a pump is regulated merely by speeding or slowing the repetition rate with no change in the quantity of liquid discharged with each stroke. The heart is remarkable in its ability to compensate to changing conditions by adjustments in heart rate, in the volume at the end of the filling period (diastolic volume) and in the volume remaining in the ventricles at the end of ejection (systolic volume). A wide variety of different factors may influence the stroke volume under various conditions which may be grouped for convenience under such headings as geometry, intrinsic properties of myocardium and external control mechanisms.

GEOMETRICAL FACTORS AFFECTING STROKE VOLUME

The architectural features of the right and left ventricles were described in Chapter 2. Neither ventricle conforms to a simple geometrical shape. In spite of the gross differences in their shape, wall thickness and outflow resistance, the two ventricles must expel precisely the same volumes averaged over any significant period of

time; otherwise large volumes of blood would be transferred between the systemic and pulmonary vascular beds.

The absolute volume of blood contained within the individual ventricular chambers can be estimated by several techniques but their results are not entirely consistent or absolute. A symposium devoted to measurement of left ventricular volume in 1966 revealed discrepancies of significant magnitude between roentgenographic and indicator-dilution techniques of measurement.[15] According to Dodge et al.,[16] the left ventricles of normal subjects contain some 70 to 80 ml. ± 10 to 20 ml. per square meter of body surface at the end of diastole with 60 to 75 per cent of that volume ejected during systole. In contrast, Rapaport[17] reported ventricular volumes estimated by thermodilution in man at about 100 ml./M^2 in normal man and about 50 per cent of the diastolic volume ejected during systole. All agree that the ventricles may fill to varying degrees during diastole and empty to varying degrees during systolic ejection. A substantial, but variable, amount of blood remains in the ventricular chambers at the end of systole.

THE DEGREE OF MYOCARDIAL SHORTENING IN DIFFERENT MUSCLES OF THE HEART. The various myocardial bundles in the ventricles are oriented in different directions (see Fig. 2–9) and describe circles of different diameters, so the degree of myocardial shortening must vary widely in different layers. In Figure 3–5B, the relative wall thickness and the radius of the left ventricular chamber at a particular size are represented by volume I. Volume II represents the same cross section with the ventricular volume reduced by half. In both cases it is obvious that the radius and

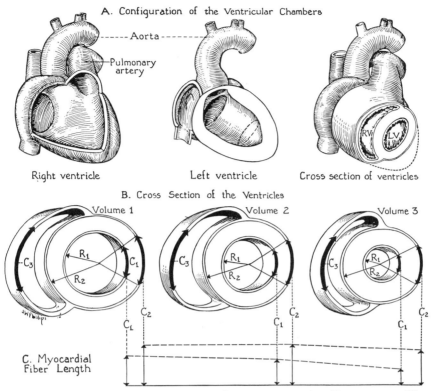

A. Configuration of the Ventricular Chambers

Aorta

Pulmonary artery

Right ventricle

Left ventricle

Cross section of ventricles

B. Cross Section of the Ventricles

Volume 1

Volume 2

Volume 3

C. Myocardial Fiber Length

FIGURE 3–5 THE DEGREE OF MYOCARDIAL SHORTENING IN THE VENTRICULAR WALLS

The right ventricular cavity is enclosed by the convex interventricular septum and the concave free wall, which may be considered a segment of a very large sphere. Very slight shortening of the fibers in the free wall of the right ventricle (C_3) will eject very large volumes (see Fig. 3–6).

The left ventricle has been compared to a very thick-walled cylinder with a conoid segment at the apex. The circumferentially arranged fibers account for most of the wall thickness which encloses the cylindrical portion of the chamber. The circles described by the inner layers have a much smaller radius (R_1) and circumference (C_1) than those described by the outer layers (R_2 and C_2). As the left ventricle contracts, the inner layers must shorten to a greater degree than the outer layers in ejecting a particular volume. On the basis of this analysis, during any normal systolic ejection the outer layers of myocardium shorten to a lesser extent and the superficial spiral muscles shorten least of all. It is possible that no two layers of myocardial fibers shorten to exactly the same extent during ejection.

circumference of the inner layers of myocardium (R_1 and C_1) are less than those of the outer layer (R_2, C_2). During contraction from volume I to volume II, the radius and circumference of the inner layer are reduced much more than those of the outer layers. This means that the inner layer of myocardium must shorten more than the outer layers. If this analysis is correct, the thickness of the ventricular walls should increase during systole and decrease during diastole.

It is apparent that during any particular ventricular contraction, the inner layers of circumferential myocardium may shorten to the greatest extent. The relative degree of myocardial shortening in the inner lining of spiral muscle (trabeculae carneae) and papillary muscles cannot be assessed by this type of analysis. The difference in degrees of shortening by various myocardial layers is diminished when the diastolic and systolic volumes remain large; the maximum difference between the shortening of the superficial spiral muscle and that of the inner layer of deep constrictor fibers would occur when the left ventricle empties maximally (see volume III in Fig. 3–5).

Relation of Diastolic Volume to the Degree of Myocardial Shortening. The degree of myocardial shortening can be reduced without changing the stroke volume if the diastolic distention of the ventricles is increased.[18]

A very slight reduction in circumference of a large sphere would eject a very much greater volume than the same reduction in circumference of a small sphere. The superficial muscles tend to conform most closely to a spherical shape, and this analysis applies within limits to these myocardial fibers (Fig. 3–6).

Deep muscles in the left ventricle are arranged circumferentially around a roughly cylindrical cavity. Here again, the reduction in volume produced by a reduction in circumference is much greater when the original circumference is large than when it is small. Thus, the degree of myocardial shortening required to eject a particular stroke volume is much less if the initial fiber length (diastolic volume) is great (Fig. 3–6).

The anatomical arrangement and orientation of the myocardial fibers in the ventricular walls was presented in Chapter 2 (Figs. 2–8 and 2–9). Close inspection revealed that virtually all fibers described helical courses conforming to neither purely longitudinal nor circumferential orientation (Fig. 2–9). A clear or concise description of contribution of the various layers to the circumferential contraction or shortening of the chambers is not yet possible. However, we may regard the deep fibers in the midportion of the ventricular wall as being roughly circumferential and the inner and outer layers as being oriented obliquely, pro-

viding a strong longitudinal pull in addition to a circumferential constriction. The layers in between appear to progressively change in orientation in intermediate stages. In subsequent discussion, the implication that the deep fibers are circumferentially oriented must be tempered with the knowledge that this is an oversimplification.

Evidence has been presented that under normal conditions, ventricular contraction generally corresponds to a reduction in the chamber from volume I to volume II in Figure 3–5. Although the same stroke volume can be ejected by a change from volume II to volume III (Fig. 3–5), the relative degree of myocardial shortening would be much greater. When the diastolic volume is large, a relatively large stroke volume can be ejected with small degrees of myocardial shortening.

Since the free wall of the right ventricle corresponds to a segment of a large sphere while the left ventricle resembles a cylinder, equal myocardial shortening in the two chambers would produce much larger stroke volumes from the right ventricle than from the left (Fig. 3–6). The right and left ventricles must eject roughly equal quantities, so the degree of myocardial shortening cannot be equal in the two ventricles.

FACTORS OPPOSING COMPLETE VENTRICULAR EMPTYING

Muscle fibers cannot shorten to an infinitely small length. If all the myocardial fibers constricted 20 per cent of their initial length, the inner layer of circumferential fibers would have attained this value and ceased contributing any tension, while the outer layers might be able to contract still more. From this point on, further shortening by the outer layers would

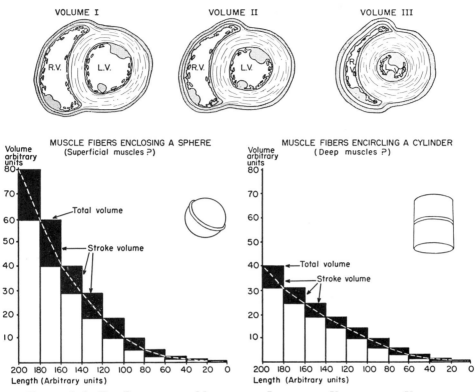

FIGURE 3–6   THE RELATION OF MYOCARDIAL LENGTH TO VENTRICULAR VOLUME

The volume of blood ejected by a ventricle (stroke volume) depends upon two factors: (a) the diastolic volume and (b) the amount of myocardial shortening. Normally, the ventricles are well distended with blood during diastole (volume I) and eject only a portion of the blood within the chambers during systole (volume II). Similar volumes of blood could theoretically be ejected from less distended ventricles (such as volume II) by much more complete systolic emptying (volume III).

The superficial spiral muscles encircle a large volume which is roughly spherical in shape. Under these conditions, very slight degrees of myocardial shortening will eject very large volumes. The larger the initial volume, the greater the volume ejected for a particular degree of myocardial shortening as indicated by the black areas on the left.

The deep constrictor muscles encircle the cylindrical portion of the left ventrical chamber. The change in volume produced by a reduction in the circumference of a cylinder is much smaller (black areas on the right) than is produced by the same reduction in circumference of a sphere (black areas on the left). Furthermore, the circumference of the left ventricle is much smaller than the circumference of the entire heart. Thus, the superficial spiral layers of myocardial fibers have a much greater initial length and enclose a sphere, so very slight shortening ejects large volumes. The deep constrictor muscles describe circles of small circumference around a cylinder, so they must shorten a great deal more to eject the same volume.

require an expenditure of energy in wrinkling and deforming the inner layers (Fig. 3–7).

The trabeculae carneae represent preformed wrinkles and combine with the papillary muscles to occupy space in the ventricles. This permits more complete systolic ejection than would be possible if the inner walls of the ventricular chamber were smooth (see Fig. 3–7). Because of the space occupied by papillary muscles and tra-

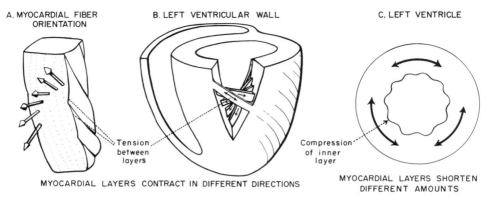

A. MYOCARDIAL FIBER ORIENTATION

B. LEFT VENTRICULAR WALL

C. LEFT VENTRICLE

Tension between layers

Compression of inner layer

MYOCARDIAL LAYERS CONTRACT IN DIFFERENT DIRECTIONS

MYOCARDIAL LAYERS SHORTEN DIFFERENT AMOUNTS

FIGURE 3–7   TENSION DEVELOPED BETWEEN MYOCARDIAL LAYERS (INTERFASCICULAR TENSION)

A, Although the right ventricular wall is quite thin, it contains myocardial fibers oriented in three different directions. Simultaneous contraction of these fibers must create tension in the fibrous and myocardial connections between the different layers (interfascicular tension).

B, The left ventricular wall is also composed of at least three layers of muscle, oriented primarily in three different directions (see Chapter 2). Interfascicular tension must develop in the connections between these layers during contraction.

C, The different layers of the thick-walled left ventricles must contract to different degrees in ejecting a particular volume of blood (see Fig. 3–5). This presumably causes tensions between layers of circularly arranged fibers, as well as compressing the inner layers.

beculae carneae, even the inner layers of circumferential fibers in the left ventricle can describe circles of reasonable diameter when the left ventricle is virtually empied. This mechanism is less important in the right ventricle because of (a) its thin wall, (b) the very long fibers which enclose the cavity and (c) the large circles described by these fibers.

The Law of Laplace. According to the Laplace formula ($P = T/R$), the pressure (P) developed by a particular level of wall tension (T) is inversely proportional to the radius of the chamber. This law was invoked to explain the difference between the wall thicknesses of the aorta and the systemic capillaries when these widely different structures sustain pressures of the same magnitude (see Fig. 1–11).

Applied to the contracting ventricle, the law of Laplace indicates that the myocardial tension required to sustain a particular level of intraventricular pressure diminishes as the radius of the chamber is reduced by ejection. In other words, this factor would tend to compensate to some extent for the loss of myocardial tension through myocardial viscosity and interfascicular tension. On the other hand, if the diastolic volume is increased, greater myocardial tension is needed to develop a particular level of intraventricular pressure.

Diastolic Recoil. The ventricular walls are composed of myocardial fibers oriented in different directions (see Fig. 2–9). Although adjacent layers appear to maintain relative orientation during systolic ejection, some fraction of the contractile tension developed by the fibers may be expended in developing tension between adjacent fibers or by producing wrinkling, distortion and compression of the inner layers of muscle (Fig. 3–7C). This tension would be stored during the systolic ejection period and released in the form of diastolic recoil when the myocardial fibers suddenly relax. At the very onset of the diastolic interval, the ventricular walls appear to spring outward to produce abrupt filling; so rapid that the ventricular pressure drops to its lowest point in the cycle. This extremely rapid filling in early diastole has important functional significance particularly in the presence of rapid heart rates with brief diastolic filling intervals. A major portion of total ventricular filling occurs during a small fraction of a second in early diastole. Rapid heart rate usually is accompanied by more complete ejection. The more complete the systolic ejection, the greater should be the amount and speed of the diastolic recoil.

After the initial rapid filling phase, the ventricle distends much more gradually until the next atrial contraction signals another cycle is beginning. The contribution of atrial systole to ventricular filling depends in large measure on the degree of ventricular distension at the time. If the ventricles approach their maximal dimensions before atrial excitation, the contracting atrial myocardium adds very little to the ventricular volume (Fig. 3–8A). This phenomenon is believed to occur

in man or animals resting quietly in the recumbent position. Under these conditions, heart rate is slow; filling pressure is ample and the ventricles may be maximally distended early in the diastolic filling period. This phenomenon is illustrated schematically in Figure 3–8 and discussed in greater detail in Chapter 6. Both the systolic and diastolic dimensions are diminished in the standing position (Fig. 3–8B), and in general the diastolic filling interval is shortened, ventricular volume progressively expands during the filling period and atrial contraction adds a significant additional increment to ventricular volume just before ventricular contraction begins. During exertion, stroke volume may remain about the same or increase slightly (see Chapter 7), in which case diastolic volume may increase slightly, systolic ejection may be slightly more complete or both. However, the changes in stroke volume during exertion are not nearly so pronounced as are the changes in the rates of ventricular performance (see Figs. 3–14, 3–17 and 3–18).

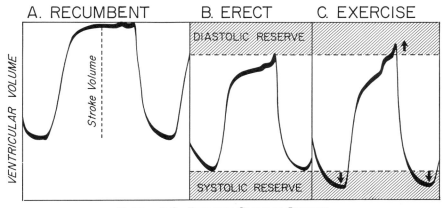

FIGURE 3–8   RESERVE CARDIAC OUTPUT

Changes in ventricular volume are represented schematically. In the supine position, the diastolic volume is approximately maximal and the stroke volume is relatively large. On standing, diastolic ventricular volume and stroke volume diminish to provide potential diastolic and systolic reserve capacity. During exertion, any increase in stroke volume may be attained by either greater diastolic filling, more complete systolic ejection or both.

Ventricular Distensibility. The architecture and geometry of the ventricular walls complicates the problem of assigning meaningful values or definitions to the term distensibility. For example, the diastolic recoil is sufficient to provide a rapid inrush of blood into the left ventricle—at effectively zero distending pressure. Under these conditions, ventricular distension is active rather than passive. The factors which terminate ventricular filling at some level below the maximal under various conditions (Fig. 3–8*B, C.*) have not been well elucidated. Furthermore, widely different ventricular volumes can be observed at the same or similar ventricular diastolic pressures in different "normal" subjects (i.e., comparing sedentary with athletic individuals) and patients with different forms of heart disease. Dodge *et al.*[16] reported ventricular volumes ranging from 100 to 400 ml. among 176 patients without consistent changes in ventricular pressure. However, in a particular normal individual, an increase in transmural pressure (intraventricular pressure minus extracardiac pressure) generally increased ventricular filling unless the heart was maximally distended as in Fig. 3–8*A*.

SHRINKAGE OF THE HEART DURING THORACOTOMY

Most profound changes in ventricular size and function occur during the administration of anesthesia and incision of the thorax as required to expose the heart.[19] This phenomenon was first noted during the recovery period following the application of various ventricular dimensional gauges to the heart of animals (see Figure 2–17). Immediately after installation of these gauges during aseptic surgery, the ventricular chambers were functioning near their minimal size even

after the chest incision had been repaired and the lungs reinflated. During the succeeding hours or days, the recorded dimensions expanded and stabilized for many days at a much larger size. Stimulated by this observation, the changes in dimensions of the ventricular chambers were studied by cinefluorographic pictures taken sequentially during anesthesia, thoracotomy and application of a cardiometer (Fig. 3–9). These studies demonstrated that under such experimental conditions, the ventricular chambers were reduced in size to levels well below those observed under any other condition or stress. These observations have extremely important significance in the interpretation of experiments on exposed hearts of animals. Investigators must constantly keep in mind that when they first expose a heart of a mammal, like a dog, the heart may have already been rendered so abnormal that its function may be outside the normal range before any experimental procedure is undertaken. Despite these reservations, observations and concepts of value can be obtained from exposed hearts and even from isolated samples of tissue. Their application to the function of organs in intact, healthy man and animals must be extrapolated with extreme caution.

INTRINSIC PROPERTIES OF MYOCARDIUM

The mechanical properties of muscle can be studied most readily and quantitatively by excising a strip and testing it under rigidly controlled experimental conditions. Such studies have demonstrated similar features in common between skeletal muscle and myocardium. If the tension exerted by a strip of resting or relaxed muscle is recorded as it is progres-

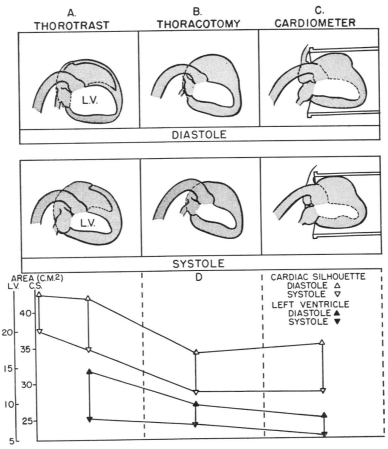

FIGURE 3-9 SHRINKAGE OF THE EXPOSED HEART

   A, Thorotrast was injected into a normal unanesthetized dog and its course through the heart was recorded cinefluorographically. The area of the cardiac silhouette and of the left ventricle during both systole and diastole are indicated in the graph, D.
   B, After anesthesia and thoracotomy, the heart definitely became smaller.
   C, The cardiac silhouette changed in configuration when the heart was placed in a loose-fitting cardiometer, but its area was not diminished. The left ventricular area was further reduced by this procedure. The left ventricle emptied almost completely at the end of systole, a situation which never was encountered among intact dogs.

sively stretched, no tension is recorded until a certain length is reached. The length at which a muscle first begins to develop tension is the "resting length." Further elongation of the muscle produces increasing resting tension, slight at first and increasing more steeply at greater lengths as illustrated schematically in Figure 3–10. If skeletal muscle is stimulated to contract without shortening (isometric contrac-

tion), it develops slight contractile tension at resting length. If the same strip is stretched and stimulated to contract at a succession of increased lengths, the contractile tension becomes very much greater, up to about 145 per cent of resting length.[20] Skeletal muscle fibers develop maximal tension at lengths about the same as they had in the animal's body, but a glance at Figures 3–5, 3–6 and 3–8 indicates

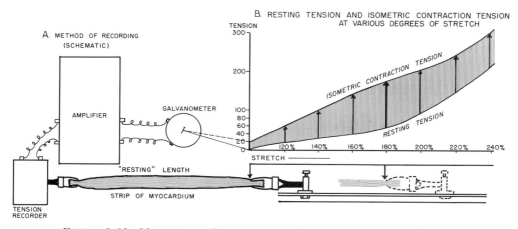

FIGURE 3–10   MECHANICAL PROPERTIES OF MYOCARDIAL BUNDLES (FROG)

A, Schematic diagram of experimental conditions employed by Lundin.[24]
B, Tension developed by a strip of frog myocardium was recorded as it was stretched from its "resting length" to 240 per cent of resting length with isometric contraction tension recorded at various degrees of stretch. The maximum contractile tension occurred at about 180 per cent of "resting length."

the difficulty of deciding what ventricular volume or dimension represents the "resting length" of myocardium.

The history of the basic concepts of cardiac function and control has been reviewed by Wiggers.[21] In 1895, Otto Frank recorded the isometric and isotonic contractions of frog myocardium and established that, within limits, myocardium resembles skeletal muscle in developing greater tension as its resting length is increased (Fig. 3–11B). Patterson, Piper and Starling[22] used the heart-lung preparation (Fig. 3–11A) to study the influence on cardiac function of variations in venous inflow, outflow resistance and heart rate.

VENTRICULAR RESPONSES IN THE HEART-LUNG PREPARATION

In the heart-lung preparation, the quantity of blood entering the ventricles could be increased by elevating the reservoir illustrated in Figure 3–11A. Experimentally induced elevation in "venous return" resulted in a higher filling pressure, a slight increase in arterial blood pressure and greater diastolic and systolic ventricular volumes. Records of this type were interpreted as follows: (a) When the reservoir is elevated, the venous pressure rises and diastolic filling is increased. (b) The myocardial fibers fail to eject as much blood as entered during diastole, so an additional increment of blood remains within the ventricle. (c) The succeeding diastolic filling is even greater, but the volume ejected remains less than that which entered. (d) The diastolic filling exceeds the systolic ejection until the ventricles become distended to a point where the energy release by the myocardium is sufficiently increased to bring the inflow and outflow into balance. (e) The equilibrium between inflow and outflow is maintained with the ventricles at their new larger diastolic and systolic size until the volume load is reduced. (f) As the reservoir is lowered, the energy released by the myocardium is excessive for the volume of inflow and the quantity ejected exceeds the volume which entered. For a few beats, outflow exceeds in-

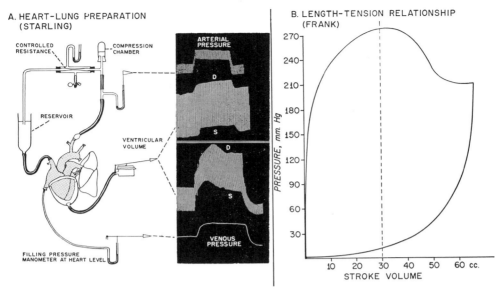

A. HEART-LUNG PREPARATION (STARLING)

CONTROLLED RESISTANCE — COMPRESSION CHAMBER

RESERVOIR

VENTRICULAR VOLUME

FILLING PRESSURE MANOMETER AT HEART LEVEL

ARTERIAL PRESSURE

VENTRICULAR VOLUME

VENOUS PRESSURE

B. LENGTH-TENSION RELATIONSHIP (FRANK)

PRESSURE, mm. Hg

STROKE VOLUME

FIGURE 3–11   THE LENGTH-TENSION RELATIONSHIP OF MYOCARDIUM

A, The ventricles in a heart-lung preparation adapt to an increased work load (either increased arterial pressure or increased stroke volume) by an increase in diastolic distention. Such experiments led Starling and his associates to postulate that the energy released by the contracting myocardium was determined by the initial length of the myocardial fibers as indicated by the end diastolic ventricular volume. (After Patterson, Piper and Starling.[22])

B, The length-tension relationship of myocardium resembles that of skeletal muscle. Progressive stretch of relaxed myocardium is attended by a progressive increase in isometric contractile tension up to some level. This length-tension diagram, derived by Otto Frank from studies of frog myocardium, was employed by Starling to illustrate his concept of the "law of the heart" by applying values of pressure and stroke volume on the ordinate and abscissa which he regarded as representative of human subjects. The use of an isometric tension curve is not appropriate for illustrating changes which would occur with ejection of stroke volumes (see Fig. 3–12).

flow until the systolic and diastolic ventricular volumes return to a lower level, actually smaller than during the control period in Figure 3–11.

The increased distention of the ventricles in response to a sudden increase in outflow pressure was explained as follows: The systolic increase in intraventricular pressure is not sufficient to eject all the blood that entered during the previous diastole (Fig. 3–11A). The succeeding diastolic filling remains the same, so an additional increment of blood remains within the ventricle. The systolic and diastolic volumes expand until the energy released by the lengthened myocardial fibers is sufficient to

meet the greater requirements for intraventricular pressure during each cycle.

THE FRANK-STARLING MECHANISM

Starling and his associates[22] confirmed Frank's general conclusions except for one crucial point, namely, that an increased diastolic volume was usually, but not always, associated with a corresponding increase in filling pressure. They stated, "We thus find no constant connection between the diastolic tension and the succeeding contraction, though as a rule these two quantities will be altered together.

But we do find a direct proportion between the diastolic volume of the heart (i.e., the length of its muscle fibers) and the energy set free in the following systole.

"The law of the heart is therefore the same as that of skeletal muscle, namely that the mechanical energy set free on passage from the resting to the contracted state depends on the area of 'chemically active surfaces,' i.e., on the length of the muscle fibres."[22]

According to these data, the normal response to either a greater volume load or a greater pressure load is an increase in both the diastolic and systolic ventricular volumes. A heart which becomes distended with a small or normal load is considered fatigued or depressed even though it may maintain a "normal" output while operating at this larger size.

Wiggers and Katz (see Ref. 21) repeated these experiments using improved techniques. Their results confirmed those of Starling and his associates that an increase in stroke volume was attended by an increase in diastolic volume (greater initial length of myocardial fibers). However, they concluded that "such changes were never dissociated from changes in initial intraventricular pressures." Apparently, Starling was not convinced by this evidence because in subsequent publications he restated his belief that diastolic volume may change without corresponding alterations in filling pressure.[23]

For half a century variations in stroke volume were most frequently explained by a few fundamental rules which were generally held to apply so long as the functional condition of the myocardium remains within physiologic limits: (a) The *cardiac output* is determined by the venous return. (b) If the heart rate is constant, the *stroke volume* is determined by the

venous return. (c) *Stroke volume* of the ventricles depends directly on the diastolic filling. (d) The *tension* of resting myocardial fibers depends upon their length. (e) *Diastolic filling* (and diastolic volume) of the ventricles is determined by effective filling pressure. (f) *The mechanical energy set free on passage from the resting to the contracted state depends on the length of the myocardial fibers.*

A number of these concepts were derived from Starling's experiments, and most of them have been erroneously cited at one time or another as "Starling's law of the heart." A far more realistic notation would have been the Frank-Starling application of the length-tension relation of myocardium. The concept that the diastolic volume is always determined by the effective pressure (e) is contrary to both the results and the conclusions of Starling and his associates. By the same token, belief in a constant relation between length and tension of resting myocardial fibers (d) cannot be attributed to these investigators.

Assumptions Implicit in the Frank-Starling Mechanism. In retrospect, the unquestioning acceptance and durability of the Frank-Starling mechanism as the "law of the heart" seems difficult to reconcile with certain obvious weaknesses. It is now clear that the ventricles are normally maximally distended in the resting recumbent individual and become smaller on standing or during virtually any other cardiac compensation. In contrast, the exposed heart of the anesthetized dog approaches its minimal diastolic and systolic dimensions. It seems quite possible that the ventricles of the heart-lung preparation became distended in response to volume or pressure loads in part because they were about as small as they could get during the "control" periods.

One very significant conceptual

deficiency in the Frank-Starling approach is the assumption that the relation between muscle fiber length and *isometric* contractile tension would permit prediction of changes in stroke volume, stroke work or external energy release by the contracting myocardium. By definition, isometric contraction means that shortening of the muscle is prevented, a situation which precludes ejection of blood or accomplishing external work. For this reason, the responses of ventricular chambers and muscle strips must also be studied under conditions in which shortening can occur.

LOSS OF MYOCARDIAL TENSION DURING SHORTENING

To study the dynamic properties of contracting myocardium, Lundin[24] utilized a strip of myocardium arranged as indicated in Figure 3–12 but equipped with a release mechan-

ism which permitted the muscle to shorten during its contraction period. The loss of tension during shortening by 20 per cent was represented schematically by the downward slanting arrows. The maximum tension developed when shortening was prevented as completely as possible. If the muscle was permitted to shorten slowly, the loss of tension was slight. Rapid shortening was accompanied by profound reduction in contractile tension. This reciprocal relation between the contractile force and the velocity of shortening has been known for many years. Such a velocity dependent relationship might be ascribed to a form of "viscosity" by which much of the applied force is dissipated as heat due to friction. Greatly increased forces are required to displace or propel a viscous fluid at higher and higher velocities. Imagine for a moment, the amount of force required to propel a paddle through water as compared to thick paint or molasses. In a contract-

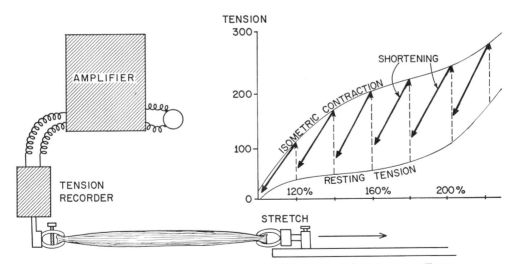

FIGURE 3–12 EFFECTS OF SHORTENING ON MYOCARDIAL CONTRACTILE TENSION

The increase in tension above resting tension developed by myocardial strips contracting under isometric conditions increased progressively from resting length to about 160 to 180 per cent of resting length, then diminished. If the myocardial strips shorten by 20 per cent during contraction, the contractile tension falls off sharply. (After Lundin.[24])

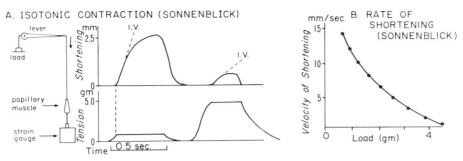

FIGURE 3–13   CONTRACTION OF EXCISED PAPILLARY MUSCLES

Isolated papillary muscles, contracting isotonically, begin to shorten after they have developed sufficient tension to elevate the load. The rate of shortening is greatest at the onset. The rate of shortening is diminished with an increasing load. (After Sonnenblick.[26])

ing muscle, internal viscosity might be visualized in terms of the forces developed by the contractile mechanism which fail to appear as external work because of dissipation of energy producing internal rearrangement within the muscle fiber. This is an attractive concept, but measurements of heat produced during muscular contraction indicate that the velocity of contraction is not limited by a passive internal viscosity in the muscle.[25] An alternative proposal is that the force on the muscle directly or indirectly influences the chemical reactions which produce the contractive forces.

Sonnenblick and his collaborators[26, 27] studied contraction of excised papillary muscles during shortening against a constant load as indicated in Figure 3–13. The rate of shortening is indicated by the slope of the shortening curve occurring under large and small load conditions. The initial portion of the curve is always steepest, indicating that the initial rate of shortening is the greatest during an isotonic contraction. By progressively increasing the load in a stepwise manner and noting the maximal velocity of shortening (steepest slope for each contraction), a curve can be drawn like that shown in Figure 3–13B. This graph demonstrates how

myocardial fibers shorten at their maximal rate and to a maximal extent under minimal load. By varying the rate of shortening, the load, the time elapsing between the onset of contraction and shortening and the initial length of the muscle, one can obtain a bewildering array of curves. Clearly, myocardial performance cannot be judged from studies of isometric contraction alone. The myocardial strips (i.e., in Figs. 3–12 and 3–13) were necessarily deprived of their blood supply. It is of importance to determine whether similar force-velocity relationships are apparent during contraction of the intact ventricles. For example, Fry *et al.*[28] conducted studies on a whole animal preparation in which left ventricular flow and pressure were varied independently. They reported that the velocity relationships in cardiac muscle appear to be much more dependent upon muscle length than is the case for skeletal muscle. A complex three-dimensional relationship between tension velocity and length was proposed as a preferred graphical method for analyzing myocardial function.

Functional Significance of Intrinsic Myocardial Properties. The applicability of concepts derived from observations under abnormal experimental conditions must ultimately be confirmed by appropriate measurements on intact animals and man functioning as nearly normally as possible. The Frank-Starling length-tension relationship appears to be manifest during certain spontaneous adaptations in intact, healthy animals (and apparently in man as well). For example, studies on the heart-lung preparation suggest that an increase in diastolic volume would be accompanied by increased energy release as expressed by increased outflow and increased stroke work. (See Fig. 3–14A). When a dog reclines from the sitting position, the ventricular diameter increases over a few beats until it appears to plateau at a maximum level. During the increase in diastolic diameter, the aortic outflow rate increases and the stroke volume (area under the flow curve) also increases. In a resting dog with spontaneously fluctuating heart rate (sinus arrhythmia), acceleration of the heart is accompanied by smaller diastolic dimensions and smaller stroke volume; slowing of the heart rate is associated with an increase in diastolic diameter and increased stroke volume (see also Fig. 3–27).

In contrast, certain other cardiovascular responses in normal animals and man do not apparently conform to the predictions implicit in the Frank-Starling length-tension relationship. For example, the left ventricular response to exercise (Fig. 3–14) reveals that when the animal stood up, the expected response occurred. However, rather drastic changes in many of the cardiac performance characteristics occurred during the period of exercise that do not appear to conform to any simple intrinsic control mechanism. The nature of these changes will not be considered in detail in this text. The exercise response is one of many normal and pathological responses which do not conform to predictions from the Frank-Starling length-tension relationship. This suggests that external mechanisms can override or modify the intrinsic properties of the myocardial fibers. The most common and most extensive functional changes are induced by stimulation of the sympathetic nerves which are distributed to the ventricular myocardium (see Fig. 3–4).

Extrinsic Control of Cardiac Function. The heart is strongly influenced by the powerful controls exerted by the autonomic nervous system. The heart rate is influenced by the balance between the slowing effects of the parasympathetic nerves in the vagus and the accelerating effects of the sympathetic nerves. Stimulation of the vagus nerves to the heart have little effect on ventricular function if changes in heart rate are prevented. In fact, there is little direct evidence that parasympathetic nerves are distributed to the ventricular myocardium (see Fig. 3–4). Sympathetic nerves distributed throughout the heart act by the release of a chemical transmitter (norepinephrine) at the nerve endings. When the adrenal gland is stimulated, it secretes a combination of norepinephrine (20 per cent) and 1-epinephrine (80 per cent) into the blood stream. Although intravascular injection of these substances was utilized for many years as a substitute for direct stimulation of sympathetic nerves to the heart, it is now generally recognized that circulating neurohormones are probably of little significance in normal cardiovascular control. Thus, the most important external control mechanisms affecting cardiac function are the parasympathetic and sympathetic effects on the myocardium.

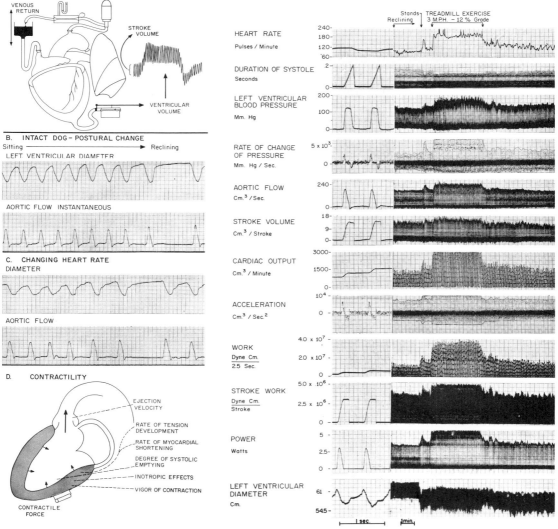

FIGURE 3–14   VENTRICULAR ADAPTATIONS DURING SPONTANEOUS ACTIVITY

A, In the heart-lung preparation, the ventricle responds to an increase in either volume load or pressure load by diastolic distension and increased energy release (Frank-Starling mechanism).

B, In intact dogs, the Frank-Starling mechanism is readily demonstrable in the increase in energy release associated with increased diastolic distension as the animal reclines.

C, This mechanism also occurs during spontaneous changes in heart rate (i.e., sinus arrhythmia) which represent variations in vagal discharge.

D, Changes in ventricular performance which do not conform to the Frank-Starling mechanism are commonly attributed to changes in "contractility," a term which has so many connotations that it is relatively meaningless.

E, The ventricular responses to exercise by healthy active dogs correspond to the changes induced by sympathetic stimulation. (From Rushmer *et al., Circulation,* 1963, *17*:118–141.)

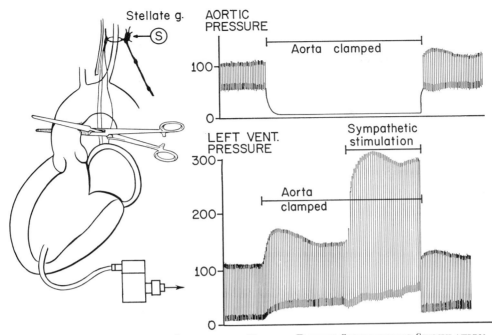

FIGURE 3–15 **VENTRICULAR CONTRACTILE TENSION DURING SYMPATHETIC STIMULATION**

Ventricular pressure is elevated during each systolic contraction by clamping the aorta so that the myocardium contracts more nearly isometrically. A very large additional increase in contractile tension can be produced by stimulating sympathetic cardiac nerves. This observation demonstrates a direct effect of the sympathetic nerve activity on myocardial contractile force, independent of any peripheral vascular effects of such stimulation.

Effects of Sympathetic Cardiac Nerves. The effects of the sympathetic nerve discharge to the heart are dramatically demonstrated by restricting the degree of myocardial shortening (see Fig. 3–15). Clamping of the aorta restricts ejection to the coronary outflow so that the myocardium contracts almost isometrically. The intraventricular pressure rises as aortic pressure rapidly drops toward zero. Ventricular systolic pressure is almost doubled when the ventricular contraction is rendered almost isometric (Fig. 3–15). If the sympathetic cardiac nerves on the left are stimulated when the ventricles are contracting almost isometrically, the ventricular pressure rises to extremely high levels, reaching 300 mm. Hg as in

Figure 3–15 and up to 500 mm. Hg in other experiments. The cardiac sympathetic nerves on the left side profoundly affect the maximum tension which can be developed by the ventricular myocardium. The cardiac nerves descending on the right side generally produce a greater change in the heart rate and a smaller increase in contractile tension. The sympathetic nerves to the heart on the right apparently converge on the S-A node to act on the pacemaker, while the left sympathetic nerves are more widely distributed to the atrial and ventricular myocardium (see Fig. 3–4).

Although the sympathetic innervation of the heart apparently induces changes more closely resembling those observed during spontaneous cardiovascular responses, such conclusions can be based only on more direct comparisons than can be achieved in the anesthetized, thoracotomized dog. Instead, the changes in cardiac performance must be studied continuously during various kinds of activity in healthy unanesthetized dogs (i.e., Fig. 3–14).

EFFECTS OF SYMPATHETIC NERVES ON VENTRICULAR EJECTION

The very great increase in ventricular systolic pressure accomplished during sympathetic discharge to an almost isometrically contracting myocardium is superimposed upon the intrinsic isometric length-tension relation of the muscle. In addition, sympathetic nerve activity also affects profoundly the velocity of shortening

of myocardium and the resulting ejection rates. A flowmeter mounted on the aorta consistently demonstrates the marked increase in peak outflow rate from the ventricle with the steep initial upslope indicating a characteristic increase in the acceleration of the blood during the powerful impulse produced by the contracting ventricular myocardium (Fig. 3–16). The same type of phenomenon is readily observed during spontaneous cardiac adaptations like exercise (see also Fig. 3–14). The typical response to sympathetic stimulation also includes a more rapid deceleration of outflow and a shorter systolic interval so that the stroke volume may be increased but little or not at all, in spite of transiently higher peak outflow rates during each cycle.

A comprehensive description of the effects of sympathetic discharge to the heart involves numerous aspects of

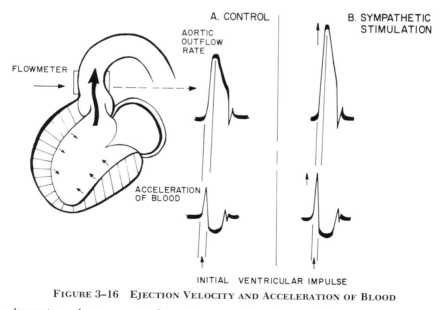

FIGURE 3–16   EJECTION VELOCITY AND ACCELERATION OF BLOOD

An ultrasonic or electromagnetic flowmeter mounted on the root of the aorta indicates the typical changes in ejection velocity, reaching a high peak flow early in systole. The steep initial upslope indicates very high acceleration of outflow. Sympathetic stimulation increases peak acceleration and elevates peak flow rates with reduced period of ejection to provide about the same stroke volume ejected in shorter time.

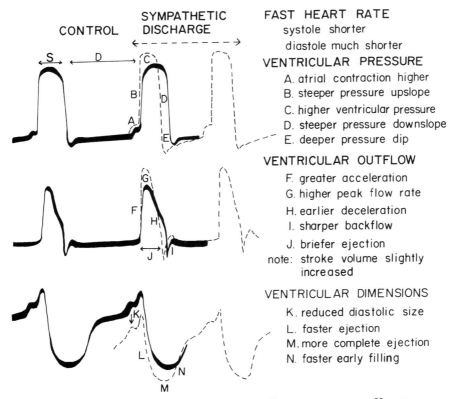

CONTROL   SYMPATHETIC DISCHARGE

FAST HEART RATE
  systole shorter
  diastole much shorter

VENTRICULAR PRESSURE
  A. atrial contraction higher
  B. steeper pressure upslope
  C. higher ventricular pressure
  D. steeper pressure downslope
  E. deeper pressure dip

VENTRICULAR OUTFLOW
  F. greater acceleration
  G. higher peak flow rate
  H. earlier deceleration
  I. sharper backflow
  J. briefer ejection
  note: stroke volume slightly increased

VENTRICULAR DIMENSIONS
  K. reduced diastolic size
  L. faster ejection
  M. more complete ejection
  N. faster early filling

FIGURE 3–17   EFFECTS OF SYMPATHETIC DISCHARGE TO THE HEART

The many changes in left ventricular function produced by sympathetic discharge to the heart are indicated in relation to heart rate, ventricular pressure, outflow and dimensions. The principal effects are on the *rates* of ventricular function, including heart *rate*, *rate* of rise and *rate* of fall of ventricular pressure, ejection *velocity*, *rate* of change of velocity (acceleration), *rate* of deceleration and *rate* of change of dimensions.

the pressure, flow and dimensional changes during the cardiac cycle (Fig. 3–17). The faster heart rate signifies a reduced duration of each cardiac cycle accomplished by a moderate reduction in the duration of systolic interval and a much greater shortening of the diastolic filling interval. The ventricular pressure record exhibits a larger pressure effect from atrial contraction, a much steeper upslope at the onset of ventricular systole. The peak ventricular pressure is somewhat increased. The downslope of the pressure record is very steep, terminating in a deeper early diastolic trough associated with the diastolic recoil, followed by more

rapid rise in diastolic ventricular pressure. Manifestations of greater acceleration to a higher peak outflow rate, earlier deceleration of flow and shorter ejection period are all found in records from both the flow sensors and the dimensional gauges. This array of changes in ventricular performance has an important unifying feature which is summarized in Figure 3–18. The most significant effect of sympathetic discharge is to cause the myocardium to function more rapidly. For example, the *rate* of rise and the *rate* of fall of pressure are increased to a greater extent than the absolute value of peak pressure. The heart *rate* in-

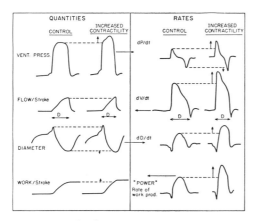

FIGURE 3–18   COMPONENTS OF INCREASED CONTRACTILITY

The changes in ventricular performance induced by administration of *l*-epinephrine demonstrate that the increased "contractility" involved predominantly increased in the rates at which the variables change (dP/dt, dV/dt, dD/dt, and "power") without necessarily increasing the quantities (ventricular pressure, flow/stroke, diameter or work/stroke). The increase in systolic ventricular pressure is primarily the result of increased ejection velocity (dV/dt).

creased; the duration of systole decreased. The peak outflow *rate* or ejection velocity is greatly increased but the volume flow per stroke (stroke volume) is increased but slightly if at all. The *rate* of change of velocity (acceleration) is greatly and consistently increased. The *rate* of change of dimensions is increased while the absolute dimensions remain about the same or diminish. The net effect of all these changes is to eject about the same stroke volume in a shorter systolic interval, permitting an increase in heart rate with a sustained or increased stroke volume and greater cardiac output.

The changes in ventricular performance illustrated in Figures 3–17 and 3–18 can be consistently induced experimentally by direct stimulation of sympathetic nerves to the heart in dogs[29, 30] and by reflex stimulation of these nerves in man.[31] Of even greater interest is the fact that changes of the same kind can be produced by selective stimulation of discretely localized sites at the base of the brain, in the diencephalon. In fact, it is possible to reproduce quite accurately the left ventricular responses to exertion without body movement by stimulating electrically very small diencephalic areas in the unanesthetized dog.

DIENCEPHALIC INFLUENCES ON VENTRICULAR PERFORMANCE

Neural pathways pass from the hypothalamus and subthalamus to and through the medullary region to terminate at the intermediolateral cell columns of the spinal cord (see Fig. 3–4). The hypothalamus has long been regarded as the font of the autonomic nervous system and has been repeatedly explored by neurophysiologists using changes in arterial pressure as their principal criterion of sites of cardiovascular control. Thus, various regions in the diencephalon have been labeled "pressor" or "depressor areas" on the basis of elevation or reduction of systemic arterial pressure.[32] Although the anterior hypothalamus is generally regarded as being the site of predominantly depressor areas and the posterior hypothalamus as being largely pressor in its influence, recent exploration of these areas[33, 34] has demonstrated that powerful depressor responses can be induced easily and consistently from many locations (Fig. 3–19). For example, a very pronounced reduction in heart rate and systolic ventricular pressure and reduced rates of change in pressure and cumulative aortic flow were produced by stimulation in the ventral nuclear group of the thalamus. After the electrode tip was

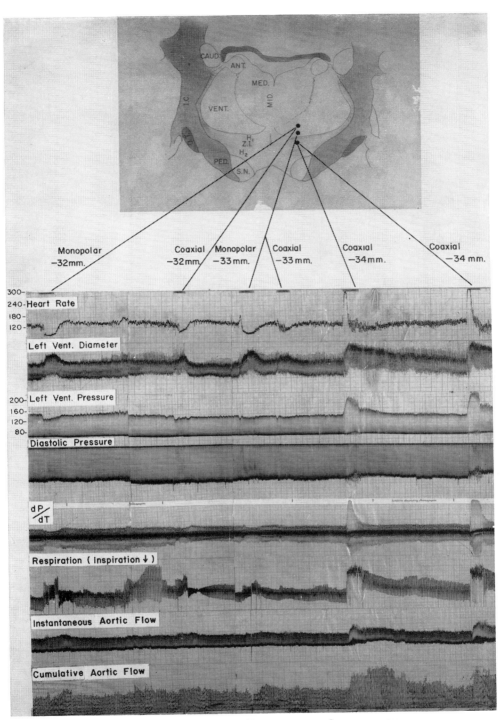

FIGURE 3-19   EFFECTS OF DIENCEPHALIC STIMULATION

Changes in ventricular performance in terms of the multiple variables. At the upper point, stimulation produced reduction in heart rate, increased ventricular diameter, reduced ventricular systolic pressure, diminished rate of change of pressure (dP/dt), altered respiration and little change in aortic flow. Two millimeters lower, the electrode was in the zona incerta and stimulation produced an extremely high transient tachycardia, increased diameter, increased ventricular systolic pressure, increased diastolic pressure, greatly increased rate of change of pressure and increased aortic flow. The sites producing these profound changes are apparently discretely localized in the diencephalon.

95

moved 2 mm. ventrad in the H_2 field of Forel, stimulation resulted in a very powerful pressor response (Fig. 3–19). This response included a transient, explosive acceleration in heart rate, greatly elevated systolic ventricular pressure and rate of change of pressure and augmented aortic peak flow rates and accumulated flow (cardiac output). Marked changes in respiratory patterns —panting—accompanied these cardiovascular changes.

Stimulation of selected areas of the brain stem quite easily produced cardiovascular changes much greater than any seen during spontaneous activity in these dogs.[35] Moreover, a very wide variety of cardiac responses has been produced by stimulation at different sites during exploration of these central regions (Fig. 3–20). At the sites indicated by the histologic sections, virtually every conceivable response was elicited and could be repeatedly induced. Of considerable interest was the fact that by selecting records from

a rather large collection, examples could be found in which the changes were almost completely restricted to a single feature of cardiac function: heart rate, left ventricular diameter or left ventricular systolic pressure and left ventricular diastolic pressure. Despite the variation in the kinds of cardiovascular responses which are apparently embodied in the diencephalic mechanisms, stimulation of the same site in different animals consistently produced the same pattern of response. In fact, a cardiac response closely simulating the changes typically observed during treadmill exercise can be quite consistently reproduced by electrical stimulation in the H_2 field of Forel.

HYPOTHALAMIC FUNCTION IN CARDIAC CONTROL

A wide variety of different autonomic functions are represented in the base of the brain. For example, the

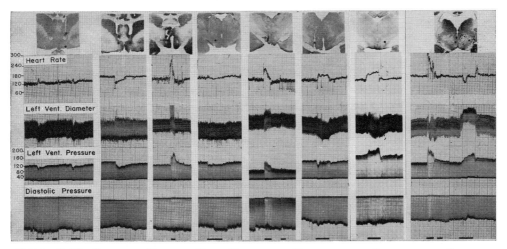

FIGURE 3–20   VARIABLE EFFECTS FROM DIFFERENT DIENCEPHALIC STIMULATION POINTS

Exploration of various sites in the diencephalon with stimulating electrodes demonstrated that many distinctive patterns of ventricular response can be elicited from different regions. Note that in some sites more or less isolated changes occur in one variable with little change in the others. However, repeated stimulation of a particular site consistently produces similar responses in the same or in different animals.

hypothalamus plays an extremely important role in the regulation of body temperature in both animals and man. Heat loss mechanisms (panting and sweating) can be induced by local heating of the preoptic and supraoptic regions in cats. The hypothalamus is apparently involved in sleep and waking; decreased activity of the hypothalamus results in somnolence and increased activity in this region leads to increased bodily activity. Somatic movements, including changes in posture and even running movements, can be produced by stimulating certain regions in the diencephalon. Many forms of overt sexual activity involve stereotyped behavior of a sort which may be influenced by the hypothalamus. This region also serves outward expressions suggesting rage. Each of these responses involves compensatory adjustments in the peripheral blood flow and also in cardiac function. Thus, it is not surprising to find that different portions of the hypothalamic region can induce such varied cardiovascular responses as are illustrated in Figure 3–20.

CEREBRAL CONTROL OF CARDIAC FUNCTION

Activity of portions of the cerebral cortex induces changes in overt behavior, and stimulation in these areas also results in some form of cardiovascular response. Thus, motor areas of the cerebral cortex, from which voluntary motion apparently stems, can also induce changes in the distribution of blood flow and increased cardiac activity. Excision of orbital surface of the frontal lobe produces extreme hyperactivity, including continuous pacing. Stimulation of this region has often been reported to induce pressor responses.[32] The cingu-

late gyrus has been implicated in the control of emotional behavior and apparently is a potent autonomic effector area. These few examples serve to emphasize the general principle that those portions of the central nervous system in which stimulation produces behavioral responses are also capable of causing cardiovascular effects.[35] This statement does not imply that the cardiovascular responses are necessarily appropriate for the type of behavior produced, because this correlation has not been demonstrated. However, the incorporation of nervous pathways capable of influencing autonomic function appears to represent an important feature of the organization of the central nervous areas controlling behavior. This type of architecture represents a potential mechanism by which patterns of autonomic adjustment may be automatically associated with particular types of behavior.

SUMMARY

The quantity of blood pumped by the heart per unit time (cardiac output) is determined by two main factors: (1) the heart rate and (2) the stroke volume. Normally each heart beat is initiated by a conducted wave of excitation generated by pacemaker cells in the S-A node. The frequency of discharge of the pacemaker is determined by the balance between the retarding effect of nerve impulses descending the vagus nerve and the acclerating effect of the sympathetic nerve impulses reaching this region. If the heart rate is increased experimentally by an artificial pacemaker directly exciting the atrium at a progressively greater rate, the stroke output of the ventricles diminishes and the cardiac output may not increase. Thus, acceleration of the heart rate alone is not necessarily an effective means of increasing cardiac output.

The quantity of blood ejected by the ventricles is represented by the difference between the volume at the end of diastolic filling and the volume at the end of systolic ejection. An increase in the diastolic distention of the ventricles produces an increase in the energy released during the subsequent systole in accordance with the Frank-Starling concept, derived and confirmed by studying the isolated or exposed hearts of dogs under rigid experimental conditions in which the investigator assumed complete control. The ventricular myocardium derives several advantages from function at large diastolic dimensions in addition to the well known increase in isometric contractile tension attained through the increased elongation of the muscle fibers. The tension developed by myocardium contracting without a change in length falls off sharply as the muscle is permitted to shorten (during systolic ejection). The contractile tension is more depleted by either a greater amount of shortening or a faster rate of shortening. To eject a particular volume the amount of myocardial shortening is greatly reduced when the ventricles function at large diastolic and systolic dimensions. The contractile tension which is lost and stored in the form of tension between layers of muscle fibers is also diminished by a reduction in relative myocardial shortening. On the other hand, the contraction tension required to elevate ventricular pressure to a particular level is increased by diastolic distention in accordance with the law of Laplace. Thus, the dimensions at which the ventricles function must represent the resultant of several interacting factors.

In addition to the functional and architectural factors indicated previously, the contractile properties of the myocardium can be greatly influenced by the stimulation of sympathetic nerves to the heart. Under the influence of these nerves, the ventricles develop tension more rapidly, shorten more rapidly, eject blood more rapidly, develop more power and can attain a much higher maximum contractile tension. The duration of systole is shortened so that, in spite of greatly accelerated ejection, the volume ejected may be not greater than during the control period. On the other hand, increased stroke volume may be produced by greater systolic ejection, by more diastolic distention or by a combination of both factors. Changes in ventricular performance are achieved by variations in sympathetic, but not by parasympathetic, discharge to the ventricles.

The cardioregulatory areas in the medulla influence the autonomic discharge to the heart as a portion of the pressoreceptor mechanism for maintaining systemic arterial pressure (see Chapter 6). The diencephalic and hypothalamic regions contain cardiovascular controls in complex neural mechanisms involved in temperature regulation, the intake of food and fluid, emotional and sexual behavior and many other patterns of behavior. It follows, then, that a wide variety of cardiovascular responses can be induced by electrical stimulation at various sites in the brain stem. Also areas of the cerebral cortex where stimulation induces changes in overt behavior also induce cardiovascular adaptations of one sort or another. Thus, there exists the possibility that the architecture of the central nervous system provides for combined patterns of somatic and autonomic adaptations.

II. CLINICAL ESTIMATION OF CARDIAC OUTPUT

Since the maximum capability of the heart can be evaluated only by determining the cardiovascular response to a load, a method for directly measuring cardiac output during exertion would be very valuable in cardiac diagnosis and prognosis. Unfortunately, direct measurements of cardiac function in man, although desirable, are virtually impossible because the heart is quite inaccessible for the determination of either stroke volume or absolute volume. Perhaps the most direct method is the calculation of changes in cardiac volume from the cardiac silhouette on roentgenographic plates. In recent years, a wide variety of techniques has been proposed to determine cardiac output by indirect methods. The basic principles and limitations of some of the techniques currently in vogue will be described.

From the foregoing discussion, it is clear that measurement of either cardiac output or stroke volume may not be sufficient to permit adequate evaluation of ventricular performance. Profound changes in the rates of change of various features of ventricular function may occur with little or no influence in stroke volume (see Figs. 3–17 and 3–18). In addition to techniques for measuring cardiac output, efforts must be directed toward devising methods of assessing the dynamic properties of ventricular performance. Some of the methods which are currently available will be presented along with some predictions for the future.

THE FICK PRINCIPLE

Blood flow through an organ can be determined if a substance is removed from or added to the blood during its flow through the organ. Applied to the lungs, the Fick principle is used to calculate the volume of blood required to transport the oxygen taken up from the alveoli per unit time. The fundamental concept is deceptively simple and can be illustrated schematically by representing the oxygen-carrying capacity of the blood as beakers on a conveyer belt (Fig. 3–21).

MEASUREMENT OF OXYGEN CONSUMPTION

Of necessity, the oxygen consumption is generally measured over a period of several minutes. The accuracy of oxygen uptake determinations from the clinical B.M.R. apparatus is generally inadequate for this purpose. A preferred technique consists of collecting in a spirometer all the air expired during carefully timed intervals and analyzing samples for oxygen content (Fig. 3–22). Comparing the oxygen content of the total exhaled volume with a similar volume of ambient air provides the data required to compute the oxygen uptake accurately.

THE ARTERIOVENOUS OXYGEN DIFFERENCE

The arterial blood throughout the body normally has a uniform oxygen content. However, to determine a significant A-V oxygen difference, it is necessary to obtain samples of *mixed* venous blood. The quantity of oxygen contained in venous blood depends upon the vascular bed from which it is returning. For example, blood from the kidneys and skin remains well satu-

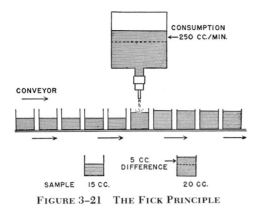

FIGURE 3–21   THE FICK PRINCIPLE

If each beaker on a conveyer belt receives 5 cc. of fluid as it passes under a dispenser delivering 250 cc. per minute, the beakers must pass the dispenser at a rate of 50 per minute (250/5) to carry that quantity of fluid. Similarly, if each 100 cc. of blood takes up 5 cc. of oxygen from the lungs (A-V oxygen difference) and 250 cc. of oxygen are consumed each minute, 50 increments of 100 cc. (5000 cc.) of blood must have passed through the lungs each minute. This is the Fick principle as it is applied to the calculation of cardiac output (see Fig. 3–22).

rated with oxygen while blood from the coronary vessels and exercising muscle is largely depleted of oxygen. The oxygen contents of venous blood from other tissues vary between these extremes. Due to laminar flow in the venous channels, currents of blood with a relatively high oxygen content may accompany streams with lower values in the same vein. The oxygen saturation of blood in the superior vena cava differs from that in the inferior vena cava and these two streams of blood do not mix completely within the right atrium. The Lipiodol streamers in Figure 2–15 graphically illustrate this fact. Mixing of blood does occur in the right ventricle and is almost complete by the time the blood has entered the pulmonary arteries. The oxygen content of a sample of blood obtained from the pulmonary artery represents an average value for

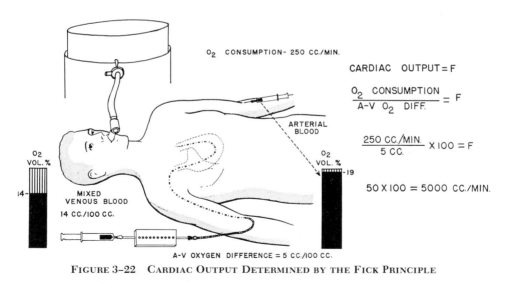

FIGURE 3–22   CARDIAC OUTPUT DETERMINED BY THE FICK PRINCIPLE

Computing cardiac output according to the Fick principle requires simultaneous determination of oxygen consumption and the arteriovenous oxygen difference. Exhaled air is collected to measure oxygen consumption per minute. Blood is withdrawn from the pulmonary artery through a catheter into a cuvette oximeter, so that the oxygen content of mixed venous blood can be read from a galvanometer. Arterial oxygen content is measured in a sample of blood from any systemic artery. The A-V oxygen difference in cubic centimeters of oxygen per 100 cc. of blood is obtained by subtracting the oxygen content of the mixed venous sample from the arterial oxygen content.

venous blood which can be used to establish the arteriovenous oxygen difference for calculating cardiac output by the Fick principle.

Cardiac Catheterization. In 1929, Forssmann[36] demonstrated that a catheter can be passed through the venous channels into the right chambers of the human heart (Fig. 3–22). Cournand and his associates[37, 38] established the safety of the procedure and stimulated widespread utilization of the method. The technique of cardiac catheterization and its sources of error have been described in detail by Cournand,[39] Warren,[40] Visscher[41] and Stow.[42]

Measurement of Blood Oxygen Content. Arterial and venous oxygen content can be directly measured with the Van Slyke apparatus, which is a time-consuming but accurate procedure in the hands of highly qualified technicians. For rapid determinations of blood oxygen content, a photoelectric method has been developed and compares favorably with Van Slyke determinations. Blood for analysis is drawn through a cuvette oximeter (Fig. 3–22), where it is transilluminated by a constant intensity light source, and the transmitted light is registered simultaneously in two spectral regions: approximately 750 to 900 millimicrons and 600 to 750 millimicrons, respectively. The former is near infra-red light in wave length and is transmitted by both oxyhemoglobin and reduced hemoglobin to approximately equal degrees. The other photocell responds to red light, which is transmitted well by oxyhemoglobin and to a very slight degree by reduced hemoglobin. The ratio between the light intensities recorded from the two wave lengths can be read in terms of absolute percentage of oxygen saturation after the apparatus has been satisfactorily calibrated by means of Van Slyke analysis. Various spectrophotometric techniques have been successfully employed for the measurement of blood oxygen content. In experienced hands, these devices more than make up for the slight reduction in accuracy through the ease with which serial determinations can be obtained in rapid sequence while the patient is being studied.

Objective determinations of cardiac output have been of great value in advancing our knowledge of circulatory dynamics, with particular reference to pulmonary function in health and disease. However, the search for an objective test of cardiac reserve was not ended by the development of cardiac catheterization, because the procedure is too complicated for routine clinical use and is not entirely suitable for use during strenuous exertion. A normal value for cardiac output at rest is often obtained even when the cardiac reserve is seriously depleted. If cardiac catheterization provided no information beyond the resting cardiac output, its utilization would be largely limited to fundamental investigation. However, several additional types of information can be gained from catheterization which are particularly useful in the diagnosis of congenital malformations of the heart.

THE STEWART PRINCIPLE

The volume of fluid in a container can be calculated by adding a known quantity of dye and measuring the concentration of the material after it has become evenly dispersed through the fluid (Fig. 3–23A). The volume is calculated according to the formula $V = A/C$, where V is the volume of fluid, A is the amount of dye added and C is the concentration of the dye in

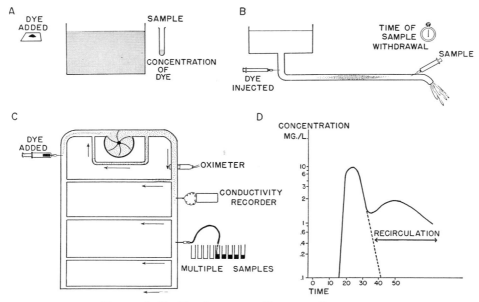

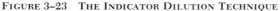

FIGURE 3–23   THE INDICATOR DILUTION TECHNIQUE

A, The volume of stationary fluid in a reservoir can be determined by completely mixing a known amount of dye and analyzing a sample for the concentration of the dye.

B, The volume flow through a simple tube can be estimated by injecting a known quantity of dye, withdrawing a sample at constant rate during the passage of the dye-containing fluid and determining the mean concentration of the sample.

C, A hydraulic model simulating the circulatory system illustrates the fact that an indicator substance may pass through short circuits and begin to recirculate before the mass of dye has passed the sampling point. Therefore it is necessary to devise means by which the amount of recirculating dye can be separated from the amount of dye sampled during its initial passage to arrive at a reliable mean concentration.

D, If the concentration of the dye passing a sampling point is plotted on semi-log paper, the descending limb after the peak can be extended to the baseline as a straight line. The area under the initial curve can be used to derive the mean concentration of the dye during its first circulation.

each cubic centimeter of the fluid. Stewart[43, 44] demonstrated that his method can also be applied to fluids in motion. Hamilton and his associates[45, 46] verified the usefulness of the method in calculating the flow through glass models and in the circulation.

GENERAL PRINCIPLES

The computation of a volume of stationary fluid by determining the dilution of a known quantity of dye is perfectly straightforward (Fig. 3–23). Similarly, the volume flow through a simple tubular system can theoretically

be determined with considerable accuracy by determining the average concentration of a known quantity of dye and the time during sampling according to the formula $F = A/Ct$, where F is flow, A is quantity of dye injected, C is the average concentration of dye in the sample and t is the duration of sample withdrawal (Fig. 3–23A). Under these conditions, the Stewart principle is quite as accurate as the Fick principle. However, conditions in the human circulation are more complex, as indicated by the hydraulic model in Figure 3–23C. Part of the dye injected at one point in this model has completely traversed the short circuits and begun to recirculate before the material has reached the more distant regions. The average concentration of the indicator substance can be measured by (1) collecting multiple samples in rapid succession, (2) continuously recording blood conductivity after saline injections or (3) making oximeter or densitometer recordings when dyes are injected. In any case, the concentration of indicator flowing past the point of recording reaches a peak, begins to descend and then increases again owing to recirculation. If the once-circulated dye can be separated from the recirculated dye, cardiac output can be computed with considerable accuracy.

The fundamental requirements for this method are (1) the injection of a material which can be accurately analyzed and which does not leave the blood during the test and (2) a sample of arterial blood which indicates the average concentration of the material during its first circulation through the arterial tree. Various dyes as well as saline solutions have been used with varying degrees of success and the average concentration has been determined either by repetitive sampling or by continuous recording.

BALLISTOCARDIOGRAPHY

The concept that a sudden motion of the blood in one direction must produce a recoil of the body in the opposite direction is not a new idea. In 1887, Gordon[47] compared the ballistic forces of the body to the recoil of a gun. In 1905 Henderson[48] used a "swinging table" to record the movements along the longitudinal axis of a patient reclining on its surface. The changing velocity of the moving blood

within the circulatory system caused the table to oscillate during each successive cardiac cycle.

GENERAL PRINCIPLES

The recoil of a rifle is frequently employed as an analogy to explain the basic principles of ballistocardiography. If a rifle is rigidly fastened on a spring-mounted table, a discharging cartridge propels the bullet out of the barrel and displaces the rifle in the opposite direction (Fig. 3–24A). Recording the movements of the table in these circumstances might provide information concerning the magnitude of the powder charge (energy release) if other conditions are known. If the magnitude of the powder charge and the muzzle velocity were unknown, the weight of the bullet (mass ejected) could not be computed from the recorded deflections. The analysis would be seriously complicated if, during the recoil of the rifle, the speeding bullet struck a steel plate mounted on the same table. Since the blood does not leave the system, the recoil of the heart and body from ejection of blood into the arteries is even more complex. For example, the blood ejected from the two ventricles moves simultaneously in several directions after leaving the heart. Its energy is imparted to the body at every turn. Routine ballistocardiograms indicate movements of the body in only one direction. Simultaneous recordings in three dimensions are extremely difficult to analyze. Finally, the records may be seriously distorted by such factors as the coupling between the body and the table. The elasticity of the skin acts as a spring interposed between the moving body and the table top and may profoundly influence the recorded deflections.

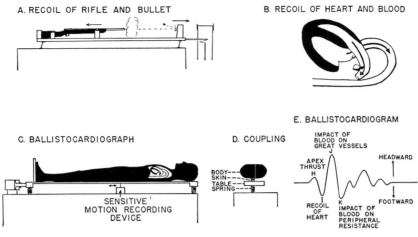

FIGURE 3–24   BALLISTOCARDIOGRAPHY

A, The recoil of a rifle during discharge of a cartridge can be recorded by attaching it rigidly to a spring-mounted table. The record would become seriously distorted if the bullet ricocheted from a barrier on the table during the recoil of the rifle.

B, The blood ejected by the ventricles travels in several directions simultaneously, imparting its energy to the body at every turn. For this reason, measurements of the recoil of the body in one direction only are inadequate.

C, A low-frequency spring-mounted table which has been critically damped has been recommended for ballistocardiography because the body cannot be rigidly fastened to the table. The tissues in contact with the table have an elasticity which is equivalent to interposing a spring between the body and the table top.

D, If the springs supporting the table are stiff in relation to the elasticity of the tissues, the recorded patterns tend to reflect the elastic properties of the tissues supporting the body as the forces are imparted by the heart and blood.

E, Ballistocardiographic records consist of a series of deflections which have been related to the events of the cardiac cycle. Although the forces developed by the heart and blood affect the recorded patterns, a consistent relationship between these deflections and stroke volume is probably fortuitous for the most part.

EVALUATION OF BALLISTOCARDIOGRAPHY

Starr and his associates[49] extended Henderson's observations and reawakened interest in the recoil phenomena by stating that the size of the initial waves, I and J, is related to the cardiac output, and that the form of the ballistic curve is determined by the shape of the curve of blood velocity in the great vessels.[50] Actually, the size of the initial deflection is determined by the acceleration of the fluid (the rate at which velocity of ejection is built up) and not by the total stroke output. The recorded oscillations are the resultant of vascular and body movements as they may be in phase and reinforce one another or be out of phase and cancel each other. Reconstruction of the ballistocardiographic records led to the following description of the causes of the various oscillations. The H wave begins with movements that take place during isometric contraction and are the most variable. The I wave is the result of a partly cancelled footward thrust developed as blood is ejected from the heart into the ascending aorta and pulmonary artery. The J wave has a complex origin, including the deceleration of blood in the heart, ascending aorta and pulmonary artery and the acceleration of blood in the descending aorta.

The obvious limitations of the method do not preclude the recognition of empirical relationships between various types of cardiac dysfunction and characteristic ballistocardiographic patterns. Since the amplitude of the deflections is influenced by the rate at which blood is accelerated, variations in the pattern should reveal alterations in the force of ventricular ejection. It may have value as a source of information about the dynamic performance of the heart (see Fig. 3–26).

PRESSURE PULSE CONTOUR METHOD

THE RELATION OF PULSE PRESSURE TO STROKE VOLUME

Erlanger and Hooker[51] recognized that the product of the pulse pressure and the heart rate indicated cardiac output, with the following reservations: "In order to be able to obtain a knowledge of the absolute velocity of blood flow from a knowledge of the pulse-pressure and pulse rate, it is necessary to know:

"1. The rate of systolic output. For if a given amount of blood be driven into the aorta with different rates the maximum pressure would be higher when this rate is rapid than when it is slow.

"2. The rate of flow from the arteries into the veins. For this flow continues during cardiac systole and consequently variations in the rate of this flow would vary the height to which the force of the heart would raise the systolic pressure.

"3. The distensibility of human arteries at different pressures. The distensibility diminishes as the pressure increases; consequently at a high pressure it would require a smaller systolic output to produce a pulse-pressure of a given magnitude than at a low pressure.

"4. The amount of blood in the systemic arteries under various conditions. The fall of pressure during diastole depends upon the relative amount of blood that escapes into the veins, not upon the absolute amount.

"We do not know how large any one of these factors is, but it seems probable that, under more or less normal conditions, none of them would produce a very large error. Upon this assumption we are perhaps justified in using the product of the pulse-pressure by the pulse rate as an index to the relative velocity of blood flow."

Clearly the stroke volume would be directly proportional to arterial pulse pressure only if the pressure-volume relations of the arterial system were not only constant and uniform among individuals, but linear from high pressure to low. Remington[52] presented a set of volume factors from known stroke volumes and pulse pressures, corrected for body size and distensibility curves. From this table, stroke volume/sq. m. body surface could be predicted with an error of about 25 per cent. According to Hamilton and Remington[53] pulse pressure correlates roughly with stroke volume determined by the dye dilution technique (r = 0.88). Over the normal pressure range, a pressure rise of 1 mm. Hg was equivalent to about 1 cc. of stroke volume/sq. m. For some purposes, this degree of accuracy might be quite sufficient. However, a great deal of effort has been expended in attempts to increase the precision with which stroke volume is derived from the pressure-pulse contour. This is no simple matter, considering the complexity of the situation.

ANALYSIS OF PULSE CONTOURS

If fluid is injected into a distensible container with fixed volume elasticity, the volume in the system can be calibrated in terms of the internal pressure (Fig. 3–25A). Once the volume-pressure relations are established, the volume contained can be determined by noting the pressure in the system. However, if fluid can escape from the system (Fig. 3–25B), the elastic chamber will remain dis-

tended only if fluid is pumped in at the same average rate as it leaks out. Under these circumstances, the pressure will increase as the chamber is distended and will decrease between pumping strokes as the fluid leaves the system. The difference between the maximal and minimal pressures indicates the amount of fluid injected at each stroke less the amount which left the system during the ejection period. If the distensible chamber is a long, narrow cylinder with elastic

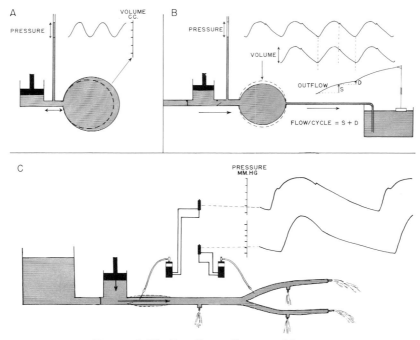

FIGURE 3–25   THE PULSE CONTOUR METHOD

A, The changes in the volume of the balloon can be determined by measuring the pressure if the pressure-volume relations are constant.

B, If fluid is pumped into a balloon and flows out through a tube offering some resistance, the flow through the system can be estimated from the pressure fluctuations. The volume and pressure within the balloon increase during ejection from the pump, but outflow occurs throughout the entire cycle. If pressure fluctuations are used to indicate changes in volume, the flow from the system can be estimated by determining the flow out of the system during diastole (D) and adding a computed value for outflow from the system during the stroke (S).

C, In the circulatory system, the pulse of pressure does not reach all parts of the elastic pressure reservoir simultaneously and its contour changes as it passes through the system (see also Fig. 5–3). Under these conditions, the volumes entering and leaving various portions of the system must be considered individually to reach maximum accuracy. Since this is not practical in intact animals or man, the computation of cardiac output from pressure pulses has been greatly simplified. However, each step toward simplification of the method involves sacrifice of accuracy.

walls, the fluid ejected by the pump is not instantaneously distributed through the system and the recorded pressure will be distorted by reflected waves. A similar situation obtains within the arterial system of the body.

Hamilton and Remington[53] recognized that prediction of stroke volume from pressure pulses must depend upon evaluation of the "individual arterial distensibility, knowledge of the pulse pressure in the arterial tree and its several parts, and the estimation of arteriolar drainage." They developed a table indicating the capacity of the various portions of the arterial tree at different pressures and another showing the pulse wave transmission times to the parts of the arterial tree at various diastolic pressures. These data were employed in the analysis of pressure pulses. Remington *et al.*[54] and Warner[55] subsequently reported a simplified technique which facilitates analysis of the pressure pulse with little increase in the error. The pulse contour method has one very important potential advantage. It permits computation of the stroke volume of individual cycles even though its accuracy may be limited.

COMPUTED AORTIC FLOW VELOCITY FROM THE PRESSURE GRADIENT

The mathematical relationship between pressure, viscosity and density expressed by the Navier Stokes equation is a fundamental and general expression describing fluid flow. Fry and his associates[56, 57] developed a modification of this relationship, which with suitable restrictions can be expressed as

$$-dp/dz = 1.1 \ (\rho/g) \ (d\omega/dt) + a\omega$$

where p is the lateral pressure in cm. H_2O, z is the distance between the pressure points in cm., ρ is the blood density in g/cm.^{3}, g is the acceleration of gravity in cm./sec.^{2}, t is time in seconds, 1.1 is an experimentally determined constant taking into account the nonuniform velocity distribution across the lumen and a is a frictional coefficient. By feeding into a computer the pressure difference between two points along the stream, the solution of the equation indicates the blood velocity from the pressure gradient continuously measured between two points a known distance apart. For this purpose, a double lumen catheter was fitted to a pair of carefully matched pressure gauges so that a very accurate recording of the instantaneous pressure difference between two points some 4 to 5 cm. apart was continuously registered. This pressure difference was fed into an analogue computer continuously solving the simplified equation to provide a flow velocity waveform, basically similar in shape to those recorded by other techniques (i.e., Fig. 3–16), often with superimposed high frequency noise. Practical difficulties result in part from the fact that the pressure difference at two points 5 cm. apart in the aorta rarely exceeds 1 or 2 mm. Hg even at high flow rates. For example, a 1 per cent error in estimating one of the two pressures would produce an error in the range of 10 per cent error in estimating the pressure gradient. High frequency "noise" often appears as spikes on an otherwise smooth flow wave form. Other problems related to drift of the baseline of the pressure gauges can produce gross distortion of the computed flow contour. Designation of zero flow is a problem except at the aortic arch where it is assumed that flow is zero at the end of diastole. Despite these technical difficulties, the pressure-gradient technique merits serious consideration because it represents one of the few methods by which instantaneous flow velocity can be estimated in man.

Jones[58] has advocated a further simplification of the basic flow formulae by substituting the time derivative of pressure (dp/dt) at a single site rather than the pressure gradient (dp/dz) described previously. Although waveforms resembling directly recorded flow records can be obtained, the theoretical validity of the method remains questionable despite reports of reasonably high correlation coefficients in comparisons with results from Fick or dye dilution techniques.[59]

Cardiac Evaluation from Dynamic Performance. Patients with very severe heart disease may have perfectly normal cardiac output and stroke at rest. The comprehensive recording of many simultaneous variables during spontaneous and induced cardiovascular responses (see Fig. 3–14, 3–17, and 3–18) have demonstrated

that the most sensitive indicators of performance are the *rates* of change, including the rate of change of pressure (dp/dt), rate of ejection (outflow velocity) and rate of change of velocity (acceleration). During normal everyday stress, which provokes sympathetic discharge to the heart, the acceleration of outflow and the peak ejection velocity of both ventricles are accentuated. This is a primary mechanism for autonomic control of the heart. On the contrary, experimental procedures believed to depress ventricular function were also found to reduce peak ejection velocity and acceleration of the blood out of the ventricles. For example, experimental coronary occlusion was followed within 15 to 20 beats by increased heart rate and reduced peak flow velocity curve with more gradual upslope (Fig. 3–26). Similar changes were noted during experimental exsanguination severe enough to depress

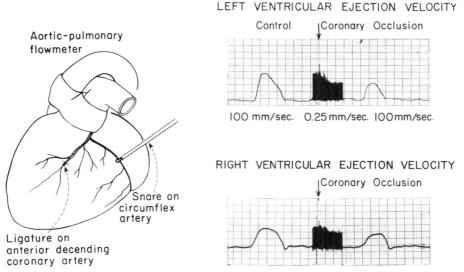

FIGURE 3–26   ACUTE CORONARY OCCLUSION

Acute ligation of the circumflex coronary artery by tightening a snare in a conscious dog with a previously ligated anterior descending coronary artery is promptly followed by a rapid reduction in the initial upslope in ejection velocity of both left and right ventricles. Peak outflow rate is depressed, and stroke volume is diminished. (From Rushmer.[60])

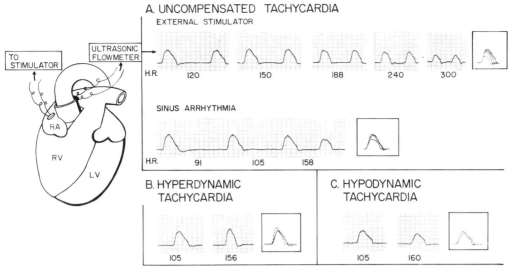

FIGURE 3–27   EJECTION VELOCITY AND ACCELERATION (SLOPE) WITH TACHYCARDIA

A, Increased heart rate, occurring spontaneously or from external stimulation, produces lower peak flow rates and smaller stroke volumes, but the initial upslope (maximal acceleration) is changed little or not at all.

B, Sympathetic stimulation produces increased acceleration, higher peak flow and shorter ejection.

C, Conditions depressing ventricular function characteristically produce marked reduction in maximal acceleration along with reduced peak flow and stroke volume. Such observations suggest that maximal acceleration may be a most valuable indicator of cardiac performance. (From Rushmer.[61])

the systemic arterial pressure. General anesthesia induced by pentobarbital or halothane produces corresponding effects.

If these experimental techniques are applicable to the appraisal of cardiac function in man, they require recording techniques which are sensitive to changes in dynamic events which transpire during the rapid acceleration of blood out of the ventricles at the onset of systole.[61] The rates of rise of ventricular and central aortic pressure are becoming widely recognized as important criteria of ventricular performance and capability. Acceleration of the blood out of the ventricles may prove to be an even better indicator of ventricular function. Changes in stroke volume and peak outflow rate can be observed during spontaneous and experimentally induced changes in heart rate (Fig. 3–27). When these waveforms are superimposed, the ini-

tial upslope appears to be unaffected. Stimulation of sympathetic nerves produces tachycardia accompanied by much higher peak outflow rate and steeper initial upslope on the flow records as indicated previously. In contrast, many conditions that depress ventricular performance, such as coronary obstruction (Fig. 3–26), produce tachycardia, lower peak outflow rate and more gradual upslope (diminished acceleration). These phenomena have also been observed by Noble, Trenchard and Guz,[62, 63] who concluded that maximum acceleration was closely associated with the maximum force in early systole and to the maximum initial velocity of shortening. They concur in the view that maximum acceleration is little affected by changes in posture or heart rate.[63] All these observations indicate the potential utility of directly measuring the dynamic properties of ventricular performance as criteria for evaluating the state of the ventricular myocardium. Information of potential value is embodied in several indicators employed in the past—the initial rate of rise of ventricular or central aortic pressure, the apex cardiogram and the ballistocardiogram. However, none of these has achieved general use for cardiac evaluation. The maximum acceleration of outflow from the ventricles may be the most important basis for cardiac evaluation proposed thus far.

Projections for the Future of Cardiac Evaluation

Outflow acceleration can be detected only by a flow sensing device. Among all the flow detectors presented in Figure 2–19, the techniques adaptable for use on man are the pressure gradient technique, the arterial pressure pulse analysis and the transcutaneous Doppler flow velocity sensor. In its simplest form, this device has provided useful clinical information regarding flow velocities in peripheral arteries. The newly developed pulse Doppler technique[64] permits sampling of flow velocity from a designated distance below the skin. This means that peak flow velocity and acceleration may well be sensed by a transducer positioned on the skin and receiving signals only from the axial stream in the aortic arch. If this prospect materializes, ventricular performance may be critically and objectively evaluated, without pain or hazard, directly through the skin of the thorax on normal subjects and patients alike.

SUMMARY

Cardiac output can be determined through the use of cardiac catheteriza-

tion according to the Fick principle. The theory is basically sound. The accuracy of the determinations depends upon the cumulative errors caused by deviations from the "steady state" conditions required for application of this theory. Very significant errors result whenever respiratory or circulatory conditions are inconstant.

The indicator-dilution technique is also basically sound for computing flow through simple tubular systems. In the circulatory system, application of the Stewart principle is complicated by problems related to recirculation of the indicator. With proper precautions, this technique affords values comparable to those derived from cardiac catheterization.

Theoretically, stroke volume can be determined from an analysis of the arterial pulse contour. However, many sources of error are present, including intangible factors such as differences in arterial distensibility among individuals. If the pulse contour method can be calibrated by the Fick principle in a particular subject, it becomes much more reliable. If the magnitude of the potential errors is recognized, the pulse contour method has considerable practical value since stroke volume of individual cycles can be estimated.

Ballistocardiography has been widely used to compute values presumed to represent stroke volume or cardiac output. Reliable recordings of body movements in response to ballistic forces during the cardiac cycle may be related to the rate or force of ventricular ejection, but even the basic principles of the method fail to reveal any direct relationship between the magnitude of the deflections and the volume of blood ejected. This fact does not preclude the establishment of empirical relations between specific ballistocardiographic patterns and certain forms of cardiovascular disease.

REFERENCES

1. BOZLER, E. The activity of the pacemaker previous to the discharge of a muscular impulse. *Amer. J. Physiol.*, 136:543–552, 1942.

2. WEST, T. C., FALK, G., and CERVONI, P. Drug alteration of transmembrane potentials in atrial pacemaker cells. *J. Pharmacol. Exp. Ther.*, 117:245–252, 1956.

3. HUNT, R. Direct and reflex acceleration of the mammalian heart with some observations on the relations of the inhibitory and accelerator nerves. *Amer. J. Physiol.*, 2:395–470, 1899.

4. ALEXANDER, R. S. Tonic and reflex functions of medullary sympathetic cardiovascular centers. *J. Neurophysiol.*, 9:205–217, 1946.

5. RANDALL, W. C., MCNALLY, H., COWAN, J., CALIGUIRI, L., and ROHSE, W. G. Functional analysis of the cardioaugmentor and cardioaccelerator pathways in the dog. *Amer. J. Physiol.*, 191:213–217, 1957.

6. RUSHMER, R. F. Autonomic balance in cardiac control. *Amer. J. Physiol.*, 192:631–634, 1958.

7. BRONK, D. W., PITTS, R. I., and LARRABEE, M. G. Role of hypothalamus in cardiovascular regulation. *Res. Publ. Ass. Res. Nerv. & Ment. Dis.*, 20:323–341, 1940.

8. STEVENSON, I. P., and DUNCAN, C. H. Alterations in cardiac function and circulatory efficiency during periods of life stress as shown by changes in the rate, rhythm, electrocardiographic pattern and output of the heart in those with cardiovascular disease. *Res. Publ. Ass. Res. Nerv. & Ment. Dis.*, 29:799–817, 1950.

9. HICKAM, J. B., CARGILL, W. H., and GOLDEN, A. Cardiovascular reactions to emotional stimuli; effect on the cardiac output, arteriovenous oxygen difference, arterial pressure, and peripheral resistance. *J. Clin. Invest.*, 27:290–298, 1948.

10. FEIL, H., GREEN, H. D., and EIBER, D. Voluntary acceleration of heart in a subject showing the Wolff-Parkinson-White syndrome. *Amer. Heart J.*, 34:334–348, 1947.

11. DOWLING, C. V., SMITH, W. W., BERGER, A. R., and ALBERT, R. E. The effect on blood pressure in the right heart, pulmonary artery and systemic artery of cardiac standstill produced by carotid sinus stimulation. *Circulation*, 5:742–746, 1952.

12. RUSHMER, R. F. Circulatory collapse following mechanical stimulation of arteries. *Amer. J. Physiol.*, 141:722–729, 1944.

13. LEWIS, T. Lecture on vasovagal syncope and carotid sinus mechanism with comments on Gowers' and Nothnagel's syndrome. *Brit. Med. J.*, 1:873–876, 1932.

14. BAZETT, H. C., and MCGLONE, B. Note on pain sensations which accompany deep punctures. *Brain*, 51:18–23, 1928.

15. DAVILA, J. C. Measurement of left ventricular volume; a symposium. *Amer. J. Cardiol.*, 18:1–47, 208–252, 566–593, 1966.

16. DODGE, H. T., SANDLER, H., BAXLEY, W. A., and HAWLEY, R. R. Usefulness and limitations of radiographic methods for determining left ventricular volume. *Amer. J. Cardiol.*, 18:10–24, 1966.

17. RAPAPORT, E. Usefulness and limitation of thermal washout technics in ventricular volume measurement. *Amer. J. Cardiol.*, 18:226–230, 1966.

18. RUSHMER, R. F., CRYSTAL, D. K., and WAGNER, C. The functional anatomy of ventricular contraction. *Circulat. Res.*, 1:162–170, 1953.

19. RUSHMER, R. F., FINLAYSON, B. L., and NASH, A. A. Shrinkage of the heart in anesthetized, thoracotomized dogs. *Circulat. Res.*, 2:22–27, 1954.

20. WILKIE, D. R. The mechanical properties of muscle. *Brit. Med. Bull.*, 12:177–182, 1956.

21. WIGGERS, C. J. Determinants of cardiac performance. *Circulation*, 4:485–495, 1951.

22. PATTERSON, S. W., PIPER, H., and STARLING, E. H. The regulation of the heart beat. *J. Physiol.*, 48:465–513, 1914.

23. STARLING, E. H. *Principles of Human Physiology*, 3rd ed. Philadelphia, Lea & Febiger, 1920, 315 pp.

24. LUNDIN, G. Mechanical properties of cardiac muscle. *Acta physiol. scand.*, 7 (Suppl. 20): 7–86, 1944.

25. HILL, A. V. The heat of shortening and the dynamic constants of muscle. *Proc. Roy. Soc.*, 126:136–195, 1938.

26. SONNENBLICK, E. H. Force-velocity relations in mammalian heart muscle. *Amer. J. Physiol.*, 202:931–939, 1962.

27. DOWNING, S. E., and SONNENBLICK, E. H. Cardiac muscle mechanics and ventricular performance; force and time parameters. *Amer. J. Physiol.*, 207:705–715, 1964.

28. FRY, D. L., GRIGGS, D. M., and GREENFIELD, F. C. Myocardial mechanics: tension-velocity-length relationships in heart muscle. *Circulat. Res.*, 14:73–85, 1964.

29. SHIPLEY, R. E., and GREGG, D. E. The cardiac response to stimulation of the stellate ganglion and cardiac nerves. *Amer. J. Physiol.*, 143:396–401, 1945.

30. KELSO, A. F., and RANDALL, W. C. Ventricular changes associated with sympathetic augmentation of cardiovascular pressure pulses. *Amer. J. Physiol.*, 196:731–734, 1959.

31. KJELLBERG, S. R., RUDHE, U., and SJÖSTRAND, T. The influence of the autonomic nervous system on the contraction of the human heart under normal circulatory conditions. *Acta physiol. scand.*, 24:350–360, 1952.

32. FULTON, J. F., RANSON, S. W., and FRANTZ, A. M. The hypothalamus and central levels of autonomic function. *Res. Publ. Ass. Nerv. & Ment. Dis.*, 20:1–980, 1940.

33. SMITH, O. A., JR., JABBUR, S. J., RUSHMER, R. F., and LASHER, E. P. Role of hypothalamic structures in cardiac control. *Physiol. Rev.*, 40 (Suppl. 4): 136–145, 1960.

34. SMITH, O. A., JR., RUSHMER, R. F., and LASHER, E. P. Similarity of cardiovascular responses to exercise and diencephalic stimulation. *Amer. J. Physiol.*, 198:1139–1142, 1960.

35. RUSHMER, R. F., and SMITH, O. A. Cardiac control. *Physiol. Rev.*, 39:41–68, 1959.

36. FORSSMANN, W. Probing of the right heart *Klin. Wschr.*, 8:2085–2087, 1929.

37. COURNAND, A., and RANGES, H. A. Catheterization of right auricle in man. *Proc. Soc. Exp. Biol. Med.*, 46:462–466, 1941.

38. COURNAND, A., RILEY, R. L., BREED, E. S., BALDWIN, DEF., and RICHARDS, D. W. Measurement of cardiac output in man using technique of catheterization of right auricle or ventricle. *J. Clin. Invest.*, 24:106–116, 1945.

39. COURNAND, A., BALDWIN, J. S., and HIMMELSTEIN, A. *Cardiac Catheterization in Congenital Heart Disease.* New York, The Commonwealth Fund, 1949.

40. WARREN, J. V. Determination of cardiac output in man by right heart catheterization. *Meth. Med. Res.*, 1:224–232, 1948.

41. VISSCHER, M. B., and JOHNSON, J. A. The Fick principle: analysis of potential errors in its conventional application. *J. Appl. Physiol.*, 5:635–638, 1953.

42. STOW, R. W. Systematic errors in flow determinations by the Fick method. *Minnesota Med.*, 37:30–35, 1954.

43. STEWART, G. N. Researches on the circulation time and on the influences which affect it. *J. Physiol.*, 22:159–183, 1897.

44. STEWART, G. N. The output of the heart in dogs. *Amer. J. Physiol.*, 57:27–50, 1921.

45. HAMILTON, W. F., and REMINGTON, J. W. Comparison of the time concentration curves in arterial blood of diffusible and nondiffusible substances when injected at a constant rate and when injected instantaneously. *Amer. J. Physiol.*, 148:35–39, 1948.

46. KINSMAN, J. M., MOORE, J. W., and HAMILTON, W. F. Studies on the circulation: injection method: physical and mathematical considerations. *Amer. J. Physiol.*, 89:321–330, 1929.

47. GORDON, J. W. On certain molar movements of the human body produced by the circulation of the blood. *J. Anat., Lond.*, 11:533–536, 1877.

48. HENDERSON, Y. The mass-movements of the circulation as shown by a recoil curve. *Amer. J. Physiol.*, 14:287–298, 1905.

49. STARR, I., RAWSON, A. J., SCHROEDER, H. A., and JOSEPH, N. R. Studies on the estimation of cardiac output in man, and of abnormalities in cardiac function, from the heart's recoil and the blood's impacts; the ballistocardiogram. *Amer. J. Physiol.*, 127:1–28, 1939.

50. STARR, I., and SCHROEDER, H. A. Ballistocardiogram. II. Normal standards, abnormalities commonly found in diseases of the heart and circulation, and their significance. *J. Clin. Invest.*, 19:437–450, 1940.

51. ERLANGER, J., and HOOKER, D. R. An experimental study of blood-pressure and of pulse-pressure in man. *Johns Hopk. Hosp. Rep.*, 12:145–378, 1904.

52. REMINGTON, J. W. The relation between the stroke volume and the pulse pressure. *Minnesota Med.*, 37:105–110, 1954.

53. HAMILTON, W. F., and REMINGTON, J. W. The measurement of the stroke volume from the pressure pulse. *Amer. J. Physiol.*, 148:14–24, 1947.

54. REMINGTON, J. W., HAMILTON, W. F., WHEELER, N. C., and HAMILTON, W. F., JR. Validity of pulse contour method for calculating cardiac output of the dog, with notes on effects of various anesthetics. *Amer. J. Physiol.*, 159:379–384, 1949.

55. WARNER, H. R. Quantitation of stroke volume changes in man from the central pressure pulse. *Minnesota Med.*, 37:111–115, 1954.

56. FRY, D. L. The measurement of pulsatile flow by the computed pressure gradient technique. *IRE Trans. Med. Electron.*, ME6:259–264, 1959.

57. GREENFIELD, J. C. Pressure gradient technique. Pp. 83–93 in *Methods of Medical Research*, Vol. 11, R. F. Rushmer, Ed. Chicago, Yearbook Medical Publishers, Inc., 1966.

58. JONES, W. B., HEFNER, L. L. BANCROFT, W. H., and KLIP, W. Velocity of blood flow and stroke volume obtained from the pressure pulse. *J. Clin. Invest.*, 38:2087–2090, 1959.

59. JONES, W. B., RUSSELL, R. O., and DALTON, D. H. An evaluation of computed stroke volume in man. *Amer. Heart. J.*, 72:746–750, 1966.

60. RUSHMER, R. F. Initial ventricular impulse; a potential key to cardiac evaluation. *Circulation*, 29:268–283, 1964.

61. RUSHMER, R. F. Recent advances in cardiovascular physiology. *Anesthesia and Analgesia*, 45:383–389, 1966.

62. NOBLE, M. I. M., TRENCHARD, D., and GUZ, A. Left ventricular ejection in conscious dogs; measurement and significance of the maximum acceleration of blood from the left ventricle. *Circulat. Res.*, 19:139–147, 1966.

63. NOBLE, M. I. M., TRENCHARD, D., and GUZ, A. Effect of changing heart rate on cardiovascular function in the conscious dog. *Circulat. Res.*, 19:206–213, 1966.

64. RUSHMER, R. F., BAKER, D. W., and STEGALL, H. F. Transcutaneous Doppler flow detection as a nondestructive technique. *J. Appl. Physiol.*, 21:554–566, 1966.

CHAPTER 4

PERIPHERAL VASCULAR CONTROL

The human body is composed of billions of cells, variously specialized, grouped and organized to perform many different functions. They can survive and function only so long as their immediate environment contains an adequate supply of essential nutrient materials and a limited concentration of waste products.

The capillaries permeate every tissue of the body, and the blood is rarely more than 0.1 mm. from any cell. The capillaries are only about 0.017 mm. in diameter, but their total length is almost 60,000 miles.[1] Thus the blood and tissue fluids are exposed to a tremendous expanse of capillary surface through which materials may be exchanged. Cells which consume essential materials rapidly must either be situated near capillaries or operate effectively at low concentrations of the various vital materials.

The Circulations of the Body. Blood flows through the systemic and pulmonary circulations of the body, impelled by the pumping action of the heart in an amount of about 5000 cc./min. in an average man at rest. (Cardiac output in Figure 4-1). This is not the only circulation involved in the delivery of oxygen and nutrients to the body cells. Filtration through the capillary walls occurs at rates ranging around 14 cc./min. of which about 11 cc./min. is resorbed back into the venous capillary blood in accordance with the Starling Hypothesis (see Chapter 1). The unresorbed fluid (about 3 cc./min.) is transported by the lymphatic system and restored to blood in the systemic veins near the heart. The process of diffusion is far more important to the circulatory process than the bulk filtration process as illustrated in Figure 4-1. For example, the exchange of water by diffusion back and forth across the capillary membrane actually exceeds the cardiac output. It amounts to more than 5000 cc./min., but how much more no one is certain. Similarly, the transfer of electrolytes, small organic molecules and gases occurs rapidly and in large quantity over the very small distances across endothelial barriers and between tissue cells (see Fig. 1-2A).

In tissues with very great or variable metabolic demands, the capillaries are arranged in close proximity to every tissue cell. For example, the number of capillaries in skeletal muscle is reported to be related to the

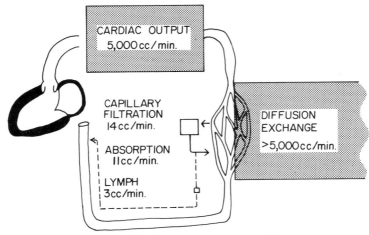

FIGURE 4-1   CIRCULATIONS IN THE BODY

The blood circulation delivers nutrients to the vicinity of the body cells in the microcirculation where local circulation involves filtration-reabsorption through capillary walls with lymphatic return of the residue and a very large exchange of water by diffusion.

oxidative activity of the individual fibers,[2] but only a fraction of the available capillaries in the myocardium is perfused at rest.[3] The high metabolic rate of tissues in small animals requires a higher rate of oxygen delivery than in larger animals; this rate of oxygen delivery accomplished by both a higher capillary density and higher unloading tension for oxygen in small animals.[4]

Oxygen Diffusion in Tissues. Each capillary subserves a volume of tissue immediately surrounding it since oxygen and other nutrient materials have highest concentration in blood and move outward along concentration gradients. Adjacent parallel capillaries (e.g., in striated muscle) supply cylindrical volumes of tissue around each capillary (Fig. 4-2A). As oxygen moves outward from the capillaries, the gas tension in the blood diminishes in the capillary blood flowing toward the venules, diminishing the unloading tension along the capillary. Theoretically the lowest oxygen tension in the vicinity of a particular cylinder occurs at the periphery of the cylinder near the venule, sometimes called the "lethal corner" (Fig. 4-2A). Two adjoining tissue cylinders (e.g., in the brain) are illustrated with corresponding oxygen tension values in the capillaries and tissues shown in relief below (Fig. 4-2B). The oxygen partial pressure decreases from the arterial to the venous end of the cylinder and from the center to the periphery so that at the "lethal corner" the tension in the tissue is only about 17 mm. Hg or even somewhat less.[5] In exercising muscle and myocardium, the oxygen tension at its lower point apparently approaches the vanishing point since the venous oxygen tension is very low (see Figure 4-3). The consequences of diminished blood oxygen are illustrated in Figure 4-2C. Three levels may be distinguished below the normal. Reaction threshold occurs when vasodilation results from lowered venous oxygen pressures of 25 to 28 mm. Hg, and a "lethal level" is illustrated at 12 mm. Hg since the oxygen tension drops to 0 (Fig. 4-2C).

Thus, tissues with high metabolic rates (brain, muscle, kidney, and so forth) characteristically have dense capillary networks through which blood flows rapidly. By this mechanism, high concentrations of essential substances are maintained near the capillary walls, providing steep gradients for diffusion. Cells with lower requirements lie farther from the capillaries and are less affected by cessation of blood flow (Fig. 4-3A). Elimination of waste products proceeds in the reverse direction propelled by diffusion gradients with maximum concentrations at the site of production in the cells.

The delivery of substances to the tissues thus involves two steps: transportation by the blood to the capillary beds and local delivery by diffusion. The efficiency of the circulatory apparatus depends upon the success with which it provides adequate diffusion gradients within the tissues.

If, for example, the metabolic activity of skeletal muscle suddenly increased without a change in blood flow, the concentration of oxygen in and around the cells would drop, the diffusion gradient would steepen, the rate of diffusion would accelerate and the arteriovenous oxygen difference would widen (Fig. 4-3B). On the other hand, if an increased blood flow completely compensated for the increased oxygen utilization, oxygen delivery would be increased without a change in the arteriovenous oxygen difference and with little drop in tissue oxygen tension. Circulatory adjustment to the varying metabolic demands of skeletal muscle is never adequate to prevent a reduction in the oxygen content of venous blood, i.e., an increase in the arteriovenous difference.

Influenced by common personal experience, we are inclined to view peripheral vascular control primarily in terms of delivery of oxygen to the tissues, as is implied by Figure 4-3. When the circulation is restored after occluding the arterial supply to the arm or leg for a few minutes, the flushing of the skin, the throbbing of the limb and the return of the power of contraction all attest to the essential role of the blood supply in the function of muscles and skin.

Functional Anatomy of Peripheral Vascular Control. Zweifach[6] has described two distinct types of capillaries: arteriovenous capillaries and "true" capillaries. The A-V capillaries are "thoroughfare" channels with fairly direct courses from the arterioles to the venules. In general, blood flows continuously through the A-V capillaries, the rate of flow being varied through the changes in the caliber of the muscular arterioles and of the A-V capillaries themselves. A-V capillaries are invested with smooth muscle, which is abundant at the arteriolar end and more diffusely distributed toward the venular regions (Fig. 4-4). Branching from the A-V capillaries are the "true" capillaries, which are intricately joined to form complex networks lying between adjacent thoroughfare channels. The "true" capillaries have no smooth muscle except for muscular cuffs (precapillary sphincters) at their points of origin from the A-V capillaries. Capillaries from the vascular network rejoin the A-V capillaries near the venular end, but there are no smooth muscle sphincters at these junctions. If all the precapillary sphincters serving a capillary bed closed simultaneously, blood would not flow through these channels. However, at any one instant, some precapillary sphincters are open and others are closed. At intervals of one-half to three minutes some sphincters

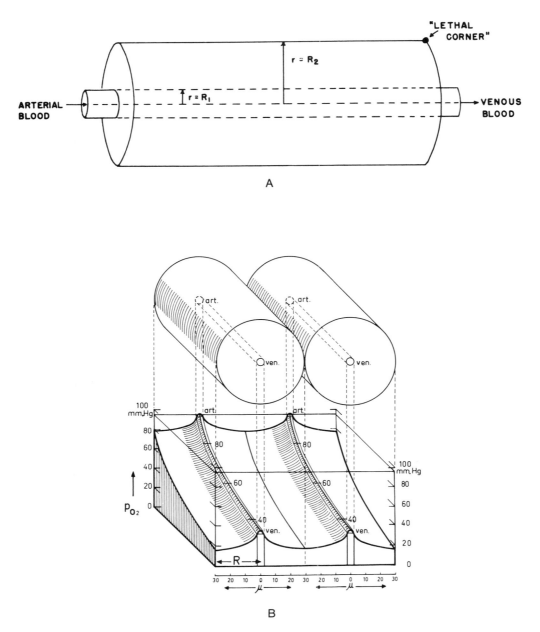

FIGURE 4-2   CONCENTRATION GRADIENTS NEAR CAPILLARIES

A, Each capillary delivers oxygen to a roughly cyclindrical volume of surrounding space by means of diffusion along concentration gradients.

B, The concentrations of oxygen along two parallel capillaries are displayed in three dimensions to show the progressive reduction in oxygen pressure during flow from arteriole to venule and at the periphery of the cyclindrical zones. (From Thews.[5])

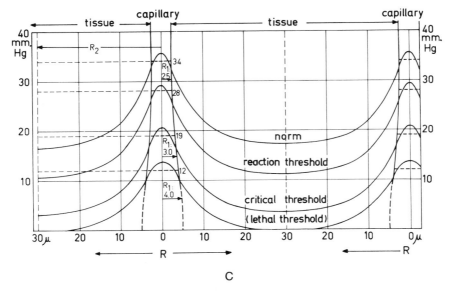

C

FIGURE 4-2 *Continued.*

C, The concentration of oxygen around capillaries under conditions of progressively greater hypoxia (see text). (From Thews.[5])

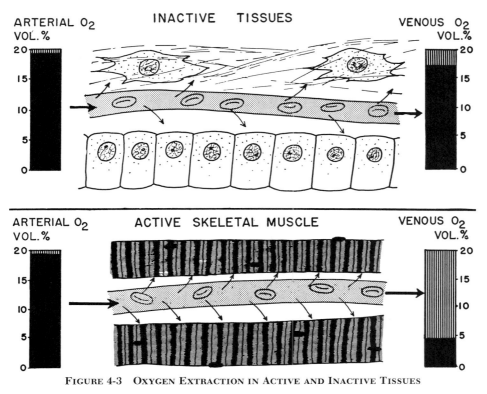

FIGURE 4-3   OXYGEN EXTRACTION IN ACTIVE AND INACTIVE TISSUES

The quantity of oxygen extracted from the blood during its flow through capillaries is determined by the relationship between the rate of oxygen utilization and the blood flow.

A, Slight oxygen extraction and small arteriovenous oxygen differences occur in tissues with relatively small oxygen requirements and active blood flow, e.g., skin.

B, Tissues which release energy at rapid rates, e.g., contracting muscle, extract a major portion of the oxygen from the blood.

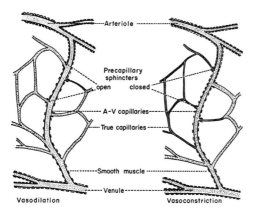

FIGURE 4-4   VASOMOTION IN A CAPILLARY NETWORK

Capillary networks, in some tissues at least, consist of arteriovenous capillaries (thoroughfare channels) and "true" capillaries. The blood flow through the different portions of the capillary bed is affected by contraction and relaxation of smooth muscle in the arterioles, A-V capillaries and precapillary sphincters. Phasic changes in the caliber in these regions produce cyclic alterations in the amount and distribution of blood flow through the various true capillaries (vasomotion).

close and others open. The caliber of the A-V channels also fluctuates asynchronously.

Dilatation and constriction of the A-V capillaries and the different combinations of dilated precapillary sphincters produce a continuously changing pattern of flow through the capillary networks. In a particular segment of the capillary bed, the blood may flow rapidly through one channel for a period of time, then cease to flow or even flow in the opposite direction, depending on which sphincters are open. The phasic changes in the caliber of the arterioles, A-V capillaries and precapillary sphincters have been termed "vasomotion" (Fig. 4-4). The rate of blood flow through the individual channels is an expression of a gradient in capillary pressure. Blood flow is rapid when capillary pressure in the arteriolar end of an A-V capillary is high in relation to venular pressure. When flow ceases, the pressure throughout the capillary approximates that in the venules.

The functional significance of vasomotion is being intensively investigated. It is apparent that this aspect of vascular control has important implications for normal function. For example, phasic vasomotor activity is expressed in periodic changes in the volume of the finger and in fluctuations in the arterial blood pressure. The existence of vasomotion implies a more precise regulation of capillary blood flow in response to local tissue demands than could result if control were exerted only by the arterioles. At the same time, descriptions of capillary blood pressure become more complicated because the pressure levels and gradients are continuously changing. However, certain generalizations can be made. If the pressure in the venules remains constant, vasomotion would affect only the pressure

gradients from arterioles to venules. When the arterioles, A-V capillaries and precapillary sphincters are dilated, the pressure gradients along the channels are steep and blood flow is rapid. When the caliber of these channels is reduced by constriction, more potential energy is lost as friction before the blood reaches the capillaries. The pressure at the arteriolar end of the capillaries is thus lowered, the pressure gradients become shallow or are eliminated and blood flow diminishes or ceases. Total blood flow through a tissue is increased by prolonging the intervals of vasodilatation and reducing the periods of vasoconstriction. The organization of capillaries illustrated in Figure 4-4 is believed to occur in those tissues which have widely varying levels of activity. Vasomotion, as a characteristic pattern of peripheral circulatory control, has been observed in a number of tissues, including rat mesentery, bat wing, subcutaneous connective tissues and canine and human hearts.

Capillary Morphology in Various Tissues. The functional requirements and environmental conditions of capillaries are not the same in different tissues. Contracting skeletal muscles, as compared to connective tissues or glands, have grossly different requirements for blood flow through their capillary networks (see Fig. 4-3). Similar diversity is readily demonstrated in the structural relationships of the capillary tubes as well. The capillaries in skeletal muscle, myocardium and skin consist of endothelial cells joined firmly at their edges with no evidence of pores or fenestrations (Fig. 4-5A, B). Pericapillary cells enclose the capillary but the investment seems incomplete, and perivascular spaces are not generally observed in fixed specimens on either light or electron microscopy.

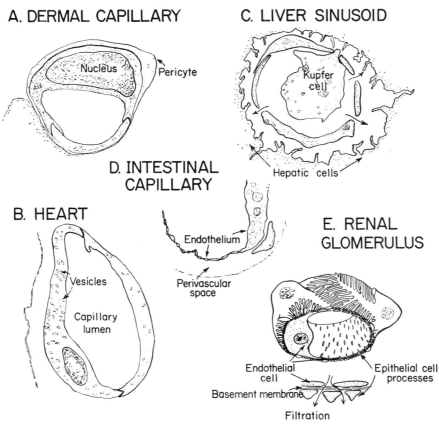

FIGURE 4-5   VARIATIONS IN CAPILLARY STRUCTURE

Schematic diagrams of electron micrographs indicate the extent to which capillaries display different characteristics in various tissues.

A, Dermal capillaries appear to be formed by endothelial cells joined at their edges without visible spaces between. Such capillaries may be enveloped by pericytes.

B, Capillaries in the heart also consist of continuous membranes of endothelial cells. Capillary endothelial cells characteristically contain large numbers of vesicles which have been implicated by some investigators in active transport of substances across the capillary membrane (Bennett et al.[8]).

C, Liver sinusoids are discontinuous membranes with large spaces between cells through which cellular elements can pass freely.

D, Intestinal capillaries may exhibit very thin regions in endothelial cells which may not be a continuous barrier between the capillary lumen and perivascular space (after Bennett et al.[8]).

E, The renal glomerulus is a complex structure composed of endothelial cells, basement membrane and epithelial cells through which filtration occurs (after Yamada[7]).

Openings or fenestrations between the processes of endothelial cells are found in several tissues such as liver sinusoids (Figs. 4-5C) or intestinal capillaries (Fig. 4-5D). The capillaries in the renal glomerulus are extremely complex as illustrated in a composite drawing by Yamada.[7] Bennett, Luft and Hampton[8] proposed a rather complicated classification of various types of capillaries based on the basement membranes, porosity or perforations and pericapillary investment:

Type:

A With complete continuous basement membrane

B Without complete continuous basement membrane

1 Without fenestrations or pores

2 With *intra*cellular fenestrations or perforations

3 With *inter*cellular fenestrations or perforations

α Without a complete pericapillary cellular investment interposed between parenchymal cells and the capillary

β With a complete capillary cellular investment interposed between parenchymal cells and capillary

Majno[9] presented a comprehensive description of the ultrastructure of capillaries, including a pictorial classification based on the continuity of the main filtration barrier: the endothelial sheet (Fig. 4-6). On this basis three main types are designated: continuous, fenestrated and discontinuous. For each of these categories, the endothelial cells may be high or low (thin). The low variety of continuous endo-

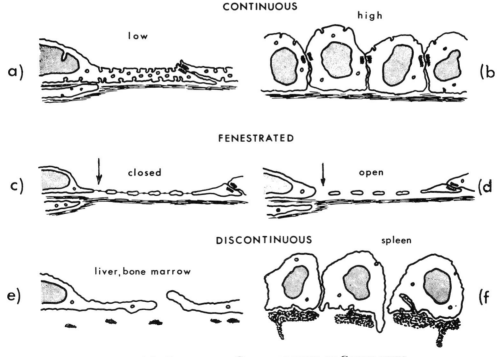

FIGURE 4-6 FUNCTIONAL CLASSIFICATION OF CAPILLARIES

The capillaries in various tissues have widely different architecture which can be distinguished in terms of the degree and type of fenestration in the endothelial cells and the height or thickness of the endothelial cells. (From Majno, G.[9]).

thelium (Fig. 4-6A) is found in striated muscle, myocardium, central nervous system, smooth muscle of digestive and reproductive systems and subcutaneous and adipose tissues.

Postcapillary venules of lymph nodes and thymus had high endothelial cells (Fig. 4-6B). Endothelial cells with intracellular fenestrae may be closed in endocrine glands, choroid plexus, ciliary body and intestinal villi (Fig. 4-6C). In the renal glomeruli, the fenestrae appear to be open (Fig. 4-6D). Sinusoids of liver, bone marrow and spleen have gross intercellular gaps as shown in Figures 4-6E and F. Clearly, the barrier to bulk flow, filtration and diffusion offered by endothelial cells must be very different in capillaries as varied in structure as those illustrated in Figures 4-5 and 4-6. The differences in function of various tissues and organs are also clearly represented by differences in blood flow and oxygen extraction.

NORMAL OXYGEN DISTRIBUTION

In most tissues other than skeletal muscles and myocardium, adjustments of blood flow in relation to oxygen consumption or metabolic activity would be inappropriate. For example, the oxygen consumption in skin is quite trivial and yet extremely large amounts of blood may flow through this organ to support its function of dissipating heat. Similarly, the amount of blood flowing through the kidney is very large in relation to its metabolic activity. Thus, only a small fraction of the oxygen presented to the kidney substance is taken up and the blood leaving the kidney does not differ greatly from arterial blood.

To illustrate these points, the quantity of blood flowing each minute

through several organs is plotted on the abscissa in Figure 4-7. The quantity of oxygen presented to the tissues in the arterial blood was 19 cc. per 100 cc. of blood (ordinate in Fig. 4-7). Thus, the area of each rectangular figure represents the quantity of oxygen presented to each organ each minute. The stippled area represents the quantity of oxygen in the venous blood leaving the organ, and the remaining area (vertical lines) indicates the amount of oxygen extracted by the tissue. Note the very small quantity of oxygen extracted from blood in the kidney. Myocardium extracts about 70 per cent or more of the oxygen presented to it. Resting skeletal muscle utilizes only about one third of the oxygen in the blood it receives, but contracting skeletal muscle extracts about three fourths of the oxygen from the blood. Thus, the difference between the oxygen contents of arterial and venous blood (A-V oxygen difference) varies widely from tissue to tissue. The average A-V oxygen difference at rest, based on mixed venous blood, ranges around 4 to 6 cc. per 100 cc. of blood.

RESISTANCE TO BLOOD FLOW

The blood pumped by the heart is distributed to the various tissues according to their functions. The rate at which the blood flows through the vascular channels is dependent upon the energy lost in the form of friction. Little pressure energy is dissipated in the long arterial conduits (Fig. 1-7), but the pressure gradient becomes steeper as the blood flows through the smaller and smaller branches toward the periphery. Thus, a substantial fraction of the pressure head available in the aorta is dissipated as the blood flows through the terminal arteries, arterioles and capillaries. The amount of pressure dissipated is regulated by

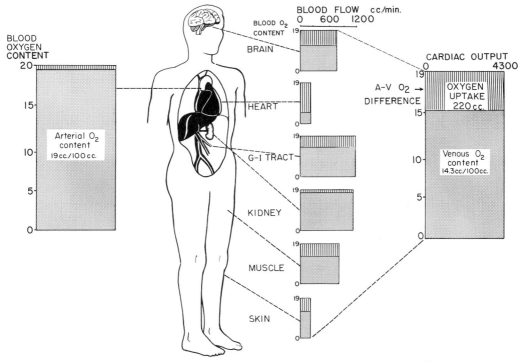

FIGURE 4-7   THE ARTERIOVENOUS OXYGEN DIFFERENCES IN VARIOUS TISSUES

The blood flow through some tissues is voluminous in relation to the oxygen requirements (kidney and skin). In contrast, the myocardium extracts most of the oxygen from the blood. The arteriovenous oxygen differences represent the relationship between blood flow and oxygen utilization in various tissues.

variations in the caliber of the vascular channels. The extent to which the vessels change their diameters for this type of regulation becomes progressively greater and more significant toward the peripheral ramifications of the arterial tree. The wall of the aorta contains a substantial quantity of elastic tissue (about 40 per cent by weight). The proportion of elastic tissue diminishes and the proportion of smooth muscle is greater in the more peripheral arterial branches (Fig. 4-8).

The pressure within the lumen of the blood vessels must be supported by tension in their walls in accordance with the law of Laplace $(P = T/r)$; so that the greater the radius of the tube,

the greater the wall tension required to support a given internal pressure (see Fig. 1-11). The tension supported by various components of the vascular wall has been analyzed by Burton.[10] The tensile strength of the elastic tissue in the aorta is capable of supporting three times the normal aortic pressure, providing a good margin of safety. The force required to break the collagenous tissue in the aorta is so great that in most experiments the clamps holding the tissue slip before breakage occurs. The caliber of the vascular channels is adjusted by changing tension exerted by smooth muscle (see Fig. 4-8), which can maintain tension for a long time with a very small expenditure of energy.[10]

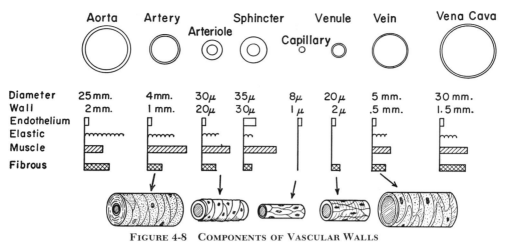

FIGURE 4-8 COMPONENTS OF VASCULAR WALLS

The relative amount of elastic tissue and fibrous tissues is largest in the aorta and least in small branches of the arterial tree. Smaller vessels have more prominent smooth muscle in the media. Capillaries consist only of endothelial tubes. The walls of the veins are much like the arterial walls but are thinner in relation to their caliber.

Critical Closing Pressure. By virtue of Laplace's law, active tension exerted by smooth muscle in the wall of a cylindrical tube may produce a fundamental instability. Suppose that when the wall tension is precisely balanced against the pressure in a blood vessel ($P = T/r$) the tension exerted by the smooth muscle is slightly increased. The radius of the vessel decreases slightly, and the tension required to maintain the pressure is further reduced so that the radius continues to shrink. If this occurred, the caliber would progressively diminish until the lumen of the vessel closed. Thus, if smooth muscle predominates in the wall, as in arterioles, precapillary sphincters and arteriovenous shunts, the vessels would tend to be either fully open or fully closed. Burton proposed the concept of a *critical closing pressure* at which the lumina of such small vessels would close because the wall tension was being supported predominantly by smooth muscle. According to this con-

cept, the sites of controlled resistance in the terminal vascular networks should be either wide open or closed. Microscopic examination fails to confirm this prediction completely since graded variations in the caliber of vessels and sphincters can be observed. However, the control of capillary flow distribution clearly involves changing patterns of closure of the vascular sphincters.

The concept of critical closing pressure neglects the influence of the thickness of the vascular walls. In vessels with walls which are thick in relation to the radius, $P = T\delta/r$, where P is the pressure, T is the tension in the wall, δ is the thickness of the wall and r is the radius of the tube. With constriction of the vessel, the wall becomes thicker. Internal stresses develop in the wall as the lumen is progressively constricted until extremely great tension must be developed to obliterate the lumen completely.

Mechanisms of Vascular Constriction. The lumina of larger arteries can be reduced but are not completely obliterated by contraction of the smooth muscle in the walls. Reduction in the caliber of such arteries involves severe deformation of the smooth muscle cells, the internal elastic membrane and the endothelial cells. The forces required to completely occlude the lumen can be simulated by encircling a piece of gum rubber tubing with a strong ligature or string and pulling on its two ends in an attempt to close the lumen. The smallest terminal arteries, arterioles and precapillary sphincters can be completely constricted by contraction of the layers of smooth muscle. In the transition from the normal dilated state to maximal constriction, the wall components of small arteries and arterioles are greatly distorted. Van Citters et al.[11] studied serial histological sections of mesenteric arteries (about 1 mm. O.D.) in which a localized constriction was produced by local application of a drop of epinephrin. Quick freezing preserved the normal relationships disclosing a wall thickness only about 1/30 of the radius in the normal dilated state (Fig. 4-9). Sections obtained in the maximally constricted regions showed the lumen reduced to about 25 per cent of the total diameter, with a wall-to-lumen ratio of about 1:2. The endothelial cells were rounded and perched on the folds of a highly convoluted internal elastic membrane. The smooth muscle cells were severely distorted and the nuclei rounded. Similar histological changes were subsequently reported by Hayes.[12] Measurements of various components of the walls in contracted small arteries and arterioles were examined as potential objective criteria for the degree of vasoconstriction by Stromberg et al.[13]

Complete occlusion of the lumen of small arteries was not observed in the studies just described. In contrast, the terminal branches or arterioles may become completely obstructed by smooth muscle contraction and deformation of the rounded endothelial cells[14] which serve as a plastic plug as illustrated by three examples on the right of Figure 4-9.

BASIC REQUIREMENTS FOR CARDIOVASCULAR CONTROL

The tissues and organs served by the vascular system have widely varying functions and ranges of activity. If the changing requirements of tissues for blood flow had no priority or coordinating mechanism, the circulatory responses might easily become chaotic and break down, e.g., during running on a hot day after a full meal. At the risk of oversimplification, the fundamental requirements for cardiovascular regulation can be described in terms of uncomplicated hydraulic systems.

A common form of such systems consists of a large tank supported at sufficient height to give a head of pressure. In such a system, the pump can be set to operate at constant speed, variations in demand being accommodated at the expense of the reserve volume in the tank. However, this type of system could not easily be adapted to man or animals because a large quantity of blood would have to be carried around above the head. Portability can be achieved only if the capacious storage tank is replaced by a small pressure tank. In this case, however, an increase in outflow from the system must be rapidly and precisely compensated by adjusting the output of the pump.

Consider a model circulation consisting of a pump, a compression chamber and several variable orifices (Fig. 4-10). By adjustments in stroke vol-

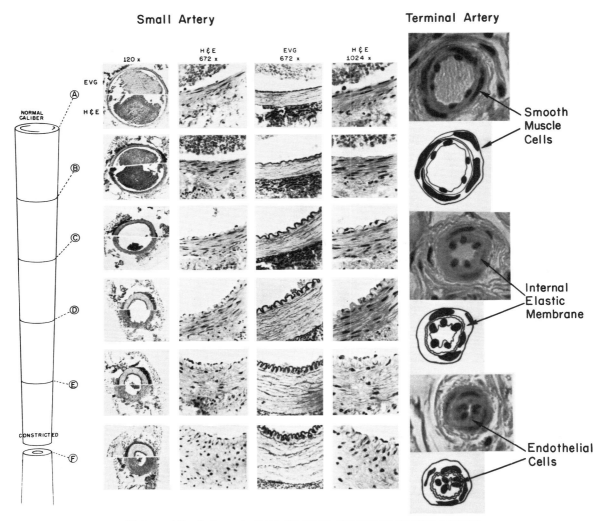

FIGURE 4-9   ARCHITECTURAL CHANGES DURING VASOCONSTRICTION

Left, The wall of a small artery (about 1 mm. outside diameter) is very thin in the dilated state (upper figure) and the components are stretched out circumferentially. As the artery constricts, the wall thickens and the components become rounded and deformed. Such vessels do not become occluded at maximal constriction. (From Van Citters, Wagner and Rushmer.[11])

Right, Terminal branches may become occluded by the endothelial cells, which have become rounded, tending to serve as a plastic plug. (From Ruch and Patton, *Physiology and Biophysics,* 19th Ed., W. B. Saunders Co., 1965.)

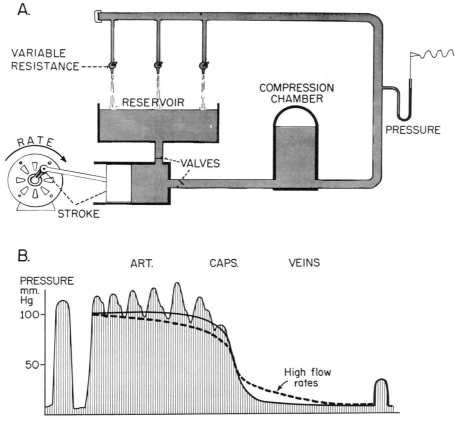

FIGURE 4-10   PRESSURE GRADIENTS

A, The principles of cardiovascular control can be illustrated by a simple hydraulic model. In this system, the pressure head is determined primarily by the relation between the resistance to outflow and the pump output (stroke volume × heart rate). To maintain the pressure at a constant level, any change in outflow resistance must be promptly compensated by an adjustment in the pump output. The pressure head, outflow resistance and pump output are so intimately related that none can be altered without effect on the others.

B, The pressure gradient along the arteries and veins is very shallow under resting conditions. However, if the blood flow is greatly acelerated, the pressure gradient in the terminal arteries and veins becomes steeper, diminishing the pressure gradient along the small vessels (arterioles, capillaries and venules). The magnitude of the change is exaggerated in the figure.

ume, stroke frequency and total outflow resistance, the mean pressure in the system can be maintained at constant levels for indefinite periods of time. If the stroke frequency and outflow resistance are properly set, the pressure in the system never drops to zero between strokes. Once such an equilibrium is established, alterations in any one of the three variables will

be immediately reflected in changes in pressure within the system. To maintain a constant pressure, any alteration in one variable must be simultaneously balanced by adjustments in the others so that inflow always equals outflow. For example, if the stroke frequency is increased and the outflow resistance is not changed, the stroke volume must be reduced until pump output is restored to previous levels. Similarly, opening one outflow orifice more widely would produce a fall in pressure unless the resistance to outflow from other valves was increased or the pump output was rapidly augmented by an increase in either stroke volume or stroke frequency. In this system, maintenance of a constant mean pressure automatically provides a precise balance between inflow and outflow. This schematic model illustrates the fundamental principle by which the cardiac output is continuously adjusted to compensate for changes in peripheral resistance. The mean arterial blood pressure tends to stay within a relatively narrow range both at rest and during activity. To the extent that the requirements of the tissues for blood flow are reflected by their changes in peripheral resistance, cardiac output is continuously adjusted to equal the total blood flow in all the tissues.

The quantity of blood flowing through a set of vessels per unit of time is determined by two factors: (1) the pressure gradient from the arteries to the veins and (2) the resistance of the vascular bed as influenced by constriction in the smaller and terminal branches. The mechanisms by which the systemic arterial blood pressure is maintained within a reasonable range despite wide fluctuations in the distribution and total quantity of blood flowing through the peripheral tissues are described in Chapter 5. In the following discussion of the mechanisms of vascular control, the arterial pressure head will be considered to be relatively fixed.

Pressure Gradients at High Flow Rates. Despite the gradual reduction in the caliber of the long arterial trunks, the pressure drop along them is very slight (2 to 4 mm. Hg from the axillary to the radial arteries) at rest in a cool environment. As a result, flow along the arteries is normally slow (Fig. 4-10B). However, peripheral vasodilation in the extremities of man during reactive hyperemia may accelerate the flow rates as much as ten times. Under such conditions, the pressure drop between the brachial and radial arteries increases from 5 mm. Hg to 25 mm. Hg.[15] The rate of pressure drop along the terminal branches of the arterial system also steepens so that the pressure at the arterioles is markedly depressed. The increased pressure required to propel the increased flow along the veins also results in a high pressure head at the venules because central venous pressure cannot be greatly depressed. Thus, in the presence of high flow rates through a segment of the vascular tree, the arterial and venous pressure gradients are steepened and the pressure drop across the arterioles and capillary networks is reduced far below the normal resting conditions. Under these conditions, the resistance to flow through the larger arterial and venous conduits assumes major importance in the dissipation of pressure energy during flow.

MECHANISMS OF VASCULAR REGULATION

The quantity of blood flowing through various vascular beds and its distribution among the myriad vascular channels depend primarily upon smooth muscle contraction at the sites of controlled resistance. Histologic examination of vascular smooth muscle fails to reveal structural differences from one vessel to another. Yet the functional disparity between the vessels of different organs is so great that a single substance may produce constriction in one organ and dilation in another.

The Role of the Nervous System.
In a hydraulic system like that in
Figure 4-10 there must be sensitive
and responsive controls to quickly
adapt to abrupt changes in levels of
activity of the various tissues without
precipitous or soaring changes in arterial blood pressure. The involve-
ment of the nervous system in such
control is a matter of everyday experience. Individuals with impairment of
the sympathetic nervous system are
subject to fainting merely on assuming
the erect position. Obvious flushing or
pallor of the skin can develop rapidly
in response to emotions (embarrassment or fear) as well as by changes in
environmental temperature. The functional role of neural control of the vascular system is to adjust the cardiac
output and the distribution of this total
flow to meet the varying needs of
tissues, maintain systemic arterial
pressure and still preserve the essential functions of the heart, brain and
other vital tissues. The specifications
for such a system have been presented
in an engaging and imaginative summary by Burton.[16] To preserve the vital
functions, the neural controls are generally powerful enough to override
hormonal mechanisms.[17] These vascular adjustments are effected involun-
tarily by the sympathetic nervous system. Contrary to previous concepts,
the sympathetic nervous system rarely
discharges en masse but rather displays well developed functional differentiation.[18] The discharge of sympathetic nerves to blood vessels of skin,
kidney or viscera is a constantly changing pattern accompanying changes in
type and level of functional activity.
Renkin and Rosell[19] present evidence
supporting the view that arterioles and
precapillary sphincters are controlled
separately, contributing to the shifting
patterns of flow in capillary networks
like those illustrated in Figure 4-4.

According to Lutz and Fulton,[20]
however, some vascular smooth muscle has dual innervation (constrictor
and dilator), only vasoconstrictor or
vasodilator nerves serve some vascular smooth muscle and a third class
of muscle cells apparently does not receive any innervation. Vascular
smooth muscle without a nerve supply
reacts to both epinephrine and acetylcholine (the transmitter substances for
the sympathetic and parasympathetic
nervous systems, respectively), and
vessels highly sensitive to acetylcholine may have no demonstrable
cholinergic innervation. Some vascular beds respond to changes in the
carbon dioxide tension in arterial
blood; others dilate in response to
unidentified metabolites. Thus, concise descriptions of peripheral vascular
control are impossible because the system is very complex and because not
nearly enough is known about it. For
the present discussion, some of the
more important controls will be considered in terms of neural, hormonal,
chemical and physical mechanisms.
Then, the factors which appear to be
prominent in the control of certain
key organs will be discussed.

Sympathetic Vasomotor System.
Neural control over the peripheral vascular system is dominated by the sympathetic division of the autonomic
nervous system. Nerve cell bodies
lying in the intermediolateral cell
column of the thoracic division of the
spinal cord give off axons that pass out
the ventral root and synapse either in
the ganglia of the sympathetic chain or
in accessory ganglia. The postgan-
glionic axons follow the segmental
nerves to the peripheral vessels or
pass directly to perivascular plexuses
through which the fibers pass to the
periphery. The terminal branches of
the sympathetic constrictor fibers pass
to vascular smooth muscle and appar-

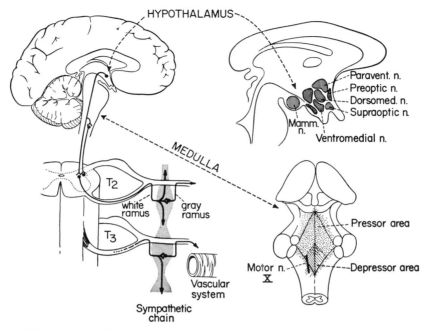

FIGURE 4-11   CENTRAL CONTROL OF SYMPATHETIC VASOCONSTRICTION

Sympathetic constrictor nerves, distributed to peripheral vascular system, originate from the intermediolateral cell column of the thoracic cord. Impulses descend from the medullary region and the hypothalamus to modulate the sympathetic nerve discharge. The hypothalamus plays an important role in autonomic control of many different visceral functions. Changes in systemic arterial pressure can be readily produced by stimulation of the "pressor" and "depressor" areas in the medulla. However, these medullary areas may actually represent pathways from higher levels down to the spinal cord, rather than "vasomotor centers."

ently release transmitter substances which induce contraction or relaxation of the smooth muscle components in the walls.

The collections of nerve cell bodies in the intermediolateral column serve as spinal vasomotor centers, receiving impulses over afferent fibers entering the spinal cord from various structures and also receiving regulatory impulses descending from higher neural structures (Fig. 4-11). Immediately after cervical spinal section in man the blood pressure tends to be poorly sustained.[21] Since the spinal lesion has interrupted descending pathways but has neither injured the cells at the thoracic level nor interfered with their afferent input, this

condition indicates that volleys of impulses descending the spinal cord normally modulate the discharges of the spinal vasomotor centers. Sometime later such patients regain vascular reactivity. This reactivity is a function of the spinal centers and is reflex in nature. For example, when the spinal cord is bombarded by impulses aroused by experimental distention of the bladder, the systemic arterial pressure may rise to 300 mm. Hg or more.[25]

MEDULLARY CENTERS. Electrical stimulation of some areas in the medulla oblongata produces prompt elevation in blood pressure (pressor areas), and stimulation of other medullary areas causes a sharp reduction in blood pressure (depressor areas; Fig. 4-11). These regions are generally termed the vasoconstrictor and vaso-dilator "center," respectively. These so-called centers are not strictly local-ized but are diffuse networks of inter-connected neuron groups. The nature of the interaction between the pressor and depressor zones is not known, and they are continuously influenced by impulses from many sources such as pressoreceptors, chemoreceptors, somatic afferent sources and the higher levels of the nervous system (see later discussion). These medullary centers of cardiovascular regulation appear to be essential to normal control of sys-temic arterial pressure (see Chapter 5).

DIENCEPHALIC CENTERS. The region of the hypothalamus contains control centers integrating reactions which involve the vascular system. These reactions include temperature regulation, water balance, thirst and hunger and cardiovascular responses to exertion. Electrical stimulation of discrete hypothalamic and subthala-mic sites produces profound changes in the heart rate, ventricular contrac-tility and arterial pressure and also dilation of blood vessels in skeletal muscle by means of the familiar sym-pathetic cholinergic vasodilator fibers (see later discussion). Supplementing such functional evidence of central nervous system control is a growing body of anatomical evidence of neural pathways descending from the dience-phalon to the midbrain and spinal cord.[22]

Impinging on the hypothalamic centers are nerve impulses from many parts of the brain, including the motor and premotor cortex, the frontal cortex, the orbital cortex, the temporal lobe, the amygdala, the insula and the cingulate gyrus.[23, 24] In general, if electrical stimulation of an area in the brain consistently yields behavior re-sponses, cardiovascular responses are also induced. Conversely, if electrical stimulation of a cerebral area does not induce cardiovascular responses, it rarely evokes behavioral changes.

SYMPATHETIC CONSTRICTOR NERVES. The sympathetic constric-tor fibers exert their most profound effects on the blood vessels of skeletal muscle, the skin and the splanchnic bed (see Figs. 4-13 and 4-14). The sympathetic constrictor nerve fibers apparently exert their action on smooth muscle at the so-called alpha (α) re-ceptor sites at which *l*-epinephrine and norepinephrine also act (Fig. 4-12A). The blood vessels of skeletal muscles are served by both adrenergic constrictor fibers and cholinergic dila-tor fibers. The constrictor fibers to the skin are involved in conservation of heat, and the direct vascular connec-tions between the small arteries and small veins (arteriovenous anasto-moses) in the skin are directly con-trolled by the hypothalamic heat loss center. Through these channels large volumes of blood pass directly from the terminal arteries into the voluminous venous plexuses for heat dissipation. The arteriovenous anastomoses are completely dominated by the con-strictor fibers, dilating maximally when the constrictor nerves are cut. In other areas, severance of the constric-tor fibers leaves the blood vessels with considerable constrictor "tone" (i.e., they are partially constricted).

SYMPATHETIC VASODILATOR SYS-TEM. Stimulation of the sympathetic chain in the lumbar region of cats or dogs may cause initial dilation fol-lowed by constriction in the vascular beds within skeletal muscle. When the constriction was eliminated by adren-ergic blocking drugs, pure vasodila-tion was obtained.[23] The vasodilator response was restricted to skeletal muscle and was potentiated by eserine

A. GENERAL VASOMOTOR CONTROL MECHANISMS

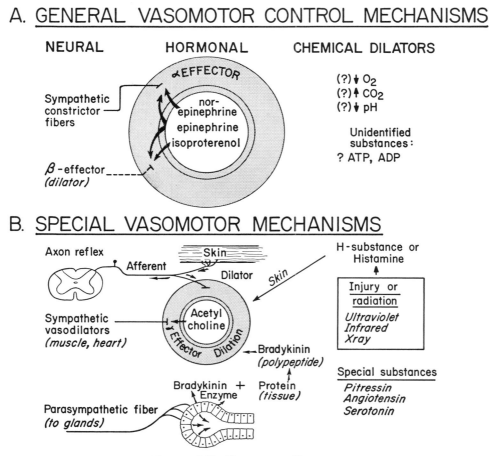

NEURAL

HORMONAL

CHEMICAL DILATORS

αEFFECTOR

nor-epinephrine
epinephrine
isoproterenol

Sympathetic constrictor fibers

β-effector (dilator)

(?) ↓ O_2
(?) ↑ CO_2
(?) ↓ pH

Unidentified substances:
? ATP, ADP

B. SPECIAL VASOMOTOR MECHANISMS

Axon reflex

Afferent

Skin

Dilator

Skin

Sympathetic vasodilators (muscle, heart)

Acetyl choline

Effector   Dilation

Bradykinin (polypeptide)

Bradykinin + Enzyme

Protein (tissue)

Parasympathetic fiber (to glands)

H-substance or Histamine

Injury or radiation

Ultraviolet
Infrared
Xray

Special substances

Pitressin
Angiotensin
Serotonin

FIGURE 4-12   VASOMOTOR CONTROL

A, Vasoconstriction or vasodilation can be produced in various tissues by means of many neural, hormonal and chemical mechanisms. Sympathetic fibers and circulating norepinephrine and *l*-epinephrine are widely believed to act at specific sites (α effectors). The β effectors are not innervated. The chemical dilators are proposed mechanisms for explaining vasodilation following temporary occlusion of blood supply to a vascular bed (reactive hyperemia).

B, The special vasomotor mechanisms are found prominently in the skin although the sympathetic vasodilators are found in skeletal muscle and heart and the postulated bradykinin mechanism affects glands. No definite role in normal vascular regulation has been assigned to the special constrictor substances, vasopressin (Pitressin), angiotensin and serotonin.

and eliminated by atropine.[23] A substance like acetylcholine was found in the effluent perfusate from such muscles.[24] These observations form the basis for the concept of a sympathetic cholinergic vasodilator system (Fig. 4-12B). It is believed that this system originates in the motor cortex and that

impulses descend from there to the hypothalamus, pass through the medullary centers and leave the spinal cord with the sympathetic nerves to induce vasodilation of the blood vessels in skeletal muscles. When the sympathetic constrictor fibers to the skeletal muscle are blocked or inactivated, the blood vessels dilate somewhat but continue to display considerable basal tone (partial constriction). Upon stimulation of the sympathetic cholinergic vasodilator system the blood flow may become five or six times greater. The evidence for active neurogenic vasodilation in muscle and skin of man has been reviewed by Greenfield.[25] Species variability has been clearly shown by Uvnäs[26] in that cholinergic vasodilator nerves have been demonstrated in dog, cat, mongoose, fox and jackal but appear to be absent in lemur, old world monkey, rabbit, badger and polecat. There may be basic differences in vasomotor mechanisms in these different animals.

Axon Reflex. Stimulation of the peripheral ends of severed dorsal roots (afferent fibers) produces vasodilation in skin vessels. This response was formerly ascribed to activity of motor fibers issuing from the spinal cord against the stream of the sensory fibers that normally enter the cord by this route. A preferred explanation for this phenomenon is the hypothetical axon reflex. According to this concept, sensory nerve fibers in the skin may have collateral fibers distributed to adjacent blood vessels (Fig. 4-12B). Impulses generated from the sensory endings may pass directly to the dilator termination in the blood vessel as well as to the spinal cord. Such a mechanism has been invoked to explain the dilatory effects of certain irritants and mechanical stimulation of the skin.

Parasympathetic Dilator Mechanism. Stimulation of the parasympathetic nerves supplying certain glands (e.g., salivary glands) induces a profuse secretion and an intense vasodilation. Existence of parasympathetic vasodilators was postulated to explain the hyperemia. Hilton and Lewis[27] presented evidence that the glandular cells, activated by the parasympathetic fibers, release an enzyme (bradykinin) into the interstitial spaces. There this enzyme acts on tissue proteins to split off a polypeptide which diffuses to vessels in the vicinity, and produces vasodilation (see Fig. 4-12B). Bradykinin was apparently recoverable from the glandular excretion, and, after saline was perfused under the skin during profuse sweating, a substance like bradykinin was recovered in the perfusate.[28] Thus, the bradykinin mechanisms may be involved in the vasodilation of the skin which accompanies profuse sweating. It is tempting to postulate that the same type of mechanism is involved in the vasodilation which accompanies other visceral activity induced by parasympathetic activity (e.g., that in the gastrointestinal tract). Bradykinin injected into arteries produces marked vasodilation in man, being among the most active on a molar basis. The observation that carboxypeptidase B, which blocks bradykinin dilatation, failed to influence exercise hyperemia or cholinergic sympathetic vasodilation serves as a note of caution in ascribing a role for kinins in these responses.[30]

Hormonal Mechanisms. Impulses arriving at the terminals of the autonomic nervous system exert their influence on the effectors by release of transmitter substances. In the parasympathetic nervous system, this transmitter is acetylcholine, a rather potent vasodilator substance in some vascular beds. Through Euler's investigations,[31] the transmitter substance for sympathetic constrictor fibers has been identified as norepinephrine, which is found in high concentration in sympathetic nerves and in tissues with an intact sympathetic innervation. This substance differs from *l*-epinephrine, which is excreted primarily from chromaffin cells in the adrenal medulla and from other chromaffin cells scattered in different parts of the body, particularly in the heart. In man, norepinephrine produces vasoconstriction in those vascular beds where it produces any response at all. In contrast, *l*-epinephrine also has a vasodilator action in skeletal muscle, and perhaps in the heart, and a powerful effect on myocardial performance.

THE CONCEPT OF VASCULAR RECEPTORS. Catechol amines exert either of two effects on the vascular beds in skeletal muscle — vasoconstriction or vasodilation. Norepinephrine is a powerful vasconstrictor, but *l*-epinephrine can have either a dilator or a constrictor action, depending upon the circumstances. Ahlquist[32] was therefore led to propose that two distinct types of receptors, or binding sites — α and β receptors — are involved at the smooth muscle. (Since the term "receptor" might be misconstrued to mean the sensory or afferent receptors of reflex activity, the word "effector" has been substituted for "receptor" in Figure 4-12.)

It is thought that norepinephrine acts only on the α receptors and that these receptors excite the constrictor mechanism. *l*-epinephrine is also believed to have the same effect when acting on α receptors. A substance called kinekard of unknown composition has been extracted from blood plasma and has been shown to produce vasoconstriction and is believed to act on adrenergic receptors.[33] If these receptors are blocked by an appropriate drug (azapetine; Ilidar), then injected *l*-epinephrine produces vasodilation by its action on the receptors. The β receptor is blocked by very large doses of adrenergic blocking agents and is believed to be without innervation. The β receptors are believed to be confined to the blood vessels in skeletal muscle and perhaps in myocardium. Gamma (γ) receptors are believed responsible for the cholinergic vasodilation initiated by the sympathetic vasodilator in skeletal muscle.

The pharmacology of vascular smooth muscle, including the concept of receptors, has been reviewed by Green and Kepchar.[34] Although existence of these receptors, or effectors, has excited much interest among physiologists, it seems doubtful that the circulating catechol amines are very important in the normal peripheral vascular control. On the other hand, the action of norepinephrine as the transmitter substance for the sympathetic constrictor nerves is undoubtedly important in the control of certain vascular beds.

ACETYLCHOLINE. The transmitter substance issuing from the parasympathetic nerve endings is quite definitely acetylcholine. If the proposed bradykinin mechanism withstands the tests of time and critical evaluation, direct action of acetylcholine in vascular smooth muscle as a normal control mechanism need be postulated only for the sympathetic cholinergic vasodilator fibers which serve skeletal muscle and perhaps the coronary vessels. Intravenously administered acetylcholine produces vasodilation in various vascular beds, but this effect is probably not a significant facet of normal peripheral vascular control. The cholinesterase levels in the blood are so high that circulating acetylcholine is rapidly destroyed. Thus, very large doses must be administered intravenously to produce vascular effects.

Chemical Dilators. It is common experience that, if the blood supply to a limb is obstructed for a few minutes and then released, the skin supplied by these vessels flushes a vivid red.

Such vasodilation induced by temporary occlusion of the blood supply is termed *reactive hyperemia*. Roy and Brown[35] studied these vascular reactions and concluded that it "seems to us to throw much light on the manner in which the local circulation is carried on under normal conditions. It shows us that there is a local mechanism independent of the centres in the medulla and spinal cord by which the degree of dilation of the vessels is varied in accordance with the requirements of the tissues." This was in 1879; the same views are widely held today, and we are still unable to identify the substance, substances or other mechanisms which actually induce the vascular dilation in reactive hyperemia or during increases in the metabolic activity of the tissues. Lewis[36] described a series of astute observations and subscribed to the view that the vasodilator substance is a normal metabolite.

UNIDENTIFIED VASODILATOR SUBSTANCES. The effects of obstructed blood flow or increased metabolism which are perhaps the most obvious include: diminished oxygen tension in the tissues, increased carbon dioxide and lowered pH due to accumulation of acid metabolic products. As a matter of fact, perfusion with arterial blood of diminished oxygen content may produce vasodilation in some organs, particularly the heart, skeletal muscles, skin and, to a lesser extent, the gastrointestinal tract. If the low oxygen were the immediate cause of the vasodilation, however, the blood flow should return to control levels by the time the oxygen debt is repaid. Evidence has been presented that the oxygen debt is overpaid in both skin[37] and muscle,[38] and the excess blood flow may vary from 50 to 200 per cent of that necessary to repay the calculated oxygen debt.[39] Furthermore the increased flow may persist after the venous oxygen content has returned to normal or even attained supernormal values. On the contrary, Hymen[40] found an exact quantitative repayment of effective blood flow debt indicating control by some unidentified vasodilator substance. The identity of such substances is clouded by evidence that potassium, ATP and lactic acid injected into arteries may have a marked effect but produce little change when injected locally by intramuscular injection.[41] Mellander *et al.*[42] showed that locally induced hyperosmolarity was associated with vasodilation in muscle.

At the present time reactive hyperemia is attributed to vasodilator metabolite(s) accumulating during hypoxia, but the cause is not histamine. In short, the vascular reaction must be attributed to *unidentified vasodilator substance(s)*.[34] To provide such a hypothetical substance with an attractive name might gain some measure of reassurance but will certainly not accelerate progress toward its identification. In fact, the label "unidentified vasodilator substance" is used in Figures 4-12 and 4-13 as a signpost directing attention to an important unsolved problem.

ADENYLIC ACID DERIVATIVES. Adenosine triphosphate (ATP) is an important source of energy for metabolism. During the release of energy, this substance is converted into adenosine diphosphate (ADP). If ADP were a strong vasodilator, it might qualify as a mechanism for adjusting the blood flow in accordance with metabolic demands. Considerable evidence has been compiled to demonstrate that ATP, ADP, adenosine monophosphate and even adenosine have vasodilator effect.[43] They all probably act on the same inhibitory sites to permit vasodilation, but ATP and

ADP are more powerful than the others. Although these substances deserve further study, there is no evidence that they are released from cells so that they might act on the vascular smooth muscle. One difficulty in such studies is that the vascular beds are so exquisitely sensitive to these substances that the concentrations necessary for vasodilation are less than can be detected with current methods.

VASOPRESSIN (PITRESSIN). The neurohypophysis excretes a polypeptide, vasopressin, which has a fairly strong vasoconstrictor action in coronary vessels. This substance does not appear to react at the effector (receptor) sites involved by epinephrine, serotonin or histamine. The close spatial and functional relations between the hypothalamic centers and the neurohypophysis certainly suggest that release of vasopressin might contribute to vascular control, but no specific action of this mechanism has ever been demonstrated. Vasopressin is composed of eight amino acids, a characteristic shared by two other substances which induce smooth muscle contraction: oxytocin, which induces contraction of the uterus, and angiotensin.

ANGIOTENSIN. Under some circumstances the kidney releases a protein, renin, that acts on a blood protein (renin substrate) to produce angiotensin I, which is composed of ten amino acids. This decapeptide does not affect the caliber of blood vessels, but under the influence of converting enzyme it loses two amino acids to form angiotensin II, which has potent vasoconstrictor qualities (see Fig. 5-19). The synthesis of these substances is a most notable achievement by Page and his collaborators.[44] This mechanism was explored in a search for the cause of systemic arterial hypertension and has been proposed as one of the mechanisms for normal peripheral vascular control which go awry in patients who developed hypertension. Since the cellular sources of renin are not known, the mechanism or mechanisms by which its production is accelerated or depressed are completely obscure. The sensing element which monitors the concentration of angiotensin I or II or renin in blood has not been discovered, and it thus seems premature to assign this mechanism a role in normal peripheral vascular control. This subject will receive more attention in Chapter 5.

SEROTONIN. The serum of clotted blood causes contraction of blood vessels. Since the substance responsible for this reaction could easily complicate research on hypertension, Page and his colleagues[45] investigated the problem and isolated a substance called serotonin or, more exactly, 5-hydroxytryptamine. When injected intravenously this substance has a very complex action on the pulmonary circulation,[46] which otherwise is quite unresponsive (Figs. 4-13 and 4-16). Serotonin also is a vasodilator in peripheral beds, notably the coronary vessels; however, under normal conditions it is confined within platelets and mast cells, and release into the blood stream has not been demonstrated. Thus, its role in normal vascular control remains doubtful.

H-SUBSTANCE AND HISTAMINE. Mechanical stimulation of the skin (e.g., by firm stroking) produces a sequence of vascular changes including local vasoconstriction, a surrounding vasodilation or flare and, finally, local swelling or edema. Lewis[36] attributed this "triple response" to the release of "H-substance" from the injured tissue. This substance is generally identified as histamine, which can be derived from histidine by splitting off carbon dioxide. Experimentally, histamine causes vasodilation in the terminal capillary beds but constriction of the larger arterial branches. Histamine-like substances are generally considered to be present during vascular responses to tissue injury caused by such forms of radiation as ultraviolet light (sunburn), infrared (thermal burns) and roentgen rays and by mechanical stress and trauma. However, this substance is not apparently involved in normal control.

MYOGENIC RESPONSES. In 1902 Bayliss[47] reported experiments which indicated that "the muscular coat of the arteries reacts, like smooth muscle in other situations, to a stretching force by contraction" independent of the nervous system. More recently Folkow[48] and others have investigated this concept that elevated internal pressure produces vasoconstriction in denervated vascular beds. The evidence of this type of reaction is quite universally indirect. Without any questioning of these observations it seems illogical, as McDonald and Taylor have pointed out, to emphasize this mechanism as the physiologically dominant one since it would appear to act as a positive feed-back loop and so to be completely unstable. "Thus, a rise in blood pressure would cause a vasoconstriction which would cause further rise in pressure."[49] If smooth muscle is indeed capable of a myogenic response, then it must act in conjunction with, and be governed by, built-in sensing and control systems.

VASCULAR CONTROL IN SPECIFIC TISSUES

The anatomic arrangement and environmental conditions of arteries, arterioles and sphincters vary from one vascular bed to another, but the smooth muscle cells which invest these vessels and induce changes in their caliber look the same in all vascular beds. Nevertheless, the vascular smooth muscle in different tissues responds in widely different ways under the influence of the mechanisms illustrated in Figure 4-12. Under these conditions, control of the vascular system cannot be considered in general terms. The characteristics of the vascular responses peculiar to each major tissue or organ must be detailed individually. In the following discussion, the organs of the body will be discussed roughly in the order of increasing reactivity or diversity of mechanisms inducing vasomotor responses. Green and Kepchar's[34] excellent review is a valuable reference to supplement the following discussion.

Brain. The cerebral vasculature is probably the most resistant to vasomotor influences to be found in the body. According to Kety,[50] the cerebral blood flow of healthy young men is about 54 ml. per 100 gm. of brain tissue per minute and the respiratory quotient is approximately unity, indicating that carbohydrate is the prime source of energy. The energy requirement of the brain is about 20 watts, compared to the thousands of watts required by electronic computors.

It is well established that autonomic nerves supply the cerebral vessels. This innervation may influence the cerebral blood flow in lower animals, but there is little evidence of its effectiveness in man. After reviewing a great many potential factors, Sokoloff[51] concluded, "an overall view of the action of drugs on the cerebral circulation is the great resistance of the cerebral blood flow to change" (Fig. 4-13). Increased carbon dioxide tension has the most potent effects on cerebral vessels, but it rarely elevates cerebral flow as much as twofold. Reduced oxygen tension in the arterial blood has also been reported to dilate cerebral vessels.[52]

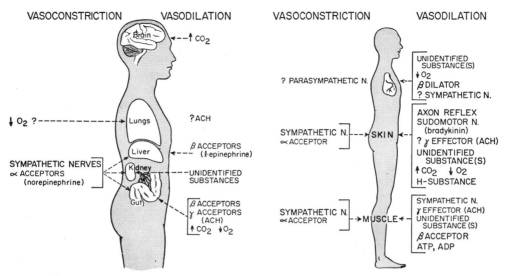

FIGURE 4-13   VASOMOTOR MECHANISMS IN VARIOUS TISSUES

Vascular beds in some tissues are very unresponsive to all normal vasomotor mechanisms; e.g., cerebral vessels are slightly affected by CO_2 and pulmonary vessels by O_2 content. The splanchnic vascular bed is quite reactive and responds to many different controlling mechanisms. The vascular reactivity of the coronary vessels is difficult to determine because most of the mechanisms affect cardiac function as well. The vessels of skin and muscle respond to a very large number of different control mechanisms and are extremely reactive.

Reflecting the constancy of the overall cerebral metabolism, the total cerebral blood flow is remarkably constant. However, the blood flow is not uniform throughout the brain substance, varying from 0.14 ml. per gram in spinal white matter to 1.8 mg. per gram in the inferior colliculus.[53] Primary sensory areas subserving visual, auditory and somatosensory functions receive significantly higher blood flows than do other cortical areas. Under thiopental anesthesia, the differences in blood flow through sensory areas disappear.

Lungs. The pulmonary circulation appears to be almost as unresponsive as the cerebral to normal controlling mechanisms (Fig. 4-13). The pulmonary vascular bed is an extremely low resistance system (Chapter 1), and its resistance readily becomes even less. Thus the amount of blood flowing through this system can increase two or three times with very little increase in the pressure gradient from the pulmonary artery to the left atrium. Because definitive demonstration of any active vasomotor change induced by neural, hormonal or chemical agents has proved very difficult, the reduction in resistance as flow increases has been ascribed to passive distention of the vascular bed. At higher pulmonary blood flow rates, however, the pressure gradient increases in direct proportion to the flow rate as though the vascular bed had reached a maximum cross-sectional area and was behaving more like a system of rigid tubes.[54]

Hypoxia apparently induces some vasoconstriction, which would tend to shunt blood from collapsed or inactive lung parenchyma toward regions where gases could be interchanged.

Fairly large concentrations of acetylcholine infused directly into the pulmonary artery produce a slight and questionable fall in pulmonary arterial pressure.[54] There is, however, no evidence that either hypoxia or acetylcholine is normally a regulator of pulmonary vessels.

The evidence on the action of vasodilator drugs on pulmonary vessels is inconclusive. They are constricted by serotonin and under these conditions respond with vasodilation to acetylcholine, histamine and adenosine triphosphate.[55] The functional significance of this observation remains obscure. Some evidence for a parasympathetic innervation of the lung activated by stimulation of the carotid chemoreceptors has been presented by Daly and Daly,[56] but such a mechanism would play little or no role in normal control.

It thus seems safe to consider the pulmonary vascular bed as one that does not share in peripheral vasomotor alterations. This attitude appears entirely logical since all of the cardiac output flows through the lungs. There is no obvious need for a means of changing the distribution of blood flow from one part of the lungs to another under normal conditions, because all parts serve the same function.

Liver. The liver, like the lung, is a low-pressure system served by two vascular systems. A major portion (about four fifths) of the blood flowing through the liver arrives by way of the portal vein under low pressure after having passed through the capillaries in the gastrointestinal tract upstream. The remainder enters under the systemic arterial pressure head by way of the hepatic artery. Both stimulation of sympathetic nerves and norepinephrine apparently produce some constriction of both the hepatic and portal arterial systems, but the effects are relatively mild. Since epinephrine, isoproterenol and acetylcholine have little or no effect on either vascular system, neither β nor γ effectors are believed to exist here. Reactive hyperemia does not follow temporary occlusion of the blood flow. Thus, the liver is a system that is quite unresponsive to the available control systems.

Spleen. Stimulation of the splenic nerve greatly increases the vascular resistance and activates the mechanism by which the cells concentrated in the spleen are dumped into the active circulation. The changes in resistance apparently are mediated by norepinephrine; the emptying mechanism by *l*-epinephrine. Dilation follows administration of extremely small concentrations of cholinergic substances, although existence of a parasympathetic innervation has not been demonstrated.

Kidney. The splanchnic sympathetic nerves exert a vasoconstrictor effect on the renal vessels. Norepinephrine and *l*-epinephrine act on effectors to produce constriction. Temporary occlusion of renal blood flow results in reactive hyperemia induced by unidentified dilator substances. Above a certain critical pressure (i.e., 70 mm. Hg) the blood flow through the kidney tends to remain quite constant in spite of progressively elevated arterial perfusion pressure. This has been termed *autoregulation* and may result from elevation of perivascular pressures in step with increases in perfusion pressure, so that flow remains relatively constant.

Gastrointestinal Tract. The splanchnic nerves are profusely distributed to the vessels of the splanchnic bed and are believed to play an important role in the maintenance of systemic arterial blood pressure. These nerves apparently act through α effectors so that administration of nor-epinephrine induces similar effects on this bed. Prolonged stimulation of intestinal vasoconstrictor fibers induces a pattern termed "autoregulatory escape," an initial constriction followed by an escape of resistance vessels from the nervous influences within 1 to 2 minutes while the perfused capillary exchange area remains reduced.[58] Significant dilation follows injection of isoproterenol, indicating the presence of β effectors. Mild dilation from administration of acetylcholine suggests the presence of γ effectors. However, according to presently available information, the autonomic nerves act on the α effectors but not on the β effectors. Since such levels are beyond the physiologic range, the resulting dilation has very limited significance.

Heart. The terminal coronary vessels penetrate the walls of the heart. There they are compressed by the contracting myocardium, particularly within the wall of the left ventricle of the heart. During ventricular systole, the outflow from the coronary veins is accelerated and the inflow through the coronary arteries is impeded. However, the pumping action of ventricular systole apparently does not facilitate blood flow. Sudden arrest of the heart immediately increases both the arterial inflow and the venous outflow, indicating that ventricular contraction impedes flow through the coronary vessels.[59] More vigorous contraction of the myocardium, induced by catechol amines or sympathetic stimulation, tends to increase simultaneously the work load on the myocardium and the impedence to coronary flow. A close relation between the cardiac effort, the myocardial oxygen consumption and the coronary flow has been repeatedly reported. Gregg[59] pointed out that most of the oxygen is normally removed from the coronary blood so that the oxygen content of coronary sinus (venous) blood cannot be reduced very much. Therefore increased oxygen delivery must be achieved primarily by increased coronary flow.

It seems likely that low oxygen tension or low oxygen content in the blood produces coronary dilation, but this dilation could reflect the effects of unidentified vasodilator substances since the coronary vessels exhibit reactive hyperemia. Carbon dioxide and altered pH apparently have no effect. According to Green and Kepchar,[34] the only agents which consistently cause constriction of the coronary arterioles are vasopressin and angiotensin. Many drugs appear to produce coronary dilation but have no known functional significance in normal control.

Skeletal Muscle. The blood vessels supplying skeletal muscles generally are now believed to have double sympathetic innervation. The sympathetic constrictor fibers activate typical α receptors and, apparently, participate in the generalized sympathetic discharges which tend to support systemic arterial blood pressure. When this sympathetic constrictor mechanism is eliminated, the blood vessels of muscle maintain a substantial degree of vasoconstriction. Sympathetic vasodilator fibers act through cholinergic γ receptors, which can produce maximal dilation and can be readily blocked by atropine. The sympathetic vasodilator system is confined to skeletal muscle and is apparently dissociated from the control of the blood pressure regulatory system of the medullary vasomotor areas. Instead, the nerve impulses which ultimately reach the sympathetic vasodilator nerve endings have been traced from the motor cortex of the cerebrum near the cruciate sulcus to the supraoptic part of the hypo-thalamus, to the collicular area and through the medullary regions, appar-ently bypassing the medullary cardio-regulator centers, to impinge rather directly on the sympathetic outflow in the spinal cord.[60]

Thus there are four postulated mechanisms by which vasodilation in skeletal muscle may be achieved: (1) inhibition of the sympathetic con-strictor mechanism (twofold to three-fold increase), (2) activation of the sympathetic vasodilator system (five-fold to sixfold increase), (3) the β ef-fectors and (4) unidentified vasodilator substances present immediately after exercise (sixfold to tenfold increase). The β effectors are not innervated but are activated by circulating l-epine-phrine or injected isoproterenol (Fig. 4-12). The function of this mechanism in normal body economy has not been established.

The skeletal muscles are prone to develop extremely intense reactive hyperemia following temporary occlu-sion of their blood supply. This state is attributed to unidentified metabolic vasodilator substances.

Extremely small quantities of adenosine triphosphate (ATP) produce profound vasodilation in skeletal mus-cle. A similar degree of vasodilation can be produced by adenosine diphos-phate (ADP). In fact, these substances are such potent dilators that the effec-tive doses for the skeletal vessels defy chemical detection. Although ATP and ADP are fine potential candidates for the position of "unidentified vaso-dilator substances," their role has not been conclusively demonstrated.

The contraction of skeletal muscle impedes blood flow just as ventricular contraction does (see previous discus-sion). Thus, the blood flow through an extremity is greater immediately after the cessation of exercise than during

the exertion itself. The compression of blood vessels by contracting muscle can actively pump venous blood against a very high resistance (see Fig. 7-8).

Skin. The skin has the most complex assortment of available con-trol mechanisms (Fig. 4-13) and con-tains a vascular bed which is very accessible for study by physiologists and clinicians. The result is an im-posing, almost overwhelming mass of literature that defies precise de-scription.

The predominant neural control is exercised by the sympathetic vaso-constrictor nerves; the mediator is probably norepinephrine. In contrast with vessels in muscle, skin vessels dilate maximally when the sympathe-tic constrictor influence on them is eliminated. Consequently, the full range of cutaneous flow can be achieved by release of constrictor tone. No sympathetic or parasympathetic vasodilator fibers directly affecting cutaneous vessels have been de-scribed. Injection of acetylcholine in-duces a slight dilation of these vessels which suggests the presence of γ ef-fectors that are not innervated. Stim-ulation of the peripheral ends of sev-eral dorsal roots produces vasodilation which can best be explained in terms of an axon reflex (see Fig. 4-12B). The normal course of impulses in such a mechanism is from sensory nerve endings in the skin to collaterals which directly impinge on blood vessels. Recent evidence suggests that the parasympathetic supply to the sweat glands (sudomotor) triggers the release of an enzyme (bradykinin enzyme) that acts on tissue proteins to form bradykinin which diffuses to adjacent blood vessels and induces a vasodila-tion of the deep and superficial vas-cular plexuses. (Fig. 4-12).

The skin exhibits severe reactive

hyperemia following temporary occlusion to blood supply. Thus, it can be postulated that unidentified vasodilator substances participate in the control of the skin vessels. A vasomotor role of low oxygen or elevated carbon dioxide has not been established.

Local warming of the skin produces a vasodilation which is believed to result from release of constrictor tone through central reflexes rather than from a direct action of the heat on the blood vessels. These reflexes probably involve the hypothalamic temperature regulating centers, acting through sympathetic vasoconstrictor nerves. Excessive cold applied to the skin may produce a brief vasodilation which may be independent of the nerve supply.

Finally, flushing of the skin from embarrassment or emotional stimuli represents vascular changes induced from higher levels of the nervous system.

EFFECTS OF CONTROL MECHANISMS ON FLOW DISTRIBUTION

When ultrasonic flowmeters are installed on arteries or veins, the instantaneous flow through these regions can be continuously registered during the spontaneous activity of healthy dogs and during reactions experimentally induced in the presence or absence of anesthesia.[61]

Flow Distribution During Spontaneous Activity. The instantaneous flow through the superior mesenteric or hepatic artery, the renal artery and the terminal abdominal aorta of intact dogs was continuously recorded while the animals were engaged in various activities, including: reacting to a startling event, standing erect with the head up (60 degrees), standing with the head down (50 degrees), sit-

ting, drinking water, entering a treadmill and exercising at 3 m.p.h. on a 12 per cent grade (Fig. 4–14). As the changes in the wave form of the instantaneous flow do not indicate the changes in volume flow per unit time, the flow records have been integrated with an analogue computer so that the flow during intervals of 2.5 seconds is accumulated. In this manner the influences of both changes in wave form and changes in heart rate are taken into account, and the height of the resulting deflection is an accurate measure of volume flow during a particular period. The contribution of each stroke can be identified from the distance separating pairs of darker spots representing diastole on the integrated flow line.

Each of the preceding spontaneous actions was associated with obvious deflections in the records of instantaneous flow. The integrated flow per unit of time through the superior mesenteric and renal arteries, however, remained remarkably constant, although slight changes accompanied the startle reaction and standing erect with the head up. In all seven dogs studied, volume flow was remarkably constant in the renal artery and in the superior mesenteric or hepatic artery during virtually all forms of spontaneous activity which were studied. On the other hand, the integrated flow as well as the instantaneous flow in the terminal abdominal aorta was very responsive to most forms of activity. During exercise the forward flow of blood through the hindquarters exceeded zero throughout the cardiac cycles, a condition indicating both a considerably reduced peripheral resistance and a greatly increased blood flow. The mean pressure in the abdominal aorta was quite constant except when standing erect with the head up. The heart

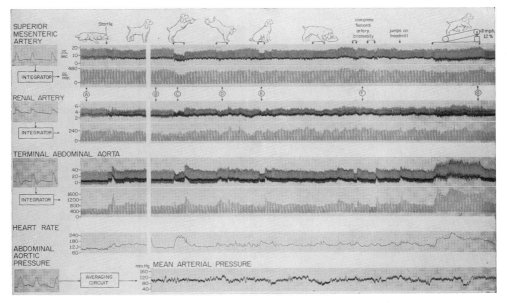

FIGURE 4-14   FLOW DISTRIBUTION DURING SPONTANEOUS ACTIVITY

Instantaneous and integrated flow through the superior mesenteric artery, renal artery and terminal abdominal aorta as recorded simultaneously and continuously in an intact dog during a series of cardiovascular adjustments to spontaneous activity including startle reaction, standing erect with head up, head down, eating, constriction of femoral arteries bilaterally, entering treadmill and exercise. Note that blood flow per unit of time (integrated) through the superior mesenteric and renal arteries changes very little during most responses except standing with head up. Flow to the hindquarters increased greatly during treadmill exercise.

rate increased notably during the startle reaction, standing erect and exercise.

Effects of Diencephalic Stimulation. Stimulation of selected sites in the diencephalon produced a wide variety of flow patterns in dogs under chloralose anesthesia. Changes in flow distribution reminiscent of those during exercise consistently resulted from stimulation in the region of the H_2 fields of Forel; stimulation of this region was already known to cause changes in cardiac function comparable to the changes accompanying exercise.[62] In the studies of blood flow, repeated stimulation as the electrode was advanced at 1 mm. increments toward this area produced the changes illustrated in Figure 4–15. No significant alterations followed stimulation at the first two points selected. After the electrode was advanced only 1 mm., the superior mesenteric and renal flows definitely decreased and the flow through the terminal aorta increased. Stimulation after the electrode was moved 1 mm. farther produced an even greater response, but, as the electrode was advanced still farther, the response lessened. The influence of diencephalic stimulation on the blood flow through these arteries and the promptness of the response indicate that their nerve supplies were intact. Thus, the relative slightness of the changes in superior mesenteric and renal flow during spontaneous activity probably cannot be attributed to damage of essential innervation during application of the flow sections.

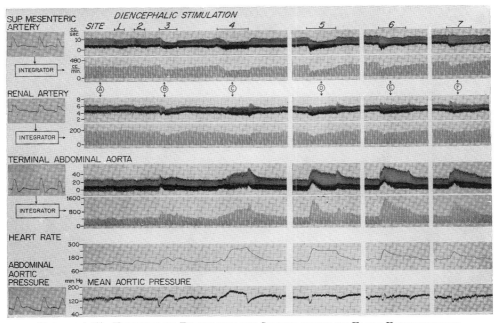

FIGURE 4-15   EFFECTS OF DIENCEPHALIC STIMULATION ON FLOW DISTRIBUTION

A series of stimuli was applied as the electrode was advanced in 1 mm. increments to and through the H$_2$ fields of Forel. The changes in flow distribution resemble those observed during spontaneous exercise by the same animal. Stimulation in this diencephalic region simultaneously produces these changes in flow distribution, changes in cardiac rate and function resembling the exercise response (see Fig. 7-4), increased respiratory ventilation and, on some occasions, running movements.

SUMMARY

The basic principles of peripheral vascular control are generally considered in terms of mechanisms by which the blood flow through various tissues are adjusted in relation to metabolism and the oxygen requirement. Actually, many tissues have functional requirements for blood flow which are unrelated to the oxygen consumption (e.g., kidney, skin, liver, and perhaps the gastrointestinal tract; Fig. 4–16). In fact, the principal tissues that require blood flow related to their metabolic rates (oxygen uptake) are the striated muscles: myocardium and skeletal muscles. After temporary occlusion of the blood supply to these tissues they exhibit a most powerful reactive hyperemia apparently caused by unidentified metabolic vasodilator substances.

The blood flow, oxygen extraction and vasomotor control are quite different in the various vascular beds. The neural control mechanisms are clearly important in the regulation of blood flow through many tissues, but not all. Neural controls are based principally on the sympathetic constrictor system, which continuously maintains varying degrees of constriction within the vascular beds. In addition there is a sympathetic vasodilator system, which is restricted to skeletal muscle (and, perhaps, the heart). Vasodilation is attributed currently to parasympathetic activation of certain structures, notably glands, with resulting formation of bradykinin by an enzyme released from the gland into the interstitial

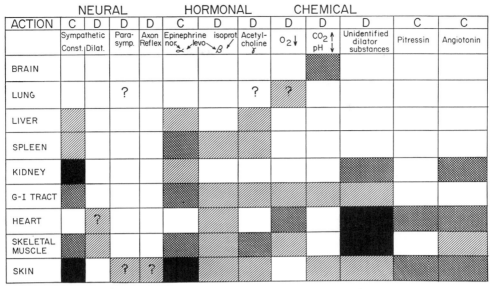
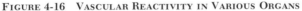

FIGURE 4-16 VASCULAR REACTIVITY IN VARIOUS ORGANS

The responsiveness of the various vascular beds illustrated in Figure 4-13 is here indicated schematically by the density of the shading under each of the neural, hormonal and chemical factors. The action of the mechanisms is indicated by *C* for constriction and *D* for dilation. The question marks indicate that the response is controversial. Note that both the diversity of the response and the intensity of the response tend to be much greater in the gastrointestinal tract, heart, skeletal muscle and skin than in the brain, lung, liver and spleen.

tissues. Circulating autonomic hormones, *l*-epinephrine, norepinephrine and acetylcholine have powerful vasomotor activity when injected, but their role in normal peripheral vascular control remains questionable. The vasodilator substances, which seem to accumulate when tissues metabolize in an environment containing inadequate oxygen, have not been definitely identified and represent an important challenge in this field.

The vascular reactivity in various organs is strikingly different (Fig. 4-16). For example, the cerebral circulation is little affected by neural or hormonal substances and is mildly dilated by increased carbon dioxide tension. Control of the pulmonary circulation is difficult to demonstrate experimentally. The coronary vessels dilate readily in response to metabolic

vasodilator substances but are otherwise quite nonreactive so far as can be determined experimentally. In contrast, the splanchnic bed, kidney, liver and spleen are fairly responsive to a variety of mechanisms, and skeletal muscles and the skin are influenced by a bewildering number of factors.

REFERENCES

1. ZWEIFACH, B. W. The microcirculation of the blood. *Sci. Amer.*, 200:54–60, 1959.
2. ROMANUL, F. C. A. Distribution of capillaries in relation to oxidative metabolism of skeletal muscle fibres. *Nature*, 201:307–308, 1964.
3. MYERS, W. W., and HONIG, C. R. Number and distribution of capillaries as determinants of myocardial oxygen tension. *Amer. J. Physiol.*, 207:653–660, 1964.
4. SCHMIDT-NIELSEN, K., and PENNYCUIK, P. Capillary density in mammals in relation to body size and oxygen consumption. *Amer. J. Physiol.*, 200:746–750, 1961.

5. THEWS, G. Gaseous diffusion in the lungs and tissues. Chapter 20 in *Physical Bases of Circulatory Transport: regulation and exchange*. E. B. Reeve and A. C. Guyton, Eds. Philadelphia, W. B. Saunders Co., 1967.

6. ZWEIFACH, B. W., and KOSSMANN, C. E. Micromanipulation of small blood vessels in the mouse. *Amer. J. Physiol.*, 120:23–35, 1937.

7. YAMADA, E. The fine structure of the renal glomerulus of the mouse. *J. Biophys. Biochem. Cytol.*, 1:551–556, 1955.

8. BENNET, H. S., LUFT, J. H., and HAMPTOM, J. C. Morphological classification of vertebrate blood capillaries. *Amer. J. Physiol.*, 196:381–390, 1959.

9. MAJNO, G. Ultrastructure of the vascular membrane. In *Handbook of Physiology, Section II Circulation*, Vol. 3. William Hamilton, Ed. Bethesda, Amer. Physiol. Soc., 1965.

10. BURTON, A. C. Physical principles of circulatory phenomena; the physical equilibria of the heart and blood vessels. In *Handbook of Physiology, Section II Circulation*, Vol. I. William Hamilton, Ed. Bethesda, Amer. Physiol. Soc., 1962.

11. VAN CITTERS, R. L. WAGNER, B. M., and RUSHMER, R. F. Architectural changes in the walls of small arteries during vasoconstriction. *Circulat. Res.*, 10:668–675, 1962.

12. HAYES, J. R. Histological changes in constricted arteries and arterioles. *J. Anat.*, 101:343–349, 1967.

13. STROMBERG, D. An index for quantitative measurement of vasoconstriction in histologic sections of blood vessels. *Vascular Surg.*, 3:68–80, 1960.

14. VAN CITTERS, R. L. Occlusion of lumina in small arteries during vasoconstriction. *Circulat. Res.*, 18:199–204, 1966.

15. WALLACE, J. M., and STEAD, E. A. Fall in pressure in radial artery during reactive hyperemia. *Circulat. Res.*, 7:876–879, 1959.

16. BURTON, A. C. Why have a circulation? In *Physiology and Biophysics of Circulation*. Year Book Medical Publishers, Inc., 1965.

17. FOLKOW, B. Range of control of the cardiovascular system by the central nervous system. *Physiol. Rev.*, 40 (Suppl. 4):93–99, 1960.

18. FOLKOW, B., JOHANNSON, B.; and LÖFVING, B. Aspects of functional differentiation of the sympatho-adrenergic control of the cardiovascular system. In *Medicina Experimentalis*, R. Domenjoz and S. Karger, Eds. Basel, New York. (*Med. Exp.* 4:321–328, 1961.)

19. RENKIN, E. U., and ROSELL, S. Independent sympathetic vasoconstrictor innervation of arterioles and precapillary sphincters. *Acta physiol. scand.* 54:381–384, 1962.

20. LUTZ, B. R., and FULTON, G. P. Smooth muscle and blood flow in small blood vessels. Pp. 13–23 in *Factors Regulating Blood Flow*, G. P. Fulton and B. Zweifach, Eds. Washington, Amer. Physiol. Soc., 1958.

21. WHITTERIDGE, D. Cardiovascular reflexes initiated from afferent sites other than the cardiovascular system itself. *Physiol. Rev.*, 40 (Suppl. 4): 198–200, 1960.

22. SMITH, O. A. Anatomy of central neural pathways mediating cardiovascular functions. In *Nervous Control of the Heart*, W. C. Randall, Ed. Baltimore, The Williams and Wilkins Co., 1965.

23. FOLKOW, B. Nervous control of blood vessels. *Physiol. Rev.*, 35:629–663, 1955.

24. ERICI, I., FOLKOW, B, and UVNÄS, B. Sympathetic vasodilator nerves to the tongue of the cat. *Acta physiol. scand.*, 25:1–9, 1952.

25. GREENFIELD, A. D. M. Survey of evidence for active neurogenic vasodilatation in man. *Fed. Proc.*, 25:1607–1610, 1966.

26. UVNÄS, B. Cholinergic vasodilator nerves. *Fed. Proc.*, 25:1618–1622, 1966.

27. HILTON, S. M., and LEWIS, G. P. The relationship between glandular activity, bradykinin formation and functional vasodilatation in the submandibular salivary gland. *J. Physiol.*, 134:471–483, 1956.

28. FOX, R. H., and HILTON, S. M. Sweat gland activity, bradykinin formation and vasodilation in human forearm skin. *J. Physiol.*, 137:43p–44p, 1957.

29. FOX, R. H., GOLDSMITH, R., KIDD, D. J., and LEWIS, G. P. Bradykinin as a vasodilator in man. *J. Physiol.*, 157:589–602, 1961.

30. WEBSTER, M. E., SKINNER, N. S., JR., POWELL, W. J. Role of the kinins in vasodilation of skeletal muscle in the dog. *Amer. J. Physiol.*, 212:553–558, 1967.

31. VON EULER, U. S. Noradrenaline. Springfield, Ill., C. C Thomas, 1956, 382 pp.

32. AHLQUIST, R. P. Adrenergic drugs. Pp. 378–407 in *Pharmacology in Medicine*, Vol. 2, V. A. Drill, Ed. New York, McGraw-Hill, 1958.

33. DOREVITCH, N., NAYLER, W. G., LOWE, T. E. The action on isolated smooth muscle of kinekard, a cardioactive fraction isolated from human plasma. *J. Pharmacol. Exptl. Therap.* 155:367-375, 1967.

34. GREEN, H. D., and KEPCHAR, J. H. Control of peripheral resistance in major systemic vascular beds. *Physiol. Rev.*, 39:617–686, 1959.

35. ROY, C. S., and BROWN, J. G. The blood pressure and its variations in the arterioles, capillaries and small veins. *J. Physiol.*, 2: 323–359, 1879–1880.

36. LEWIS, THOMAS. *The Blood Vessels of the Human Skin and Their Responses*. London, Shaw & Sons Ltd., 1927, 322 pp.

37. PATEL, D. J., and BURTON, A. C. Reactive hyperemia in the human finger. *Circulat. Res.*, 4:710–712, 1956.

38. YONCE, L. R., and HAMILTON, W. F. Oxygen consumption in skeletal muscle during reactive hyperemia. *Amer. J. Physiol.*, 197:190–192, 1959.

39. KORNER, P. I. Circulatory adaptations in hypoxia. *Physiol. Rev.*, 39:687–730, 1959.

40. HYMAN, C., PALDINO, R. L., and ZIMMERMAN, E. Local regulation of effective blood flow in muscle. *Circulat. Res.*, 12:179–181, 1963.

41. CROSS, R. B., GIMLETTE, T. M. D. The effect of intramuscular injections of K, ATP and lactic acid on muscle blood flow estimated by ^{133}Xe clearance from the point of injection. *J. Physiol.*, 189:43p, 1967.

42. MELLANDER, S., JOHANSSON, B., GRAY, S., JONSSON, O., LUNVALL, J., and LJUNG, B. The effects of hyperosmolarity on intact and isolated vascular smooth muscle; possible role in exercise hyperemia. *Angiologica*, 4:310–322, 1967.

43. FOLKOW, B. The vasodilator action of adenosine triphosphate. *Acta physiol. scand.*, 17:311–316, 1949.

44. PAGE, I. H., McCUBBIN, J. W., SCHWARZ, H., and BUMPUS, F. M. Pharmacologic aspects of synthetic angiotonin. *Circulat. Res.*, 5:552–555, 1957.

45. PAGE, I. H. Serotonin (5-hydroxytryptamine): the last four years. *Physiol. Rev.*, 38:277–335, 1958.

46. ROSE, J. C., and LAZARO, E. J. Pulmonary vascular responses to serotonin and effects of certain serotonin antagonists. *Circulat. Res.*, 6:282–293, 1958.

47. BAYLISS, W. M. On the local reactions of the arterial wall to changes of internal pressure. *J. Physiol.*, 28:200–231, 1902.

48. FOLKOW, B. Description of the Myogenic Hypothesis. *Circulat. Res.*, Supplement 1, Vols. 14 and 15:1279–1287, 1964.

49. McDONALD, D. A., and TAYLOR, M. G. The hydrodynamics of the arterial circulation. *Progr. Biophys. Biophys. Chem.*, 9:105–173, 1959.

50. KETY, S. S. The physiology of the cerebral circulation in man. Pp. 324–340 in *Circulation*, J. McMichael, Ed. Oxford, Blackwell Scientific Publications, 1958.

51. SOKOLOFF, L. The action of drugs on the cerebral circulation. *Pharmacol. Rev.*, 11:1–85, 1959.

52. LASSEN, N. A. Cerebral blood flow and oxygen consumption in man. *Physiol. Rev.*, 39:183–238, 1959.

53. SOKOLOFF, L. Factors regulating the total and regional circulation of the brain. Pp. 79–88 in *Factors Regulating Blood Flow*, G. P. Fulton and B. Zweifach, Eds. Washington, Amer. Physiol. Soc., 1958.

54. COURNAND, A. Control of the pulmonary circulation in normal man. Pp. 219–237 in *Circulation*, J. McMichael, Ed. Oxford, Blackwell Scientific Publications, 1958.

55. RUDOLPH, A. M., KURLAND, M. D., AULD, P. A. M., and PAUL, M. H. Effects of vasodilator drugs on normal and serotonin-constricted pulmonary vessels of the dog. *Amer. J. Physiol.*, 197:617–623, 1959.

56. DALY, I. DE B., and DALY, M. DE B. The effects of stimulation of the carotid body chemoreceptors on pulmonary vascular resistance in the dog. *J. Physiol.*, 137:436–446, 1957.

57. FOLKOW, B., and LANGSTON, J. The interrelationship of some factors influencing renal blood flow autoregulation. *Acta physiol. scand.*, 61:165–176, 1964.

58. WALLENTIN, I. Studies on intestinal circulation. *Acta physiol. scand.*, 69 (supplementum 279):1–38, 1966.

59. GREGG, D. W. Regulation of the collateral and coronary circulation of the heart. Pp. 163–186 in *Circulation*, J. McMichael, Ed. Oxford, Blackwell Scientific Publications, 1958.

60. LINDGREN, P., and UVNÄS, B. Vasoconstrictor inhibition and vasodilator activation—two functionally separate vasodilator mechanisms in the skeletal muscles. *Acta physiol. scand.*, 33:108–119, 1955.

61. RUSHMER, R. F., FRANKLIN, D. L., VAN CITTERS, R. L., and SMITH, O. A., JR. Changes in peripheral blood flow distribution in healthy dogs. *Circulat. Res.*, 9:675–687, 1961.

62. SMITH, O. A., JR., RUSHMER, R. F., and LASHER, E. P. Similarity of cardiovascular responses to exercise and to diencephalic stimulation. *Amer. J. Physiol.*, 198:1139–1142, 1960.

CHAPTER 5

SYSTEMIC ARTERIAL PRESSURE

The distribution of blood flow through the various peripheral vascular beds is controlled primarily by changes in caliber at the sites of resistance in the vessels leading to the capillary networks (Chapter 4). This form of flow control depends upon the maintenance at all times of an adequate pressure head within the systemic arterial system (Fig. 4–10).

FACTORS DETERMINING MEAN SYSTEMIC ARTERIAL PRESSURE

The high pressures maintained within the systemic arteries constitute a pressure reservoir to supply the driving force propelling blood through the complex networks of narrow channels in the microcirculation. This hydrostatic head of pressure is normally in the range of 120/80 mm. Hg and must not fall below some critical level (i.e., 60/40 mm. Hg) lest perfusion of the brain be insufficient to maintain consciousness or to maintain functional integrity of rapidly metabolizing tissues such as the heart and kidney. The control of the arterial pressure is a complex problem because it can be altered by a very large number of factors as illustrated schematically in Figure 5–1.

The systemic arterial pressure is ultimately determined by the relationship between the cardiac output and the total peripheral resistance. An uncompensated reduction in either can lead to reduced pressure in the arterial system. The cardiac output is, in turn, determined by the product of the heart rate and the stroke volume. Since the left ventricle does not always fill completely during diastole nor empty completely during systole, the stroke volume must be regarded as the difference between the diastolic and systolic ventricular volumes.

Numerous factors influence the stroke volume, as indicated schematically in Figure 5–1. Among the influences on diastolic ventricular volume are the effective ventricular filling pressure and the resistance of the ventricular walls to distention (distensibility). The ventricular filling pressure depends upon the total volume of blood in the cardiovascular system and the distribution of this blood as it is affected by the venous capacity in various channels and

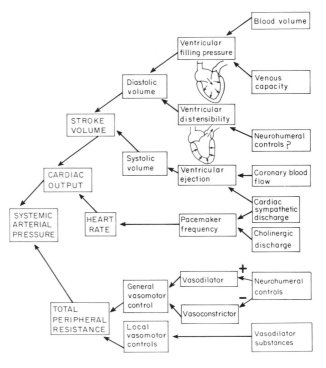

FIGURE 5-1 FACTORS DETERMINING SYSTEMIC ARTERIAL PRESSURE

The many interacting factors which determine the level of the systemic arterial pressure present a wide variety of alternative mechanisms for control. Note that each branch point represents a potential site of control or compensation for any perturbation of the system (see text).

reservoirs. The distensibility, or compliance of the ventricular walls, is not a simple elastic relation between length and tension but changes during the sequence of filling and is affected by the rate of filling. The sympathetic discharge to the ventricular myocardium affects the rate and degree of systolic ejection. The energy released by the contracting myocardium to expel the blood must be replenished continuously by processes dependent upon the continued flow of blood through the coronary arteries.

Control over heart rate can be readily traced to the balance of sympathetic and parasympathetic discharges into the region of the pacemaker. This balance is affected by a very wide variety of neural pathways. Reflexes initiated by distortion receptors in the carotid sinus and aortic arch are generally recognized as mechanisms for producing tachycardia in response to

lowered systemic arterial pressure. Spontaneous variations in heart rate apparently stem from diverse central mechanisms acting through the autonomic system as final common pathways. For example, visual images, sounds, cold, pain and cerebration can all affect heart rate. Our knowledge of these mechanisms is woefully inadequate.

General control over the peripheral resistance is exerted by the autonomic nervous system and circulating hormones, which are both predominantly constrictor in nature, except in skeletal muscles and glands. In addition, local accumulation of various chemicals (carbon dioxide, acids, adenosine triphosphate, adenosine disphosphate and histamine) have a predominantly vasodilator action.

Systemic arterial pressure could theoretically be reduced by an appropriate and uncompensated alteration in any of the controlling factors, as illustrated in Figure 5–1. It is obvious, however, that the analysis could be readily extended further to include factors controlling the total blood volume, those affecting the venous capacity, the causes of changes in coronary blood flow and so on. Even an oversimplified scheme like that in Figure 5–1 inevitably leads to the conclusion that many mechanisms are potentially capable of causing a depression of systemic arterial pressure. With but a moderate stretching of the imagination, a clinical cause of arterial hypotension was listed for virtually every mechanism indicated in Figure 5–1. Thus, either blood loss (hemorrhage) or reduced plasma volume (deshydremia) could lead to reduced blood pressure, reduced diastolic volume, diminished stroke volume, smaller cardiac output and lower systemic arterial pressure. Similarly, venodilatation could reduce ventricular filling pressure by changing the distribution of blood and lowering central venous pressure and so on down the list.

Compensatory Mechanisms

When factors that influence the systemic arterial pressure are represented schematically like the branchings of a tree, each fork in the arborization constitutes an opportunity for a functional compensation. For example, a reduction in cardiac output can be offset by a corresponding increase in total peripheral resistance, so that the systemic arterial pressure remains unchanged. Similarly, a reduction in total peripheral resistance can be completely compensated for by a corresponding increase in cardiac output (e.g., during exercise). A reduction in ventricular stroke volume can be balanced by an increase in heart rate, so that cardiac output is unchanged. A

local vasodilatation can be compensated by a generalized vasoconstriction. If the ventricular diastolic volume is diminished, the stroke volume can be maintained by more complete systolic ejection. A reduction in the sympathetic discharge to the cardiac pacemaker can be balanced by a correspondingly effective reduction in the parasympathetic discharge to prevent a change in heart rate. The ventricular filling pressure is established by the relationship between total blood volume and the capacity of the cardiovascular system, with particular reference to the venous system. A reduction in total blood volume can theoretically be compensated for by a constriction of the venous capacity, maintaining the central venous pressure unchanged. Thus, any change in arterial pressure signifies an alteration in some mechanism(s) in Figure 5–1 which was not fully compensated for by other mechanisms.

A monitoring system which senses systemic arterial pressure and induces appropriate cardiovascular compensations to maintain this pressure within a relatively narrow range will automatically adjust the balance between inflow and outflow so that the total flow through capillary networks does not exceed the capacity of the pump.

The requirements of a pressure-regulating system are indicated schematically in Figure 5–2. By adjustment of the pump motor and the resistance valves, the pressure head can be set at a predetermined level. Pressure-sensing elements which continuously monitor this pressure can act upon a black-box control system. In such a system, wider opening of one resistance valve increases the outflow from the high pressure side, dropping the pressure head. This lowers the output from the pressure transducers which in turn acts on the control sys-

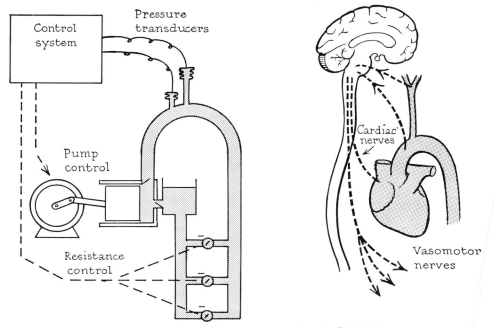

FIGURE 5-2   CONTROL OF ARTERIAL BLOOD PRESSURE

The pressure head in a simple hydraulic system could be controlled by means of pre-
sensing elements transmitting signals proportional to pressure through leads to a black-box
grating system which appropriately adjusts the pump output and valve settings in response
deviation from some preset level. The corresponding elements for the control of arterial bloo
sure include carotid sinus and aortic arch pressoreceptors feeding into the nervous system which provides integration of nerve impulses to the pump and peripheral vascular system.

tem to close other resistance valves, speed up the pump, or do both. In other words, the pressure level is set, the pressure-sensing elements detect a shift in pressure from this level as an error signal, and proper corrective adjustments to return the pressure to the "normal" level are instituted.

The systemic arterial pressure is apparently controlled essentially in this manner. There are, however, some complications. First, the process by which the "normal range" of systemic arterial pressure is originally set at a mean of about 90 mm. Hg is not obvious. Second, to detect an error, the pressure-sensing elements must continuously register actual pressure above atmospheric pressure even

though they are stretch receptors located in flexible walls apparently capable of varied distensibility. The pressure-sensing mechanism must integrate a fluctuating arterial pressure and induce responses which are related to changes in mean pressure rather than to changes in either the systolic or the diastolic pressure.

ARTERIAL PRESSURE PULSES

The principal function of the arterial system is to accept the repetitive spurts of blood injected by the heart and to convert this intermittent inflow into a relatively steady outflow through the peripheral resistance ves-

A. DISTORTION OF THE ARTERIAL PULSE WAVE ALONG THE AORTA

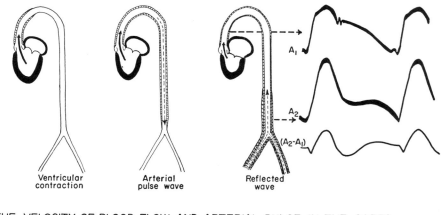

Ventricular   Arterial   Reflected
contraction   pulse wave   wave

B. THE VELOCITY OF BLOOD FLOW AND ARTERIAL PULSE IN THE AORTA

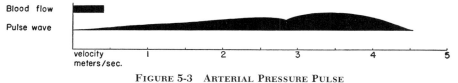

Blood flow

Pulse wave

velocity
meters/sec.

FIGURE 5-3   ARTERIAL PRESSURE PULSE

A, The arterial pressure pulse is a wave of pressure which passes rapidly along the arterial system. Blood suddenly ejected into the ascending aorta at the beginning of systole has insufficient energy to overcome all the inertia of the long columns of blood in the arteries. Therefore, blood tends to pile up and distend the ascending aorta, causing a sudden local increase in pressure. Blood is then forced into the next portion of the aorta, extending the region of distention and initiating a pulse of pressure which travels rapidly along the arteries toward the periphery. These waves of pressure, reflected by peripheral structures, travel back toward the heart and become superimposed on the advancing pulse wave. This produces a higher peak of systolic pressure, a slurring of the incisura and a lower diastolic pressure in the femoral artery. If the peripheral arterial pulse wave is subtracted from the pulse recorded at the arch of the aorta, the resulting wave form $(A_2 - A_1)$ suggests a natural frequency of the peripheral arterial system.

B, The pulse wave velocity (4 to 5 m. per second) is much faster than the velocity of blood flow (less than 0.5 m. per second). The pulse wave velocity is determined by the elasticity (compliance) of the arterial walls.

sels into the capillary networks. The geometry of the vascular bed and the visco-elastic properties of the arterial walls play important roles in conveying of blood down the long arterial channels with a minimal loss of pressure head but with a damping of the violent pressure fluctuations in the peripheral vessels.

At the onset of ventricular ejection, blood flows into the aorta faster than it leaves through the arterioles. The inertia of the long columns of blood in the arteries opposes acceleration. Blood ejected by the left ventricle

accumulates in the first portion of the aorta (Fig. 5–3A), increasing the tension in the walls of this region. The increased pressure and wall tension in the root of the aorta force blood into the adjacent segment of aorta which, in turn, is stretched and develops increased tension. In this way, a pulse of pressure moves rapidly down the aorta at a velocity which is determined by the elasticity of the walls and the pressure of the blood (Fig. 5–3B).

During the latter part of systole ventricular ejection slows, and the pressure in the root of the aorta falls.

Ventricular pressure drops rapidly to a level below the arterial pressure, and the aortic valves close.

SYSTOLIC PRESSURE

The peak systolic pressure in the central aorta is determined largely by the left ventricular stroke volume, the peak rate of ejection and the distensibility of the aortic walls. For example, the slow ejection of a small stroke volume into an easily distensible aorta produces a small elevation in systolic pressure. A rapid ejection of a large volume into a rigid aorta produces a large rise in systolic pressure, as does a normal stroke volume injected at normal velocity into a rigid atherosclerotic artery. The greatly accelerated ventricular ejection associated with sympathetic stimulation also produces greatly increased systolic pressure in the aorta (see Fig. 3–17).

DIASTOLIC PRESSURE

After ventricular systole is completed, the aortic valves are closed by a retrograde surge of blood, represented on the pressure pulse by the dicrotic notch (see Fig. 5–4). After the aortic valves snap shut, the arterial pressure gradually falls as blood flows out through the myriad of peripheral vascular networks. The rate at which the diastolic pressure falls is determined by the pressure at the end of the systolic interval, the rate of outflow through the peripheral resistances and the diastolic interval. If the next systole were delayed for 3 or 4 seconds, the arterial pressure would continue to fall, asymptotically approaching a level of about 10 mm. Hg. The minimal diastolic pressure is determined primarily by the total peripheral resistance and by the heart rate (Fig. 5–4). The pulse pressure (the

maximum systolic minus the minimum diastolic pressure) is increased by the factors that increase systolic pressure and reduce diastolic pressure.

DISTORTION OF THE ARTERIAL PULSE DURING TRANSMISSION

The form of the arterial pressure pulse changes as it passes down the arterial tree (Figs. 5–3 and 5–4). The systolic wave becomes considerably higher, is more sharply peaked and falls abruptly; the gradual decline in central diastolic pressure becomes replaced by several damped oscillations. These changes in the form of the pulse have been variously attributed to (a) pressure waves reflected from the periphery[1] or from abdominal aortic branches,[2] (b) a damping transmission line,[3] (c) the resonant frequency and damping coefficient of the arterial walls[4] and (d) highly damped steady-state oscillations. Although the exact cause has not been completely determined, it is clear that the pulse pressure becomes progressively greater as the pulse traverses the major branches of the arterial tree, so that the systolic pressure peak in the femoral or brachial arteries reaches values as much as 15 to 20 mm. Hg higher than those in the central aorta.

It is important to recognize that an increase in systolic pressure, with an increase in both pulse pressure and mean pressure, can occur without a change in peripheral resistance by three different mechanisms: (a) increased stroke volume, (b) increased ejection rate and (c) reduced arterial distensibility. These factors can be exaggerated by the distortion of the pressure pulse during its transmission to the site of measurement at the brachial artery.

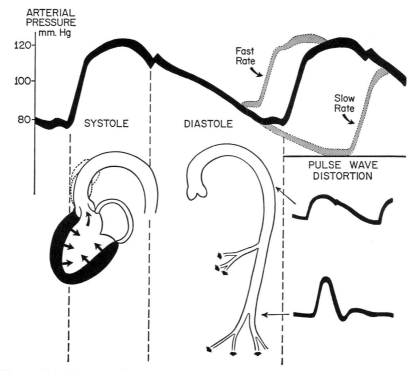

FIGURE 5-4   FACTORS AFFECTING SYSTOLIC AND DIASTOLIC ARTERIAL PRESSURE

The systolic pressure is determined primarily by the rate and volume of ventricular ejection in relation to the arterial distensibility. The diastolic pressure is determined by the rate of diastolic pressure drop (related to peripheral resistance) and the heart rate as it affects the duration of diastole. The pulse wave is distorted by damping and reflections as it travels along the arterial trunks such that the peak systolic pressure is higher and the diastolic pressure is flatter but the mean arterial pressure is only slightly less than at the arch of the aorta.

I. MEASUREMENT OF ARTERIAL PRESSURE

Measuring arterial blood pressure involves determining both the systolic and the diastolic pressure. These two pressure levels actually represent the excursions of the arterial pressure pulse at the point of measurement.

SPHYGMOMANOMETRY

Since the pulse waves rapidly spread through the arterial system and are modified to varying degrees, the arterial pressure at any instant varies throughout the arterial tree. Determinations of arterial pressure generally represent the maximal and minimal pressure of the pulse wave at the point of measurement.

The most accurate records of arterial pressure pulses are obtained through intra-arterial needles connected to suitable pressure recordings systems (see later). To reproduce the wave as it appears in the artery, the

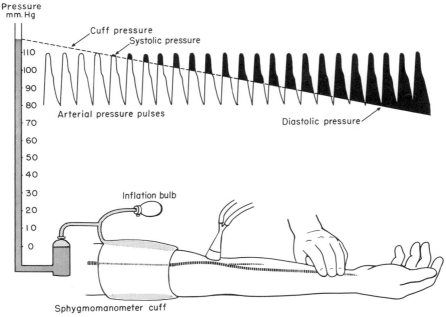

FIGURE 5-5   SPHYGMOMANOMETRY

When the pressure within the sphygmomanometer cuff is increased above arterial blood pressure, the arteries under the cuff are occluded and no pulse can be palpated at the wrist. As the cuff pressure is gradually released, the systolic peaks of pressure finally exceed cuff pressure and blood spurts into the arteries below the cuff, producing palpable pulses at the wrist. The sudden acceleration of blood below the cuff produces vibrations which are audible through a stethoscope. The pressure in the mercury manometer at the time the pulse is heard or felt indicates systolic pressure. As cuff pressure is further diminished, the sounds increase in intensity and then rather suddenly become muffled at the level of diastolic pressure where the arteries remain open throughout the entire pulse wave. At still lower pressures, the sounds disappear completely when laminar flow is re-established.

recording paper would have to move at the velocity at which the pulse travels past the needle (Fig. 5–3*B*). Since this is impractical, the records are generally obtained on paper moving relatively slowly, and the pulse waves are compressed in time (Fig. 5–5).

The arterial blood pressure is generally measured with a sphygmomanometer consisting of an inelastic cuff containing an inflatable rubber bag. The rubber bag is connected by rubber tubing to a rubber bulb and to a device which continuously records the pressure within the cuff (e.g., a mercury manometer, Fig. 5–5). When the cuff is snugly applied to the arm, inflation of the rubber bag compresses the tissues under the cuff. If the rubber bag is inflated to a pressure which exceeds the peak of the arterial pulse wave, the artery is continuously collapsed and no pulse wave can be palpated in the artery peripheral to the occlusion. If the pressure in the cuff is gradually reduced, a point will be reached at which the peak of the pulse wave slightly exceeds the pressure in the surrounding tissues and in the rubber bag (Fig. 5–5). At that level, the pulse becomes palpable and the pressure indicated on the mercury manometer is a measure of the peak of the arterial pulse or systolic pressure.

The spurt of blood flowing through the artery under the cuff rapidly accelerates the column of blood in the peripheral arterial tree, producing turbulence and distinctive sounds (Korotkoff sounds) which can be heard through a stethoscope applied over the artery just below the cuff. As the pressure in the cuff is reduced further, the difference between systolic pressure and cuff pressure progressively widens and the artery is open during a greater proportion of the time. In general, the quantity of blood surging under the cuff is similarly increased, and the sounds heard through the stethoscope tend to become louder. When the pressure in the cuff falls below the minimal pressure of the arterial pulse wave, the artery remains open continuously and the emitted sounds become muffled because the blood flows continuously and the degree of acceleration of the blood by the pulse wave is suddenly reduced. At still lower cuff pressures, the sounds disappear altogether as laminar flow is re-established.

Origins of Korotkoff Sounds. In his original publication, Korotkoff[6] described two distinct types of sounds heard over the brachial artery as the pressure was reduced in a pressure cuff above the elbow. The first "short tones" appear with passage of part of the pulse wave under the cuff. With further fall in the pressure, the "systolic compression murmurs" are heard, which pass again into "tones (second)." An experimental analysis of the mechanisms of production of these sounds[7] indicated that the first "short tones" or tapping sounds were due to acceleration transients produced by abrupt arterial wall distension as a jet of blood surged under the cuff into the distal artery. The "compression sound" appeared to stem from the turbulent jet distal to the compressed arterial segment. Criteria for measurement of

arterial pressure appear to be largely dependent upon the appearance of the acceleration transient (systolic pressure) and its disappearance to produce the characteristic muffling (diastolic pressure).

Sources of Error in Measuring Arterial Pressure. Significant errors in arterial blood pressure readings result from improper selection or application of sphygmomanometer cuffs.[8, 9] The pressure which exists in the rubber bag is transmitted to the greatest depth at the center of the cuff. If the cuff is sufficiently wide and is properly adjusted, the pressure indicated by the manometer extends to the tissues immediately surrounding the artery (Fig. 5–6A). However, if the limb is too thick in relation to the width of the cuff, the pressure around the artery may be significantly less than that recorded from the rubber bag (Fig. 5–6B). Under these conditions, the cuff pressure required to collapse the artery must exceed the pressure which exists in the artery at that point. Thus, the systolic (and diastolic) pressure readings will be too high. If the cuff is loosely applied (Fig. 5–6C) so that the rubber bag must be partially inflated before it exerts pressure on the tissues, the area of contact is seriously reduced, corresponding to a very narrow cuff.

The Auscultatory Gap. In some patients, the sounds emitted from the artery below the cuff disappear over a fairly large range in pressure between the systolic and diastolic pressures. The cause of this auscultatory gap is not known. If the cuff pressure is increased only to levels within the range of the auscultatory gap, the pressure at the lower end of this silent range may be mistaken for a normal systolic pressure when, in fact, the true systolic pressure is excessively high. Since the pulse wave persists in the

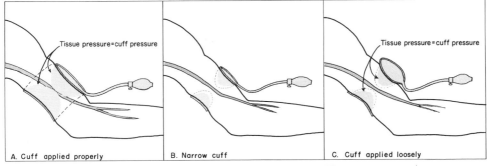

A. Cuff applied properly   B. Narrow cuff   C. Cuff applied loosely

FIGURE 5-6   TRANSMISSION OF CUFF PRESSURES TO TISSUES OF THE ARM

A, When a sphygmomanometer cuff of sufficient width in relation to the diameter of the arm is properly applied, the tissue pressure around deep arteries under the cuff equals cuff pressure. However, pressure under the edge of the cuff does not penetrate as deeply as that under the center of the cuff.

B, A cuff which is too narrow in relation to the diameter of the limb does not transmit its pressure to the center of the limb. Under these conditions, the cuff pressure must greatly exceed arterial pressure to produce complete occlusion of the artery, and erroneously high systolic and diastolic pressures will be read from the mercury manometer.

C, If a cuff of sufficient width is applied too loosely, it becomes rounded before exerting pressure on the tissues and produces the same sort of error as a narrow cuff.

range of the auscultatory gap, this source of error can be eliminated by routinely checking systolic pressure by both the auscultatory and the palpatory methods (Fig. 5–5).

Mean Arterial Blood Pressure. Since the arterial blood pressure fluctuates during each cardiac cycle, the mean arterial pressure is often used in clinical and experimental reports. The arithmetic average of the systolic and diastolic pressures would be an accurate indication of the mean arterial perfusion pressure if the arterial pressure pulse were a true sine wave (see Fig. 5–7). However, the arterial pulse wave in no way resembles a sine wave and the arithmetic average of systolic and diastolic pressures is not an accurate expression of the mean pressure. The true mean arterial pressure can be determined by damping out the pulses or by integrating the arterial pulse wave on accurate records of the pressure pulse. Vertical lines are dropped from corresponding points on arterial pulse waves to the zero pressure line. The arterial pressure pulses then correspond to a serrated upper border of a rectangular area. If the area enclosed by these lines, measured by means of a planimeter, is divided by the length of the horizontal base line (Fig. 5–7, line *L*), the quotient represents the vertical distance above the zero line (Fig. 5–7, line *H*) at which the mean arterial pressure lies. By this method the mean arterial pressure is usually about one third of the way between diastolic and systolic pressures but varies with the configuration of the arterial pulse wave.

CONTINUOUS RECORDING OF ARTERIAL BLOOD PRESSURE

Measurement of arterial blood pressures has long played an important role in cardiovascular research. Recent developments in cardiac catheterization and the pulse-contour method of

DETERMINATION OF MEAN ARTERIAL PRESSURE

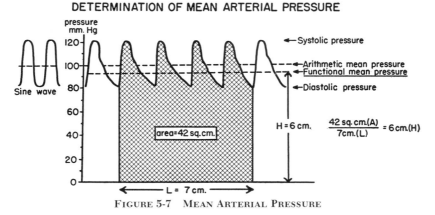

FIGURE 5-7   MEAN ARTERIAL PRESSURE

If the systolic pressure is 120 mm. Hg and the diastolic pressure 80 mm. Hg, the arithmetic mean pressure is 100 mm. Hg. If the arterial pulse wave were symmetrical (a sine wave), this value would represent the average perfusion pressure. However, the interval during which the arterial pressure is less than 100 mm. Hg is longer than that during which it is elevated above this level, so the functional mean pressure is less than 100 mm. Hg. The functional mean pressure is determined by dividing the area of the shaded region (area = 42 sq. cm.) by the horizontal dimension (L = 7 cm.) to determine the height of a rectangle having the same area (H = 6 cm.). The functional mean pressure tends to be higher than diastolic pressure by about one-third the pulse pressure, but this estimate does not apply to pulse waves having different contours, e.g., with changes in heart rate.

computing cardiac output have created widespread interest in accurately recording both pulmonary and systemic arterial pressures. Pressure transducers, suitable for recording the rapidly fluctuating arterial and intraventricular pressures, have certain essential requirements which should be understood by anyone who either uses them or wishes to appraise the multitude of clinical reports involving such equipment.

A mercury manometer is inadequate for recording pressures which fluctuate widely and rapidly, especially when the extremes of pressure are significant. The inertia of the fluid and the resistance to its flow into the manometer keep the fluid level from following the rapid changes in pressure. If a mercury manometer is connected directly to an artery through a hypodermic needle, the mercury column oscillates slightly above and below the mean pressure. The manometer obviously does not indicate the mag-

nitude of either the systolic or the diastolic pressure. The same problem arises in measuring the widely fluctuating pressures in the ventricular cavities. Thus, more complicated apparatus is required to measure arterial and ventricular pressures accurately.

Rapidly fluctuating pressures can be accurately recorded only by apparatus with an adequate frequency response. The frequency response is a measure of the rate at which a recording system responds to a sudden change in pressure. The factors which determine the responsiveness of a pressure-sensitive device can best be described in terms of simple mechanical systems.

Mechanical Pressure Transducers. A common pressure transducer consists of a tambour with a rubber membrane coupled to a writing lever. If the rubber membrane is quite flaccid, very slight pressures will stretch the membrane and displace the writing lever

MECHANICAL RECORDERS

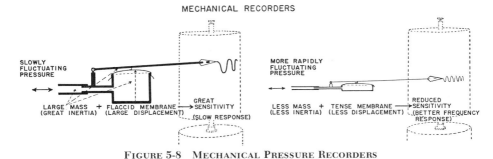

FIGURE 5-8   MECHANICAL PRESSURE RECORDERS

Pressure recording ordinarily involves the displacement of some type of elastic membrane. To displace the membrane, fluid must move into the recording capsule. The inertia of the fluid, the membrane and the recording mechanisms tends to resist displacement. When the moving mass is large and the membrane is flaccid, the recording system may be very sensitive to slowly fluctuating pressures, but will not respond to rapid changes in pressure. Reducing the moving mass and utilizing stiff membranes diminish sensitivity but improve the frequency response.

(Fig. 5–8). In response to an increased pressure, a considerable quantity of fluid must pass along the tubing and enter the tambour to produce a corresponding displacement of the membrane and writing lever. The inertia of the fluid and lever opposes a rapid response to a change in pressure, and the rubber membrane provides a relatively weak force to restore the fluid and lever to their original positions when the pressure is reduced. Clearly, such a system could not respond rapidly enough to follow the fluctuating arterial pressure. The natural frequency of a pressure transducer can be visualized in terms of a mass suspended on a spring. The smaller the mass and the stiffer the spring, the faster the oscillations which occur after a displacement from the rest position. When the mass of the fluid and of the lever is large in relation to the tension of the membrane, the oscillations are slow. If the rubber membrane is very tense, the frequency response is increased, but the sensitivity (deflection per unit of pressure) is correspondingly reduced. A more complete description of different mechanical pressure transducers was presented by Green.[10]

Electrical Pressure Transducers. In this electronic age it is not surprising that slight movements of stiff membranes should be used to affect currents or voltages which can be amplified by electronic amplifiers. Various types of electronic pressure transducers are available in which movements of membranes produce changes in (*a*) resistance, (*b*) capacitance or (*c*) inductance (Fig. 5–9*A*, *B*, *C*). In each case, stiff membranes with small fluid displacement and relatively high frequency response can be used because the output signals can be amplified enough to activate recording galvanometers of various types.

No ideal pressure recording system exists. For any particular application the transducer, amplifier and recorder must be matched to obtain optimal performance. This process invariably involves compromise of sensitivity, convenience, stability or frequency response. The nature and significance of frequency response is

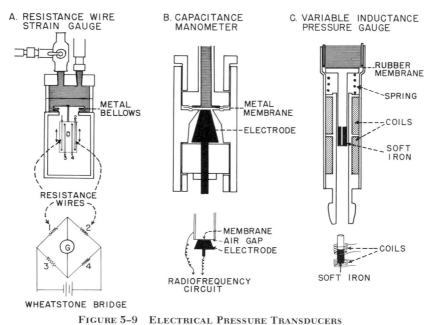

FIGURE 5–9   ELECTRICAL PRESSURE TRANSDUCERS

A, The unbonded resistance wire strain gauge (Statham gauge) consists of a metal bellows which is compressed by increased pressure within the chamber. Downward displacement of the bellows is transmitted to a metal slide supported by four sets of strain-sensitive wires wound under tension and connected to form a Wheatstone bridge. Displacement of the metal slide stretches two sets of wires and relaxes the other two. These changes in resistance imbalance the bridge in proportion to the applied pressure. The resulting voltage output from the bridge is amplified and recorded by various means.

B, The electrical capacitance diaphragm manometer is a condensor formed by an electrode (black) separated from a stiff metal membrane by a carefully adjusted air gap. Displacement of the membrane changes the thickness of the air gap. This results in a change in capacitance which is recorded by a radio frequency circuit. (From Lilly.[11])

C, Variations in magnetic flux in two coils of wire can be produced by movements of an iron slug positioned within the coils. In a differential transformer pressure transducer, the iron slug is fastened to the center of an elastic membrane so that changes in pressure produce changes in magnetic flux. (From Gauer and Gienapp, *Science*, 1950, 112:404.)

widely misunderstood even by some individuals routinely engaged in physiologic recording.

The Frequency Response of Recording Systems. It is generally agreed that a high fidelity reproduction of a wave form can be recorded by a system which has a uniform response to the tenth harmonic of its fundamental frequency. With a heart rate of 240 beats per minute, the pulse frequency is 4 per second and the tenth harmonic of this frequency is 40 c.p.s. Such a high frequency response is deemed necessary if the most rapid changes in pressure during the pulse are to be faithfully recorded.

Although it is possible to determine the frequency response characteristics of the transducer, amplifier and galvanometer individually, it is more important to test the dynamic response of the entire system assembled for use. When the transducer is connected to a fluid-filled catheter or through tubing to a hypodermic needle, the frequency response of the gauge becomes greatly reduced. The fluid in the system represents a mass which must move with changes in pressure, and its inertia markedly reduces the frequency response of the gauge. When the diaphragm is displaced by an increased pressure, its elasticity must overcome the inertia of the entire mass of fluid within the connecting tubes. The mass of fluid can be reduced by using tubing of small caliber, but only at the price of increasing the frictional resistance to movement of fluid. Thus, some of the pressure energy is dissipated as friction in fluid within narrow tubes. Increasing the frictional resistance of a system is a form of "damping." Careful matching of the frequency response of the system with an optimal degree of damping can greatly improve the response characteristics (Fig. 5–10). Damping is attained by reducing the caliber of the catheter or tube, by locally constricting the tubing with a clamp or by inserting a short section of tube with appropriate caliber.

Virtually identical arterial and ventricular pulse contours have been obtained with damped systems having uniform response to 5, 30, and 50 c.p.s.[12] The frequency response and the degree of damping of any system should be routinely established by methods indicated in Figure 5–10. Such a procedure eliminates inaccurate records caused by temporary malfunction of the system. For example, a small bubble remaining in the tubing or gauge after it is filled with fluid reduces the frequency response of the system to very low levels because air is much more elastic than the diaphragm. Additional details regarding this most important topic may be found in an excellent discussion by Fry.[13]

Artifacts from the Movement of Cardiac Catheters. Pressures from within the heart and great vessels are frequently measured through long catheters. Owing to movements of the heart, the tip of the catheter may oscillate in time with the cardiac cycle. Such movements produce artifacts which are superimposed upon the pressure pulses and often attain amplitudes equivalent to 10 mm. Hg. These motion artifacts are much more prominent when recorded with high frequency systems and are largely eliminated by using an optimally damped system responding uniformly to 5 c.p.s.[14]

The systolic and diastolic values for arterial pressure can be obtained with reasonable accuracy by a system with low frequency response, but the very rapid changes in pressure are generally slurred. With increasing interest in the dynamic properties of ventricular ejection (see Figs. 3–17 and 3–18), the rates of change of pressure as indicated by the slopes are assuming great importance. For example, Shaper et al.[15] emphasized that the maximum rate of change of left ventricular pressure in a normal resting dog varies between about 2000 and 6000 mm. Hg/sec. and under the influence of epinephrine, the upslope can reach values as high as 15,000 mm. Hg/sec. The rates of changes of pressure and flow as judged by the slopes of high fidelity records are destined to become extremely important in evaluating the dynamic performance of the ventricular myocardium in health and disease. For such purposes, recording systems must have extremely high frequency responses with proper damping and with minimal artifacts. These results can best be achieved using miniature pressure transducers located at the very tip of a cardiac catheter. These are commercially available and their clinical application will become more widespread as their cost becomes more moderate with volume production.

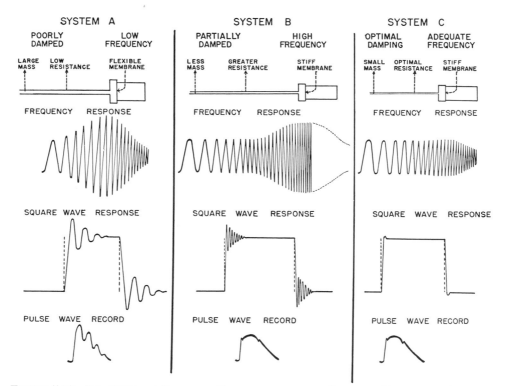

FIGURE 5-10   THE DYNAMIC RESPONSE CHARACTERISTICS OF PRESSURE RECORDING SYSTEMS

The response characteristics of a recording system should be carefully established and rechecked frequently.

System *A* has a large mass of fluid in a large caliber tube and a flexible membrane. Thus, the system is very sensitive to changes in pressure but is poorly damped. If fluctuating pressures of constant amplitude and progressively increasing frequency are applied to the end of the tube, the output from the system increases with higher frequencies up to the natural frequency of the system and then declines. The characteristics of the system can be more easily checked by suddenly raising or abruptly lowering the pressure (a square wave of pressure). In this particular system, the recorded deflection was considerably delayed in reaching the new pressure level (slow rise time). The deflection had considerable overshoot and oscillations persisted at the natural frequency of the system for a considerable time (poor damping). This system would be entirely unreliable for recording arterial pressure pulses.

System *B* has a stiff membrane and partial damping. Pressure waves of equal amplitude produced a response of uniform height over a considerable range of frequency. However, the deflections became exaggerated near the natural frequency of the system. In response to a square wave, the rise time was very short and the oscillations at the natural frequency of the system died down rather promptly. This system would be adequate for recording pressure pulses unless certain portions of the pulse had frequencies near the natural frequency of the system. The square wave response should be determined just before using such a system because a single small air bubble in the catheter or the gauge may so reduce the response characteristics that system *B* acts like system *A*.

In system *C* the membrane is more flexible than that in system *B*, but system *C* has been critically damped. In other words, the output from the system is uniform throughout a wide range of frequencies. A square wave of pressure produced a rapid response and a very slight overshoot, but no sustained oscillations. A critically damped system accurately reproduces arterial pressure pulses even though its uniform frequency response is limited to 20 or even 10 c.p.s. (From records presented by Lambert, E. H., and Jones, R. E.: *Proc. Staff Meet. Mayo Clin.*, 23:487–493, 1948.)

II. CONTROL OF SYSTEMIC ARTERIAL PRESSURE

A stabilizing mechanism must exert an overall regulation of systemic arterial pressure to prevent circulatory collapse when several major areas of the body simultaneously require increased blood flow. For example, running at full speed on a hot day after a full meal would theoretically require increased blood flow through active skeletal muscles, the skin and the gastrointestinal tract. If all these vascular beds suddenly dilated, the arterial blood pressure would drop precipitously and blood flow through vital organs (heart and brain) would be jeopardized.

ARTERIAL STRETCH RECEPTORS (PRESSORECEPTORS)

The role of receptors in the walls of cardiovascular structures in the regulation of the circulation and respiration has been studied by many investigators,[16-20] whose work has been fully reviewed by Heymans and Neil.[21] The aortic depressor nerve was discovered by Cyon and Ludwig in 1866. Since then, a great deal of information has been gathered regarding the function of neural elements in the reflex regulation of the cardiovascular system.

CAROTID SINUS

At the bifurcation of the common carotid artery into the internal and external branches there is a local dilation of the very first portion of the internal carotid artery called the carotid sinus. It has a much thinner wall than other arteries of the same size because the smooth muscle in its media is relatively sparse, particularly on the ventro-medial surface where the sinus nerve arises. In this part of the media, the smooth muscle is almost completely replaced by elastic fibers and the adventitia is fairly dense. The sensory endings in the wall of the sinus have multiple branchings like a vine (Fig. 5–11). Impulses are set off at the very fine terminations, apparently by any type of distortion. The thinning of the media seen in the carotid sinus is believed to occur at other places where such distortion receptors lie, including

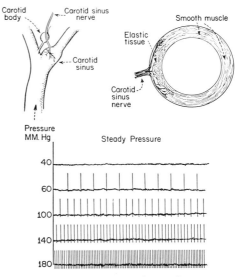

FIGURE 5-11   CAROTID SINUS STRETCH RECEPTORS

Nerve endings sensitive to stretch or distortion are located in the wall of a localized expansion at the origin of the internal carotid artery. At this site the walls contain an unusually large amount of elastic tissue and the smooth muscle of the media is somewhat deficient. Such an arrangement is particularly suited to the monitoring of pressure by these receptors, which discharge at greater and greater frequencies in response to increasing steady pressures, maintained artifically. (After Heymans and Neil.[21])

sites along the common carotid arteries, the aortic arch and the brachiocephalic artery.[21] Although these nerve endings are sensitive to any form of distortion of the wall in which they lie, they serve as pressure-sensitive elements since they are located in elastic segments of walls supporting high and fluctuating internal pressure. To be effective in regulation the receptors should monitor "absolute" arterial pressure. However, their sensitivity could theoretically be influenced by changes in the distensibility of the walls resulting from smooth muscle contraction or stiffening of the walls with aging.

Bronk and Stella[17] recorded the action potentials in single afferent nerve fibers from stretch receptors located in isolated and perfused carotid sinus. Within the sensitivity range of a receptor, an increase in distending pressure was associated with an increase in the frequency at which the receptor discharged impulses. One receptor may increase its discharge rate from zero to maximum frequency when the pressure ranges from 30 to 200 mm. Hg, and others may function within different ranges of pressure. The overlap of sensitivity between fiber groups assures responses from very low to very high pressures. If the isolated carotid sinus is distended with a steady pressure, the discharge frequency is also steady over a long period. In other words, the stretch receptors do not exhibit fatigue or adaptation. If the carotid sinus is distended by a fluctuating pressure, bursts of impulses occur during a rapid rise of pressure. Similar bursts of impulses appear during the abrupt increase in arterial pressure (Figs. 5–12 and 5–13). Thus, the discharge rate of the receptors is increased not only by the pressure in the artery but also by the rate of rise of pressure. The nerve

fibers from the stretch receptor endings in the carotid sinus travel by way of the glossopharyngeal (IXth) nerve and those from the aortic arch pass by way of the vagus (Xth) nerve to the "cardiovascular regulatory centers" in the medulla (see Fig. 3–4).

Pressoreceptor Reflexes. An increase in arterial pressure increases the rate of discharge from the stretch receptors. These impulses impinge upon the medullary centers to slow the heart by stimulating the motor nucleus of the vagus and inhibiting the "cardio-accelerator center," which acts through the cardiac sympathetic nerves. The increased sympathetic discharge also enhances atrial and ventricular contractility. At the same time, the medullary "vasoconstrictor center" is inhibited, so that the total peripheral resistance is reduced. Of all the potential mechanisms for changing peripheral resistance, the excitation or inhibition of the sympathetic vasoconstrictor outflow is the only one which has a demonstrated role in the control of arterial pressure.

Although the distortion receptors actually respond to stretch, the words "pressoreceptor" and "baroreceptor" are usually used to describe the reflexes induced by activation of these fibers. To avoid confusion, these terms will be employed in the following discussion with the reservation that they may eventually prove to be somewhat misleading.

Theoretically, the cardiovascular system can respond to an elevation in blood pressure with a reduction in heart rate, a reduction in stroke volume or a reduction in total peripheral resistance. In general, the vasomotor effects have been assigned the predominant role, and the protection of the arterial pressure level during hemorrhage has also been ascribed primarily to increased peripheral resist-

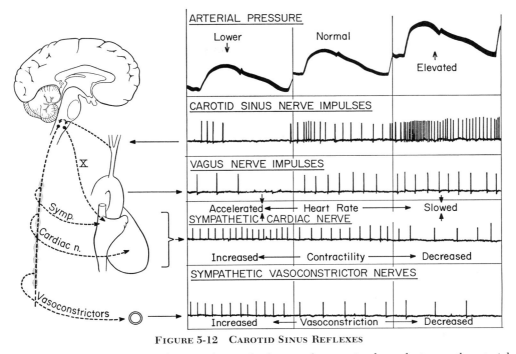

FIGURE 5-12   CAROTID SINUS REFLEXES

Single stretch receptors in the carotid sinus discharge at frequencies dependent upon the arterial pressure. When the arterial pressure is lower, the pressoreceptor impulse frequency diminishes, the vagus nerve impulses diminish and sympathetic cardiac nerve impulses increase (accelerating the heart) and the sympathetic vasoconstrictor fibers become more active and increase peripheral resistance. The net effect is to raise the blood pressure. If the arterial pressure rises above the normal set value, the impulse frequency increases on carotid sinus nerves, reducing the sympathetic discharge and increasing the vagal discharge. Slowing of heart rate and peripheral vasodilation restore the blood pressure to normal again.

ance. The growing tendency, however, is to recognize the importance of both cardiac output and peripheral resistance in such reactions. For example, Carlsten *et al.*[22] reported that direct stimulation of the carotid sinus nerve in man produced reflex bradycardia, peripheral dilation in the forearm and reduced pulse pressure—ascribed to reduced stroke volume. On the other hand, no baroreceptor effect on the pulmonary vascular system could be demonstrated.[23] This finding is consistent with the impression that the pulmonary vasculature is highly nonreactive to neural or humoral control mechanisms and does not participate in general systemic vascular responses (see Chapter 4).

The pressoreceptor mechanism illustrated in Figures 5-2, 5-12 and 5-13, acting alone, would appear to provide a simple and straightforward explanation for the maintenance of systemic arterial blood pressure within a very narrow range. Actually, the arterial pressoreceptors constitute only one of many different sources of potent influences on cardiovascular responses. Thus, the regulation of systemic arterial pressure must involve the net result of many interacting mechanisms.

Chemoreceptors.   The carotid

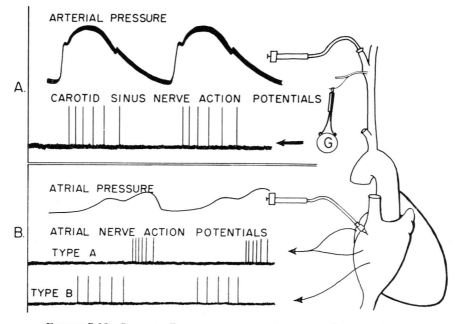

FIGURE 5-13   STRETCH RECEPTORS IN THE ATRIA AND CAROTID ARTERY

A, Individual stretch receptors in the carotid sinus discharge impulses at a frequency dependent primarily upon the arterial pressure (after Bronk and Stella[17]).

B, Stretch receptors from the atria have been divided into two groups: type A, which discharge during atrial systole, and type B, which discharge during atrial diastole (after Paintal[27]).

body, lying near the carotid bifurcation, is a reddish glomus structure which is profusely supplied with nerves and has one of the most active blood supplies in the body (equivalent to 2000 cc. per 100 gm. of carotid body tissue). The carotid bodies are stimulated by reduced oxygen, increased carbon dioxide and lowered pH in the arterial blood perfusing them. Conditions which stimulate the chemoreceptors lead to elevated systemic arterial pressure. These chemoreceptors are strongly stimulated by experimental occlusion of the carotid sinus, a fact which complicates studies of pressoreceptor mechanisms. Other chemoreceptors of similar nature are found near the aortic arch. Since the oxygen content and pH of arterial blood are diminished and its carbon dioxide content is increased only when the cardio-

vascular-pulmonary system is overtaxed or incompetent, such chemoreceptors probably have no function during normal conditions of rest. It may also be that they become involved in responses to activity only under extreme conditions.

STRETCH RECEPTORS AT VARIOUS SITES

In various experiments the results have suggested the presence of stretch receptors at many sites in the cardiovascular system including the descending thoracic aorta, abdominal vessels, cerebral vessels, lungs, atria and even the ventricular walls.[16, 24] Most of these receptors have not been implicated in the control of blood pressure. Thus, bradycardia reportedly follows distention of the left ventricular wall.[25] Rapid infusion of fluids into the systemic veins was once widely believed to be a mechanism for inducing tachycardia in association with increased venous return (Bainbridge reflex). Receptors suitable for such a response have not been found, and the original observations have not been consistently confirmed. In fact, acceleration, deceleration or no change in heart rate has recently been reported to result from intravenous infusions into isolated hearts, denervated hearts or hearts in intact animals.[26] In contrast, profound bradycardia and fainting responses, resembling the reactions induced by pressure applied to the carotid sinus in persons with hypersensitive carotid receptors, can be produced by mechanical stimulation of peripheral arteries and veins. Stretch receptors in the left atrium have been postulated as contributors to the control of blood volume. Paintal[27] has described the discharges from vagal afferent nerve fibers which fired during atrial contraction (A fibers) or during atrial filling (B fibers), as illustrated in Figure 5–13. A role for these impulses in hemodynamic regulation has not been demonstrated.

The complexity of the neural reflex mechanisms which may significantly affect the systemic arterial pressure under different conditions is illustrated in Figure 5–14. Included are the fibers from pressoreceptors and chemoreceptors, atrial afferent fibers and visceral afferents from the various organs within the abdomen and from the blood vessels throughout the body. Virtually all of these reflex actions induce lowered blood pressure and slow the heart rate. In contrast, application of cold or painful stimuli to the skin produce elevated blood pressure and tachycardia. Pathways from the higher centers of the nervous system also produce powerful vascular adaptations, associated with rage, embarrassment, fainting, and so forth. Practically all of these pathways descend through the medulla and reach the vascular system and the heart by way of the sympathetic outflow (Fig. 5–14B) plus the vagal distribution to the heart.

SUMMARY

A large number of factors and mechanisms *influence* the systemic arterial blood pressure. All the factors which affect cardiac function in terms of the heart rate, stroke volume and rate of ejection also affect the pulse pressure and, to some extent, the mean pressure. In general, the peak amplitude of the rise in systolic pressure is a manifestation of the rate and amount of systolic ejection by the left ventricle. In addition, the systemic arterial pressure is influenced by the peripheral resistance produced by all the neural, hormonal and chemical mechanisms discussed in Chapter 4. Finally, the wide variety of visceral and somatic afferent impulses converging on the medulla may significantly alter the level of the blood pressure.

Although all of these mechanisms are potentially capable of changing the blood pressure, none of them could be regarded as regulating it. Regulation of the blood pressure must involve a sensing mechanism (arterial pressoreceptors), an integrating mechanism (medullary or higher centers) and an effector mechanism (autonomic outflow), so that a deviation in arterial pressure is automatically compensated. So far as we know, only the pressoreceptor reflexes qualify as a regulatory mechanism. Such a mechanism is inherently static, tending to cause a re-

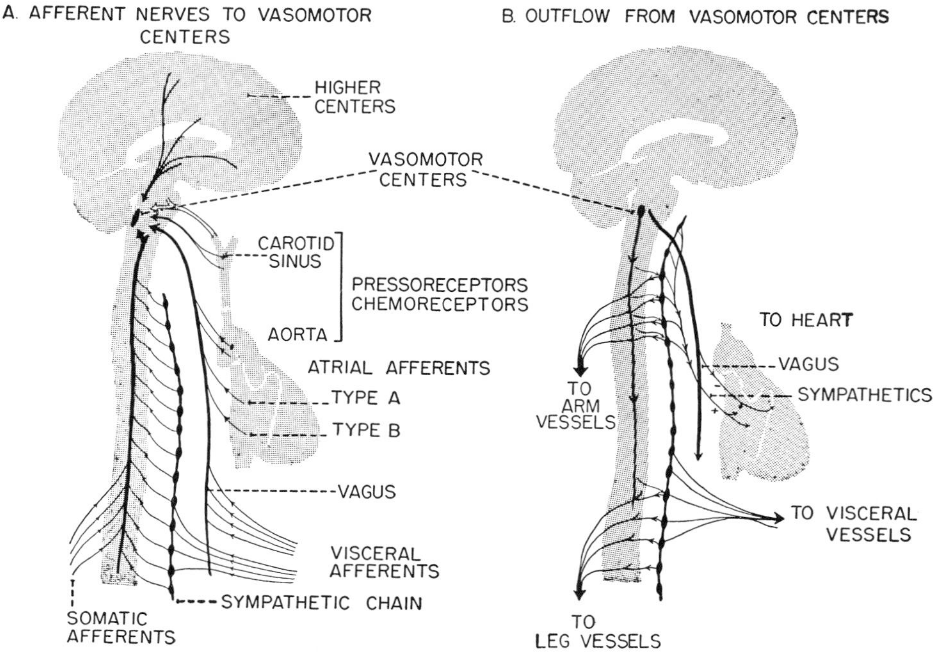

FIGURE 5-14   NEURAL MECHANISMS FOR PERIPHERAL VASCULAR CONTROL

A, The vasomotor centers in the medulla receive afferent impulses originating from many different areas in the body, including the higher centers of the nervous system, pressoreceptors from the heart and great vessels, afferent nerves from the viscera and somatic pain afferents.

B, Impulses discharged from the vasomotor centers descend the spinal cord and influence cell bodies in the intermediolateral cell column which in turn initiate sympathetic nerve impulses conducted to the blood vessels in all parts of the body.

turn to a particular level. Other factors (e.g., pain, cold, emotion) tend to produce a deviation of the blood pressure and are not known to have the sensing mechanisms required for stabilization. Whenever any of these factors causes a significant change in systemic arterial pressure, that factor must have been able to override, suppress or modify the pressoreceptor mechanism. The many mechanisms which can produce a deviation of the systemic arterial pressure from its baseline condition are unquestionably responsible for the great variation in blood pressure noted when it is repeatedly measured in one person. On the other hand, the potency of the pressoreceptor mechanism is displayed in the fact that, among most normal individuals, the blood pressure remains within a fairly circumscribed range with a fairly constant mean value. The causes of sustained variations in systemic arterial pressure should be considered from this point of view.

III. MECHANISMS OF ARTERIAL HYPOTENSION AND SHOCK

The control mechanisms which normally maintain systemic arterial pressure within a relatively narrow range despite wide variations in activity are necessarily complex. Insight into the many facets of arterial pressure regulation is provided by Figure 5–1. A failure of regulation producing low blood pressure is an important clinical problem.[28, 29] The branching representation of factors determining arterial pressure can also be employed to indicate various mechanisms which cause it to fall to abnormally low levels (right-hand column in Fig. 5–15).

The "primary" mechanisms can

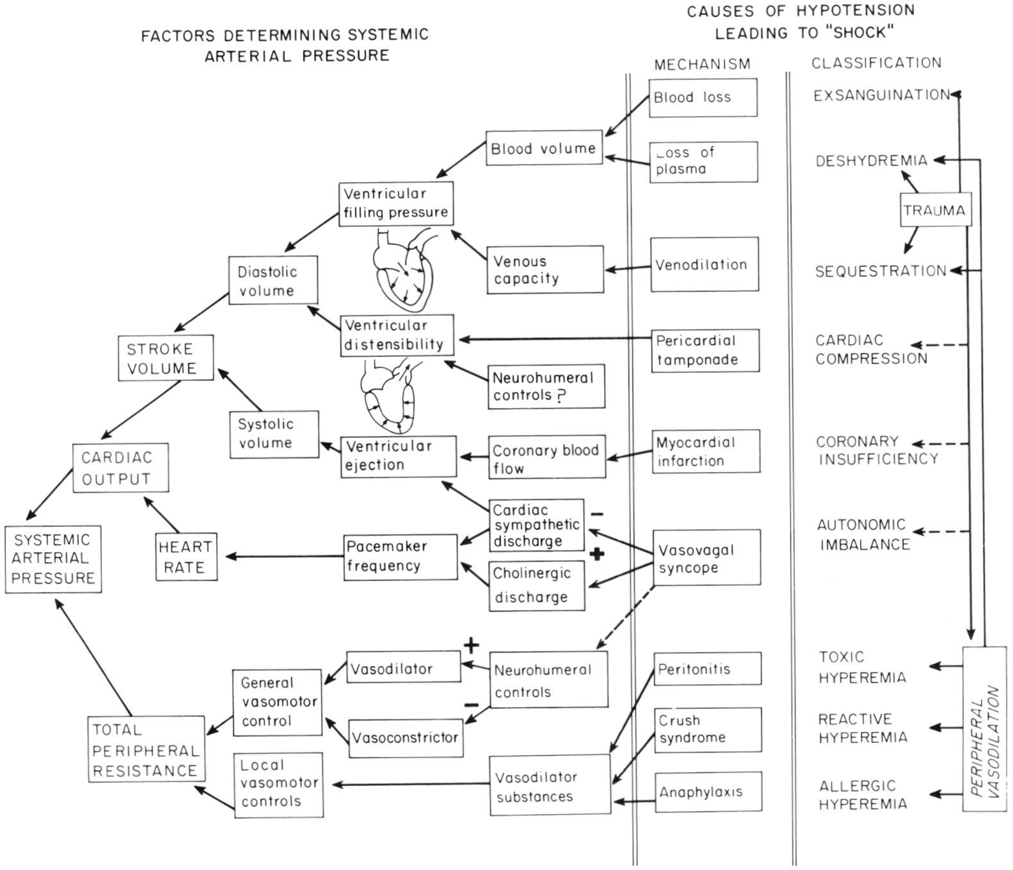

FIGURE 5-15   MECHANISMS OF ARTERIAL HYPOTENSION AND SHOCK

The various factors which determine systemic arterial pressure can be utilized as a framework for classifying causes of diminished blood pressure (hypotension) leading to a state called "shock." The mechanisms listed in the right hand column operate through the mechanisms listed to perturb the blood pressure equilibrium. Compensatory adjustments could occur theoretically at each branch point, indicating the complexity of responses even when only a single stimulus or disturbance initiated the lowered blood pressure.

affect the systemic arterial pressure only by undergoing changes that are not, or cannot be, balanced by the net effect of all the compensatory mechanisms in the chain extending from right to left in Figure 5–15. Viewed in this light, a change in any item listed under "causes of hypotension" can theoretically call forth either additive or compensatory effects among virtually all interacting factors in the chart. This does not, however, preclude identification of the initiating factors primarily responsible for the lowered blood pressure. If primary mechanisms of the sort illustrated in Figure 5–1 can ultimately be identified with specific clinical forms of shock, then an essential step in solving this complex problem can be taken by providing a group of tentative definitions of discrete forms of hypotension and shock. The classification of "shock" suggested on the right side of Figure 5–15 is intended to be only a first approximation as a basis for defining clinical disturbances of various origins.

EXSANGUINATION

The average human adult can lose somewhat more than 500 ml. of blood without significant cardiovascular disturbance, as judged by widespread experience at blood banks. If exsanguination is of such magnitude that the neural and hormonal controls fail to compensate fully, then the systemic arterial blood pressure will fall. Simple loss of blood accompanied by low blood pressure is insufficient evidence, however, to delineate exsanguination hypotension, because many people faint merely from the sight of blood. Effective criteria for the presence of exsanguination hypotension should include evidence for each step

in the functional chain of events leading from blood loss to systemic arterial hypotension in Figure 5–15. In addition, evidence for appropriate compensatory reactions should be demonstrable. Thus, a functional definition of exsanguination hypotension should include specified diminution in blood volume, ventricular filling pressure, diastolic volume, stroke volume and cardiac output. Evidence for compensatory peripheral vasoconstriction, tachycardia and increased systolic ejection (smaller end-systolic volume) would indicate that appropriate compensatory mechanisms were active.

Patients and experimental animals can survive for many hours with a mean systemic arterial pressure of 40 to 50 mm. Hg and quickly respond to restoration of the blood volume without ill effects. The term "exsanguination hypotension" should be reserved for the previously described pattern in which the blood pressure is stabilized at a low level (i.e., below a mean value of 60 mm. Hg). If the compensatory reactions begin to fail and the systemic arterial pressure is not sustained even after full restoration of the blood volume, the term "decompensating exsanguination hypotension" would appear appropriate (see *Vicious Circles in Terminal Circulatory Collapse*).

If the problem were really this simple, further research on the subject would not be needed. There is no assurance whatever that the functional definition of "exsanguination hypotension" indicated in Figure 5–15 is the correct or final one, but it is a more explicit and unique designation than is commonly employed. Some of the physiologic and semantic problems that appear during various forms of hypotension are described later.

DESHYDREMIA

The loss of large quantities of body fluids (i.e., due to cholera, burns, Addison's disease, water depletion and so forth) leads to a reduced plasma volume. Systemic arterial hypotension can also result from losses of plasma fluid into the tissues.[30] Deshydremic hypotension, characterized by increased blood viscosity and hematocrit level due to concentration of the blood cells and blood elements, theoretically can be distinguished from exsanguination hypotension with hemodilution by body fluids absorbed from the tissue spaces.

SEQUESTRATION

Nearly three fourths of the total blood volume is normally contained within the venules, venous channels and venous reservoirs. If the capacity of some large portion of the venous system suddenly increased, a substantial part of the total blood volume could be sequestered, producing effects corresponding to external blood loss. (The term sequestration is used here to denote a net increase in the quantity of blood contained within vascular channels through which forward flow may or may not persist.) For example, when a man stands, a substantial quantity of blood is displaced into his legs from the heart, lungs and upper portion of his body. During prolonged quiet standing (e.g., on parade ground) further accumulation of blood in the dependent vessels predisposes to a drop in systemic arterial pressure sufficient to cause fainting. However, sequestration of blood probably assumes far greater importance in the production of shock-like states by trauma, peritonitis or the crush syndrome (Fig. 5–15). In these conditions, sequestration probably occurs in capillaries and venules as well as in the veins and reservoirs. Lacking suitable methods of determining the amount of blood contained in various regions of the body, information concerning the incidence, significance and quantitative contribution of this mechanism is woefully inadequate.

TRAUMA

"Trauma" is a nonspecific term, and the effects of injury are so widespread and diverse that no single functional mechanism could reasonably be labeled as an initiating cause of the resulting hypotension. If blood escapes from the vascular system into the tissues or outside the body, the blood volume is diminished. Damage to capillaries may lead to loss of plasma into the tissues. Vascular distention and hyperemia in injured parts lead to sequestration of blood. In addition, hemopericardium can produce ventricular compression in some instances. Autonomic controls to heart and peripheral vessels may be disturbed by massive discharge in somatic and visceral afferent nerves. Finally, vasodilatation in the injured tissues should tend to reduce peripheral resistance. These mechanisms could contribute in various degrees to systemic arterial hypotension following injury.

CARDIAC COMPRESSION

Rapid collection of blood or fluid within the pericardial sac can be viewed as interfering with ventricular distention and preventing normal ventricular diastolic filling. Theoretically, extracardiac compression diminishes the diastolic and systolic ventricular volumes, reduces the stroke volume and lowers the cardiac output in spite of tachycardia. Systemic arterial hypotension develops when the drop in cardiac output is not adequately compensated by increased total peripheral resistance. Although pericardial tamponade may exert its effects through the same final pathway as exsanguination and sequestration, the distinction can be readily made. The total blood volume is essentially normal, and the central venous pressure should be elevated in the presence of extracardiac compression.

CORONARY INSUFFICIENCY

Acute myocardial infarction may produce severe or fatal systemic arterial hypotension by mechanisms indicated in Figure 5–15. Acute interference with the blood supply to a substantial area of the myocardium reduces ventricular ejection and the stroke volume. The infarcted myocardium not only fails to contribute to ejection, but actually expands during systole so that the effectiveness of the remaining myocardium is reduced. Under these conditions the cardiac output could be reduced in spite of increased ventricular volume and tachycardia. A full blown clinical picture of shock may then appear as compensatory mechanisms are activated in response to diminished systemic arterial blood pressure.

AUTONOMIC IMBALANCES

The sympathetic division of the autonomic nervous system directly affects the stroke volume by acting on the myocardium, affects the heart rate by acting on the pacemaker and affects the total peripheral resistance by acting on the peripheral vessels. Severe depression of arterial pressure resulting from autonomic imbalance is characterized by bradycardia and regional vasodilatation (e.g., in skeletal muscle), as though the normal baroreceptor reflexes were depressed or overridden.

The well-known syncopal reactions to carotid sinus pressure, intense visceral afferent pain or unpleasant sights exhibit transient bradycardia with peripheral vasodilatation in muscle beds. Transient autonomic imbalance frequently produces brief loss of consciousness but rarely leads to prolonged hypotension or the typical symptoms of shock. Severe disturbances of the central nervous system (e.g., head injury) may produce a shock-like state characterized by prolonged systemic arterial hypotension. The exact mechanism involved is not clear, but the importance of depression of the central nervous system in the terminal events of various kinds of shock is discussed later.

PERIPHERAL VASODILATATION

A reduction in the total peripheral resistance could be the primary mechanism producing hypotension in a number of clinical conditions. For example, peritonitis, crush injury and anaphylaxis are all characterized by extreme vasodilatation. The expected compensatory reaction to vasodilatation in one portion of the vascular system would be an appropriate increase in cardiac output, as in exercise, and vasoconstriction in other vascular areas. Severe arterial hypotension produced solely by net peripheral vasodilatation would signify that the level of cardiac output was insufficient to balance the vasodilatation. In other words, these clinical conditions should be accompained by extreme tachycardia and increased cardiac output. Sustained reduction in arterial pressure from lowered total peripheral resistance indicates either massive vasodilatation, limited compensatory vasoconstriction, or interference with a full increase in cardiac output.

VARIATIONS IN THE COURSE AND TERMINATION OF HYPOTENSION

Theoretically, effective elimination of the factor or factors that initiated the systemic arterial hypotension should be promptly followed by a return of the blood pressure to normal levels and restoration of good health. For example, exsanguination can produce an arterial hypotension lasting many hours and can be followed by a prompt return of the blood pressure to normal by restoration of the shed blood. Experience has shown, however, that most types of hypotension may be of sufficient degree and duration that deterioration and death may occur even after the apparent initiating factors are removed. Thus the condition of patients or animals suffering from protracted exsanguination hypotension may improve only transiently following restoration of the blood volume. The blood pressure returns to normal briefly and then gradually falls despite all efforts to maintain blood volume, peripheral resistance and cardiac output. This condition has been called "irreversible" shock, but should probably be considered as a group of separate entities. Just as there are many different factors capable of initiating hypotension and shock, so there are many different terminal mechanisms or pathways leading to death. An experimental example will illustrate this concept. In a healthy alert dog the mean arterial pressure was reduced to 45 mm. Hg by allowing blood to flow from the femoral artery into a reservoir slowly at first and then more rapidly (Fig. 5–16). After 2 hours about 300 ml. of blood had spontaneously returned into the dog at the same low arterial pressure. This autoinfusion was a signal of beginning cardiovas-

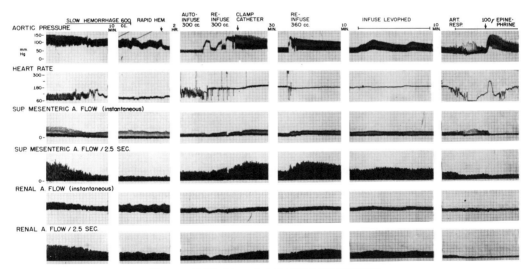

FIGURE 5-16   EFFECTS OF EXSANGUINATION

Continuous measurements of aortic pressure, heart rate and splanchnic blood flow in an intact, unanesthetized dog illustrate the effects of exsanguination (see Fig. 5–15) during a two hour period. During the period following "autoinfusion," the dog was on the brink of death from three different causes: (a) progressive fall in arterial pressure, despite restoration of blood volume, (b) respiratory arrest and (c) severe bradycardia. This example illustrates that circulatory collapse can occur from many mechanisms as suggested in Figure 5–15.

cular deterioration. An additional 300 ml. of blood was forceably reinfused, and the femoral catheter was clamped at the time indicated by the abrupt widening of the arterial pulse pressure. The arterial pressure fell progressively for 30 minutes, when the last (360 ml.) of the shed blood was reinfused. The decline persisted, but the pressure was transiently raised by the infusion of levarterenol (Levophed), without which the animal would have died from the progressive fall in pressure. Abruptly respiration ceased, but death of the animal was prevented by artificial respiration. After ventilation had been restored, the heart rate suddenly slowed, and death would surely have ensued from bradycardia had not the arterial pressure been rapidly elevated by a heroic dose of epinephrine.

The sequence of events illustrated in Figure 5–16 is representative of the common observation that the terminal patterns and final causes of death are quite variable. Prompt remedial action postponed death from one mechanism only to be followed by a different threat. In effect the animal was on the brink of death from three different causes in rapid succession: (a) progressive fall in arterial pressure in spite of restoration of blood volume and vasopressor agents, (b) respiratory arrest and (c) severe bradycardia.

Respiratory arrest might result from severe cerebral depression as indicated by other manifestations of impaired function of the brain. The animals generally remained responsive and alert until they began to exhibit autoinfusion and other signs of circulatory deterioration. Then they became unresponsive, appeared to lose consciousness and frequently exhibited depressed or absent corneal and pupillary reflexes. Severe bradycardia was a fairly common terminal event.

DEPRESSION OF CENTRAL NERVOUS SYSTEM IN TERMINAL STATES

Subnormal responsiveness or unconsciousness with sluggish reflexes has been regularly manifest when animals began to display autoreinfusion, abrupt bradycardia or respiratory arrest. In two dogs fully equipped with instruments, electrodes were chronically implanted at sites in the diencephalon where stimulation produced exorbitantly elevated heart rate and blood pressure. In these two dogs, the diencephalic sites were stimulated repeatedly during exsanguination hypotension produced in the standard manner. When autoinfusion and depression of reflexes developed, the same stimulus strength produced greatly attenuated cardiovascular response. In one of these animals, systemic arterial pressure was restored by levarterenol; the animal then lifted his head and looked around. The corneal reflex again became active and stimulation of the diencephalon again produced a response as large as during the control period. These observations were interpreted as indicating that depression of the central nervous system may be important during the terminal stages of shock, confirming the views of Ossipov[31] and Kovách and Takács.[32] The observed depression could actually occur anywhere along the relatively direct pathway from the point of stimulation to the effectors.

VICIOUS CIRCLES IN TERMINAL CIRCULATORY COLLAPSE

A reduction in blood flow through virtually all tissues is a natural result of a greatly lowered systemic arterial pressure (Fig. 5–17A). The reduced arterial pressure correspondingly di-

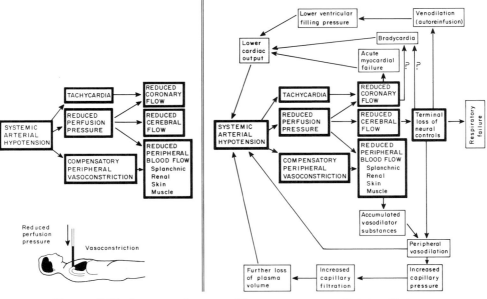

FIGURE 5-17 SYSTEMIC ARTERIAL HYPOTENSION WITH VICIOUS CYCLES

A, Some functional effects of compensation to systemic arterial hypotension include reduced coronary and cerebral blood flow as well as reduced peripheral blood flow through important visceral organs.

B, Severe and prolonged hypotension can induce vicious cycles which tend to further depress cardiac output or to induce vasodilation rendering the hypotension progressively more intractable.

minishes the arteriovenous perfusion gradient. Lower perfusion pressure tends to slow up vascular flow in every tissue, in some more than in others. The cerebral blood flow would be diminished by this mechanism primarily. In addition, a compensatory response to hypotension is a generalized vasoconstriction induced by baroreceptor reflexes. Thus, flow through the splanchnic bed, kidney, muscles and skin may be greatly curtailed. A compensatory tachycardia might also contribute to a reduction in coronary flow. No tissue would be fully spared from a diminution of blood flow.

The blood supply to the central nervous system should be adversely affected by a reduction in arterial pressure because the cerebral circulation is not very responsive to diminished blood flow. Cerebral vasodilatation is difficult to produce experimentally by neural, hormonal or chemical means except for moderate effects from increased carbon dioxide content of the blood. Thus, the cerebral blood flow is generally regarded as dependent primarily upon the perfusion pressure. A pronounced reduction in mean arterial pressure should therefore produce a corresponding reduction in cerebral blood flow (Fig. 5–17).

Respiratory arrest might result from cumulative effects of inadequate cerebral blood flow producing failure of the respiratory control centers (Fig. 5–17). On the other hand, the autoreinfusion may represent a release of the venoconstrictor tone that had caused compensatory shrinkage of venous channels and reservoirs. The relaxation of these channels could increase the capacity of the venous system and thus further diminish ventricular filling pressure and cardiac output. Abrupt appearance of bradycardia (Fig. 5–16) might signal serious autonomic imbalance from depression of the nervous system. The combined effect of lowered perfusion pressure and tachycardia could lead to acute myocardial failure with a further drop in cardiac output and lower arterial pressure.

Loss of neural controls could be expressed as a release of compensatory vasoconstriction. The resulting reduction in peripheral resistance would directly diminish arterial pressure without a further reduction in cardiac output. The compensatory constriction in peripheral vessels could be sufficiently severe and prolonged to curtail drastically flow through many vascular beds. Chemical vasodilators could accumulate and finally reach levels high enough to overcome the constrictor tone by a mechanism resembling reactive hyperemia.

The cardiovascular control could deteriorate by mechanisms like those illustrated in Figure 5–17 despite efforts at combating them. Determination of the pathways of circulatory collapse would depend upon appropriate measurements on patients in these final stages of shock. Although the difficulties involved in collecting such data are extremely severe, they must be circumvented before rational methods of therapy can be based on a full understanding of appropriate physiologic mechanisms.

SUMMARY

The first step in analyzing any clinical problem must be the identification and precise definition of the entity. An adequate definition must be based on accurate and quantitative description in terms of crucial variables. Since many of the essential variables can be measured or estimated on patients, shock can be approached in a series of logical steps for each type:

1. A discrete clinical condition currently classified under the term "shock" could be identified.

2. A specific and unique name and definition of this condition could be derived by direct and quantitative measurements of variables such as those represented in Figure 5–15.

3. The initiating factors would become apparent from these measurements.

4. The compensatory reactions that are inadequate should be distinguished from responses that are inappropriate.

5. With this knowledge at hand, a suitable model of the circulatory disturbance could be evolved and validated by quantitative measurements in experimental analysis.

6. Appropriate therapy of the defined condition could then be based on knowledge of the nature of the basic disturbance. Obviously, treatment that would effectively correct the fundamental defect from extravasation or anaphylaxis might be dangerous if applied to a patient with myocardial infarction.

7. The terminal events in fatal shock-like states can be regarded as a group of potential vicious circles that may have no obvious connection with the original cause of the systemic arterial hypotension. Effective therapy during the final stages of circulatory deterioration requires a great deal more knowledge regarding the various mechanisms of circulatory collapse than we now possess.

IV. CAUSES OF HIGH BLOOD PRESSURE (HYPERTENSION)

The cardiovascular system is equipped with a simple pressure regulating mechanism of the sort illustrated in Figure 5–2. Theoretically, such a system should ensure prompt compensation for any change in blood pressure. Such extreme stability of the systemic arterial pressure is achieved consistently in animals and men under surgical anesthesia. Under these conditions, the systemic arterial pressure remains remarkably constant over extended periods of time unless the level of anesthesia changes or external influences are introduced. The same situation is achieved in decerebrate animals, indicating that an important source of fluctuation in systemic arterial pressure stems from overriding or "resetting" of the regulating system by higher levels of the nervous system.

In normal human subjects, systemic arterial pressure diminishes more than 20 mm. Hg during sleep, reaching a minimum at 3:00 or 4:00 A.M.[33] The "basal" blood pressure has been defined as the arterial pressure present when all physical, emotional and metabolic activities are reduced to a physiologic minimum. This state is rarely achieved, so the "basal" blood pressure has been approximated with measurements made before the subject arises from a good night's sleep. This, too, is difficult to accomplish routinely, so many investigators collect their data on patients who have reclined quietly in a comfortable, soothing environment for at least 30 minutes, ten to twelve hours after the previous meal. Even under these conditions a single determination of systemic arterial pressure is almost meaningless because of fluctuations, so that average values from repeated measure-ments must be used. The emotional reaction to the act of recording the blood pressure can be alleviated by measuring blood pressure repeatedly for half an hour.[34] The difficulties involved in obtaining reproducible "basal" blood pressure values have been stressed to indicate how much caution must be used in interpreting the "casual" blood pressure recorded routinely in a physician's examining room or in a hospital.

VARIABILITY IN SYSTEMIC ARTERIAL PRESSURE

In addition to emotions, expressed or repressed, a great many factors affect the systemic arterial pressure. A complete list is beyond the scope of this book, so a few examples will have to suffice.

1. Technical Errors. The values obtained by sphygmomanometry may be in error for a number of reasons including the width of the cuff, the method of applying it, the position of the arm in relation to heart level, the rate of pressure release and the subjective nature of the end points (see Fig. 5–6).

2. Posture. Assumption of the erect posture usually produces a transient reduction in systolic pressure and a more sustained increase in diastolic pressure, with a reduction in pulse pressure (see Chapter 7).

3. Exercise. Physical exertion generally induces an increase in both systolic and pulse pressures. These increases may persist for varying periods after the termination of the exertion.

4. Eating. Ingestion of a large

meal is usually followed by a significant increase in systolic pressure.

5. Diurnal Variation. From early
morning until dinner time, the blood
pressure tends to rise progressively by
about 15 to 20 mm. Hg.

6. Temperature. In warm wea-
ther the blood pressure tends to diminish somewhat.

7. Race. Chinese, Filipinos,
Puerto Ricans, East Africans, Indians,
Arabs and aboriginal Australians seem
to have lower blood pressure than do
North American or Western European
peoples.

8. Weight. The blood pressure
tends to increase with greater body
weight. The incidence of patients with
"high" blood pressure is greater among
groups that are overweight.

9. Sex. The blood pressure is
lower among women under 40 years of
age and higher in women over 50 years
of age than in men in the corresponding age groups.

10. Age. Both systolic and diastolic arterial pressures increase with
age, so that different standards must be
established for the various age groups
(see Figure 5–18).

Additional discussion of these fac-
tors appears in the excellent texts by
Master et al.,[33] Smirk,[34] Pickering[35] and
Page.[36]

HOW HIGH IS HIGH?

The "normal" arterial blood pressure is commonly said to be 120/80
mm. Hg. This statement is clearly
meaningless from a practical point of
view if one considers all the causes of
variability listed previously and described in the first part of this chapter
(see also Chapter 4). The commonly
accepted upper limit for normal blood
pressure, 140/90 mm. Hg, has been
established largely by life insurance

companies during the past four dec-
ades. Actually, single values for the
upper limits of systolic and diastolic
pressure are unacceptable because
they fail to take into account the
sources of variability.

The problem of physiologic variability is most effectively approached
by statistical methods, based on frequency distribution. Master and his
colleagues[33] proposed new and
broader limits for the range of normal
blood pressure after studying 15,706
persons in 11 industrial plants. A frequency distribution curve of diastolic
and systolic pressures was established
for each five-year group of men and
women. A sample frequency distribution for men 40 to 44 years old is
shown in Figure 5–18A. The mean
value for systolic pressure was 130
mm. Hg. The normal range was arbitrarily set to include 40 per cent of the
subjects above and 40 per cent of the
subjects below the mean. By definition, 80 per cent of the population was
considered "normal." The borderline
range included the next 7.5 per cent of
all observations, and the remaining
values (2.5 per cent) above the borderline were regarded as "abnormally
high blood pressure." Note that this
partitioning arbitrarily defines "high
blood pressure" as the values found in
the top 2.5 per cent of each group in
Figure 5–18. The ranges of "normal,"
"borderline" and "abnormal" for men
are presented in Figure 5–18; the
ranges for women are quite similar.

The progressive rise in mean
values and borderline ranges in the
older age groups is interpreted as a
tendency for blood pressure to increase with age. However, some individuals may have little or no increase in systemic arterial pressure
with advancing age, and others may
develop high pressures more rapidly
than indicated by these figures. Pick-

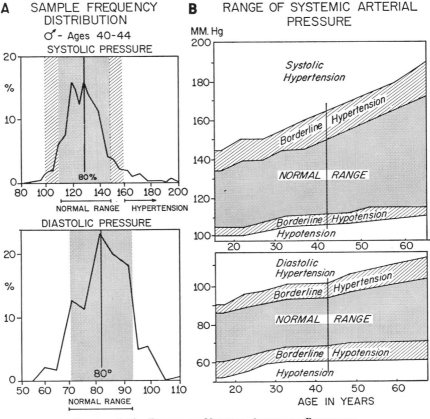

A SAMPLE FREQUENCY DISTRIBUTION

♂ - Ages 40-44

B RANGE OF SYSTEMIC ARTERIAL PRESSURE

FIGURE 5-18   RANGE OF NORMAL ARTERIAL PRESSURE

A, In males age 40 to 44, the normal arterial blood pressure is generally described in terms of range of values which will include a major portion of normal subjects (80 per cent in this graph). The "normal systolic pressure range" extends from 110 to 150 mm. Hg. Abnormal blood pressure is defined as extending above and below some borderline range.

B, Assembling the frequency distributions for various age groups demonstrates a distinct tendency for broadening of the normal systolic and diastolic pressure ranges and a tendency for higher pressures in older people. This fact must be considered in defining "high blood pressure" or hypertension.

ering[35] directed attention to the fact that the individuals with high blood pressure represent only the upper end of the frequency distribution curves and not a separate group or population. He also presented observations indicating that when high blood pressure had existed for a long time, it is not necessarily completely reversed when the original causative lesion is removed. This led him to query whether hypertension tends to produce persistent changes in vascular walls.

Since the mean systemic arterial pressure increases with age in a sample population, the number of people with blood pressures over some arbitrary level (e.g., 140/90 mm. Hg) is very great indeed. In many persons the blood pressure fluctuates more widely and tends to rise more rapidly than in the general population. In a small percentage of these people, elevation of blood pressure is obviously or suggestively associated with a recognizable disease state. However, in a vast majority of them the development of "hypertension" cannot be explained at present. In this last large category the elevated blood pressure is called "primary" or "essential" hypertension, signifying that it seems to arise without a distinctive or recognizable cause.

HYPERTENSION ASSOCIATED WITH SPECIFIC DISEASE PROCESSES

Elevated systemic arterial pressure is not a disease state; it is one sign (among many) which is common to a variety of physiologic and pathologic conditions. From the vast pool of individuals displaying this sign, a few patients may be identified in whom the elevated arterial pressure is the direct result of a specific cause and can be alleviated by removal of that cause (Fig. 5–19). A rare form of tumor consisting of chromaffin cells like those in the adrenal medulla (pheochromocytoma) provides an exceptionally good example.

ADRENAL GLAND DYSFUNCTION

Pheochromocytoma. Chromaffin cells in the adrenal medulla and elsewhere in the body normally secrete norepinephrine and *l*-epinephrine. When chromaffin cells multiply to produce a tumor or adenoma, these catechol amines are released periodically into the circulating blood to produce bouts of severe symptoms consisting of mounting hypertension, palpitation, headaches, anxiety and tremor, nausea, vomiting, blanching and coldness of the skin—in short, the signs and

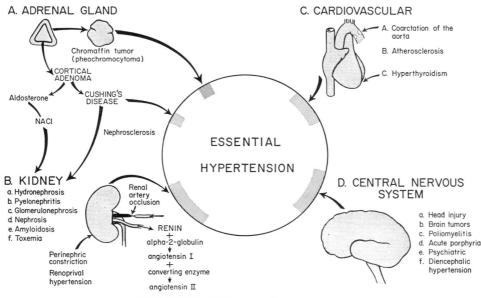

FIGURE 5-19   ESSENTIAL HYPERTENSION

Elevation of the systemic arterial pressure is a common feature in many different disease processes involving the adrenal glands, kidneys, brain and cardiovascular system (see text). Of the very large population with elevated systemic arterial pressure, only a small proportion have these specific disease processes. The very large remainder are defined as having "essential hypertension" which means that its cause is undetermined.

symptoms of a massive release of sympathetic transmitter substances. The blood pressure is elevated intermittently and tends to return toward normal in the intervals between attacks. These attacks may last for minutes or days and induce severe exhaustion. In some patients the blood pressure fluctuates widely but remains persistently elevated. The signs, symptoms, duration, course, diagnostic tests and treatment are discussed in detail elsewhere[34-36] and will not be considered here. Suffice to say that complete removal of the chromaffin tumor abolishes the symptomatic attacks. In some patients in whom the attacks have been eliminated by surgery, the systemic arterial pressure remains elevated for reasons which are not at all clear. The persistence of elevated blood pressure after elimination of its cause leads to the concept that hypertension begets hypertension (see later).

Adrenal Cortical Tumors. Changes in the blood pressure are consistently observed in patients with diseases affecting the adrenal cortex. For example, hypertension occurs in about 85 per cent of patients with Cushing's syndrome—an adrenogenital syndrome resulting from excessive secretion of adrenocortical hormones and consisting of sexual precocity, hemaphroditism, virilism of females or feminization in males and obesity. The elevated blood pressure is the most important cardiovascular manifestation of the disease. The incidence of hypertension is also high in patients with cortical adenomata but without the other signs of Cushing's syndrome.[34] At present it is impossible to identify the abnormality in cortical steroid metabolism which is responsible for the hypertension. Administration of desoxycorticosterone acetate (DOCA) produces hypertension in rats; the hypertensive effect of this hormone is accentuated by the administration of salt.[37] The same results can be achieved in human subjects. As might be expected, diminished function of the adrenal cortex (Addison's disease) is characterized by diminished systemic arterial pressure.

The potentiating effect of sodium chloride administered along with adrenal cortical hormones suggests a role for aldosterone in the induction of hypertension. Aldosterone, one of the steroid hormones normally excreted by the adrenal cortex, acts on the kidney tubules to induce retention of sodium and accelerated excretion of potassium. A few patients with primary aldosteronism resulting from tumors of the adrenal cortex have been described, and in most of them the systemic arterial pressure was above normal levels. Moser and Goldman[38] summarized a sequence following the narrowing of a main renal artery producing decreased perfusion pressure in the affected kidney and a release of renin from specialized cells within the afferent glomerular arteriole (juxtaglomerular apparatus). Renin acts on a protein substrate to produce angiotensin I which is converted into angiotensin II by an activator or converting enzyme. Angiotensin II stimulates the adrenal cortex to elaborate aldosterone which in turn causes retention of sodium and water, adding to the increase in blood pressure by a volume effect. This postulate is mentioned to indicate the degree of complexity one may encounter in such a biological control system as blood pressure regulation.

The precise mechanism by which salt excess might be linked to the development of systolic hypertension remains obscure. No single hypothesis satisfactorily explains the many conflicting observations. For example, in rats fed very large quantities of sodium chloride there is an elevation of blood pressure which correlates well with the percentage of sodium chloride in the diet.[39] Furthermore, the pathologic changes seen in rats with severe salt-induced high blood pressure resembled those observed in human patients with malignant hypertension, and the life expectancy of the animals was materially reduced. However, administration of potassium chloride along with the excess sodium chloride ameliorated the hypertension and pathologic changes, extending the life expectancy. Whereas most patients with excessive production of aldosterone exhibit elevated systemic arterial pressure, those who experience intermittent aldosteronism associated with periodic paralysis are no more susceptible to hypertension than the population at large. To confound the problem even more, hypertension can also be induced by administration of the cortical hormones which influence metabolism of glucose rather than salt, and this effect may actually be enhanced if the salt intake is reduced. Skelton[40] demonstrated that hypertension can be induced in the presence of hypofunction of the adrenal gland. For example, if one adrenal gland is excised and the medulla and most of the cortex is removed from the other, hypertension is more readily induced during the regeneration of the cortical tissue than when the regenerating gland is removed.

The kidney obviously plays an important role in the action of mineralocorticoids and in the retention or elimination of electrolytes. Thus, it is not possible to dissociate the adrenal cortical effects from kidney function. Furthermore, administration of excessive amounts of such cortical hormones leads to widespread lesions in arterial

walls within the kidney (nephrosclerosis) and pathologic degeneration of renal substance. Such changes are also prominent in Cushing's disease. Attention has therefore been directed to participation of the kidneys in provoking elevated systemic arterial pressure.

KIDNEY DISEASES

More than 100 years ago Richard Bright recognized a relation between protein in the urine and pathologic changes in the kidney with hypertrophy of the left ventricle attributable to changes in the "quality" or composition of the blood which led to constriction of the small vessels. This remains a fair description of increased peripheral resistance associated with altered kidney function.

The systemic arterial pressure is elevated during a wide variety of kidney diseases — in fact nearly all. A few of these disorders are indicated in Figure 5-19.

Interference with the arterial blood supply to the kidney or external compression of the renal parenchyma may be associated with elevated systemic arterial pressure. For example, the systemic arterial pressure may increase in patients with unilateral obstruction of the renal artery or its branches. Such lesions are commonly caused by encroachment upon the arterial lumen by local mural thickening (atherosclerosis) or by local constriction of the vessel. In a majority of such patients, successful elimination of the obstruction or excision of the affected kidney is curative. Such recovery provides strong evidence that the kidney itself is involved in the production of this form of hypertension. The number of patients with these disorders is relatively small, but they represent the counterpart in man of the experimental hypertension which Goldblatt produced years ago by graded constriction of the renal arteries of animals. It is now generally agreed that any mechanism which interferes with the blood supply to the renal parenchyma may be expected to cause elevation of systemic arterial pressure.

The renal pressor mechanism is believed to be activated by many different forms of kidney disease, most of which can be presumed to disturb renal blood flow by one means or another. Included among these disorders are hydronephrosis, pyelonephritis, glomerulonephritis, nephrosis, amyloidosis and toxemia of pregnancy. For example, obstruction of the ureter (e.g., by kidney stones) leads to expansion of the pelvis and compression of the kidney parenchyma. Pyelonephritis is stated to produce obliteration and destruction of the medium-sized renal arteries; atherosclerotic occlusion of the renal arteries may or may not be complicated by pyelonephritis. Glomerulonephritis, an inflammatory reaction in the kidney usually following streptococcal infections, causes obstruction of glomerular capillaries.

By a different mechanism, excision of both kidneys leads to a severe increase in systemic blood pressure. This increase is best demonstrated when the survival of experimental animals is being supported by means of artificial kidneys. This form of hypertension ("renoprival" hypertension) is distinctly different from that produced by the renin mechanism and is probably more closely related to the electrolyte metabolism normally involving both the kidneys and the adrenal cortical hormones. Such hypertension may be encountered in terminal states of renal disease.

CARDIOVASCULAR HYPERTENSION

Systemic arterial pressure may rise as a result of changes within the cardiovascular system itself. The cardiovascular disorders causing elevated blood pressure are exemplified by coarctation of the aorta, generalized atherosclerosis of the systemic arteries and periarteritis nodosa (Fig. 5-19).

Near the site of the ductus arteriosus a constriction of the thoracic aorta occasionally occurs as a developmental defect. This local constriction reduces the lumen of the aorta to a very small channel and greatly impedes the flow of blood from the arch to the descending thoracic aorta. Collateral channels develop around this obstruction, but blood pressure is usually far above normal in the systemic arteries arising above the constriction. In the past, this hypertension in the upper part of the body was attributed to interference with the blood supply to the kidneys, as indicated in the preceding section. However, an occasional patient develops such an obstruction below the renal arteries and still displays hypertension.[34] Moreover, the diastolic pressure in the lower extremities may be higher than normal. Surgical correction of the aortic constriction is followed by a prompt fall of blood pressure, which returns to normal over a few days.

DISEASES OF THE CENTRAL NERVOUS SYSTEM

Elevated blood pressure is associated with diverse pathologic and functional disturbances of the central nervous system such as head injury, brain tumors, selective destruction of brain tissue as in rare cases of poliomyelitis, acute porphyria, psychiatric disturbances, cardiovascular hyperreaction and disturbances of the pressoreceptor mechanism (Fig. 5–19). This list by itself indicates that hypertension can result from damage to selected portions of the central nervous system or from overactivity of other regions. To illustrate these conditions, a few will be described briefly.

Increased Intracranial Pressure. Head injuries or strategically placed brain tumors may lead to a rise in the pressure of the cerebrospinal fluid surrounding the central nervous system. Under these conditions, the systemic arterial pressure tends to increase as the cerebrospinal fluid pressure rises. This consequence is commonly attributed to compression of the brain stem in the medullary regions which contain centers of cardiovascular regulation.[34]

Destructive Lesions. Some patients with acute poliomyelitis involving the brain stem (bulbar paralysis) develop severe hypertension; the lesions lie in the medial portion of the medullary reticular substance. In general, the hypertension is transient.

Occasionally severe mental disturbances are combined with neural lesions resulting from peripheral neuritis and ascending myelitis. Examination of the urine discloses excessive excretion of porphyrin as a result of abnormal pigment metabolism. Such patients are prone to display disturbances of autonomic function (vomiting, constipation, cramping abdominal pain) as well as hypertension with tachycardia. The hypertension appears and subsides in relation to the psychoneurotic behavior.

Psychiatric Disturbances. Widespread recognition of the fact that excitement and other psychologic factors may greatly influence the level of systemic arterial pressure has led many investigators to examine the incidence of hypertension among patients with neuroses or psychoses. The results are not clear-cut because conflicting evidence has been obtained by different approaches. However, the consensus of current opinion is a conservative or doubtful attitude toward this mechanism as a dominant cause of chronic hypertension.

Diencephalic Syndrome. A labile form of hypertension associated with blotchy flushing of the face and upper chest, cold pale extremities, tachycardia and hyperperistalsis may be induced by embarrassment and excitement in young and middle-aged women. This group of symptoms and signs has been termed the "diencephalic syndrome" because it can be brought on by diffuse stimulation of the human diencephalon.

Patients with hypertension related to disturbances of the nervous system frequently display tachycardia and increased cardiac output. In patients with diseases of the adrenal glands, kidneys or cardiovascular system, on the other hand, the hypertension is generally the result of increased peripheral resistance with little or no increase in heart rate or cardiac output. This distinction should be kept in mind when attempting to assign a cause to hypertension of unknown origin.

Surprisingly enough, the wide variety of causes of elevated systemic arterial pressure discussed are responsible for a very small proportion of the cases of abnormally high blood pressure. The remainder represents patients with "primary" or "essential" hypertension (Fig. 5–19).

ESSENTIAL HYPERTENSION

The causes of sustained hypertension can be identified in only about 5 to 10 per cent of such patients; the remaining 90 to 95 per cent are generally classified as having "essential" or "primary" hypertension (see Fig. 5–19). A more realistic term would be "hypertension of undetermined origin."

THE NATURE OF ESSENTIAL HYPERTENSION

Essential hypertension is a term applied to high blood pressure which cannot be attributed to a specific lesion. Since blood pressure rises progressively with age—faster in some individuals than in others—the patients with essential hypertension are those at the high end of the frequency distribution curves for each age. Inheritance, environment and sex may affect the rate at which the blood pressure rises. In general, the higher the blood pressure, the shorter the life expectancy. Headache and vertigo are common complaints of such patients and cerebral vascular accidents (strokes) are frequent complications. The elevated systemic arterial pressure leads to left ventricular hypertrophy. Since vascular disease may interfere with coronary blood supply, congestive heart failure occurs frequently in later stages.

In most patients with benign hypertension, the blood pressure fluctuates more widely than normal, but rises progressively and slowly over many years. In a small percentage of such patients, the hypertension becomes "malignant" or rapidly progressing. Characteristic vascular changes in the retina of the eye (hypertensive neuroretinopathy) appear early in this phase of the disease, and kidney function often becomes rapidly impaired. Patients with malignant hypertension have a very limited life expectancy, usually succumbing within a few months but occasionally surviving one or two years. Left ventricular failure or cerebral vascular accidents may cause death before renal failure becomes fully developed.

CAUSES OF ESSENTIAL HYPERTENSION

The problem of establishing the cause of "essential" hypertension is comparable to attempting to determine the origin of fever in a group of patients after all known causes have been specifically eliminated. A great deal of effort has been expended in attempts to determine which of the mechanisms illustrated in Figure 5–19 might be responsible for such hypertension. The search for renal hypertension without renal disease, adrenal hypertension without adrenal dysfunction, vasomotor hypertension without central nervous system abnormality and cardiovascular hypertension without cardiovascular lesions has provided much controversy and semantic confusion but has shed little light on the subject at hand.

Exclusion of Standard Mechanisms. During the early stages of essential hypertension none of the hypertensive mechanisms illustrated in Figure 5–19 can be shown to be operative. Electrolyte metabolism and excretion are entirely within normal limits. Renal blood flow and function are normal, and the extent of atherosclerotic lesions is not greater than that among patients with normal blood pressure. The presence of neural lesions cannot be demonstrated.

Although there is considerable evidence that angiotensin may be involved in certain spontaneous and experimental hypertensive states, it seems doubtful that this mechanism is the common exciting cause of "essential" hypertension for several reasons. During the early phases of moderate hypertension in younger persons, the kidneys appear to be entirely normal functionally and anatomically. Dogs with moderate hypertension from unilateral renal ischemia may have no evident renal vascular disease in the other kidney. Abnormal amounts of renin have not been found consistently in human patients with primary hypertension. Finally, patients with congestive heart failure may have easily demonstrable increases in the amount of renin in the plasma without having hypertension. Thus it is difficult to believe renin in *undetectable* concentrations in the plasma of hypertensive patients is the cause of their high blood pressure. One of the most confusing elements in the puzzle stems from evidence that hypertension is self-perpetuating.

Hypertension Begets Hypertension. Since patients with "essential" hypertension exhibit no identifiable cause of it, the therapy of it has been largely directed toward reduction of the blood pressure by various means. Without casting doubt on the wisdom or success of this approach, one should recognize that the implied basis of this therapy is that elevated systemic arterial pressure acts in some manner to produce even greater increases in this pressure. It is true that the elevation of the systemic pressure produced by several experimental procedures may persist after the exciting cause has been removed. One explanation of this phenomenon depends upon the pronounced tendency toward development of degenerative lesions in the walls of the renal blood vessels. According to one view, this "nephrosclerosis" impedes blood flow through the renal parenchyma, exciting the renin mechanism so that the amount of circulating angiotensin II increases and produces generalized vasocon-

striction. Theoretically, then, elevated systemic arterial pressure from any cause would become self-sustaining though the development of nephrosclerosis and the original cause might disappear, effectively confounding investigators. Experimental hypertension induced by neural mechanisms (section of the carotid sinus nerves or chronic stimulation of sympathetic nerves) is not generally associated with renal lesions, nor is this type of hypertension self-perpetuating. Another mechanism for self-sustaining hypertension could be related to resetting of the pressoreceptor mechanism.

Reseting the Pressoreceptor Mechanism. Kubicek et al.[41] produced arterial hypertension which was sustained over several weeks (up to 38 days) by continuous electrical stimulation of the splanchnic nerves. Within 20 hours of sustained stimulation the systemic arterial pressure rose significantly; but the pulse rate was normal, indicating that the pressoreceptor mechanism was no longer attempting to compensate. As soon as the stimulation was interrupted, the blood pressure began to fall toward the control level and the heart rate accelerated. In other words, the pressoreceptor mechanism had been reset to the new higher level and was acting to oppose the fall of pressure. This resetting could occur at the cardiovascular control centers in the central nervous system or at the peripheral receptors in the carotid sinus.

Interestingly enough, McCubbin et al.[42] demonstrated that the frequency at which carotid sinus stretch receptors discharged in response to a given pressure was clearly lower in chronically hypertensive dogs than in normal animals (Fig. 5–20). In other words, the peripheral pressoreceptors themselves apparently can adapt to a sus-

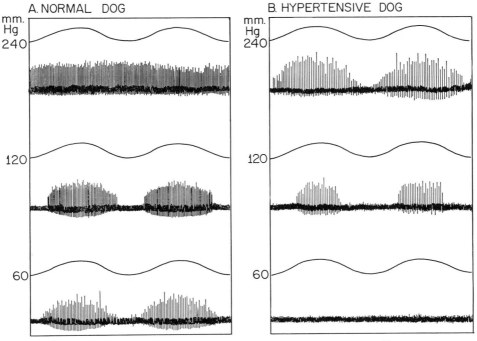

FIGURE 5-20   CAROTID SINUS SENSITIVITY IN HYPERTENSIVE DOGS

The frequency of discharge of carotid sinus stretch receptors was recorded during induced pressure fluctuations at various mean pressure levels in normal control dogs and in dogs with chronic renal hypertension. The carotid sinus discharge frequency at the same pressure levels was much lower in the hypertensive dogs suggesting reduced sensitivity of the pressure monitoring system. (After McCubbin, Green and Page.[42])

tained increase in arterial pressure, with only a slight lag. The adapted pressoreceptor mechanism would act to sustain the pressure at the higher level to which it had been reset rather than to compensate toward "normal." Adaptation of the integrating centers in the nervous system might also occur. The concept of resetting of the pressoreceptor mechanism is not a wholly satisfactory explanation of the sustained elevation of systemic arterial pressure because the blood pressure does tend to return to normal levels over longer periods of time when the stimulus to neurogenic hypertension is removed. A more sustained depression of carotid sinus pressoreceptor activity would result from pathologic changes in the walls of the vessels that would restrict their distensibility.

Atherosclerosis of the Carotid Sinus.   The carotid sinus region is a site of predilection for atherosclerosis.[43] This has been recognized since Burns first described the condition in 1811. Pathologic thickening and even calcification may occur here when other portions of the arterial tree are relatively unaffected. Such changes may begin at relatively early ages (as young as 19 years). If the wall of the carotid sinus is stiffened by this process, the amount of stretch in the wall for a particular pressure range would be reduced, curtailing the stretch on the distortion receptors in the wall. Under these conditions, the nerves might still be quite responsive to external compression and yet display greatly reduced discharge frequency from changes in internal pressure.

Generalized Vasoconstriction. Theoretically, the mean arterial blood pressure would be doubled if half of the vascular channels were completely closed or if the circumference of all the resistance vessels were reduced by only about 20 per cent. Generalized reduction in circumference is more effective than a decrease in the number of *channels* open because the pressure gradient and resistance to flow are related to the reciprocal of the radius to the fourth power $(1/r^4)$ in accordance with Poiseuille's law (see Fig. 1–6). In blood vessels with appreciably thick walls, the reduction in external circumference would be even less and would most certainly be imperceptable without the most meticulous quantitative measurements. Several mechanisms might be involved in a generalized vasoconstriction sufficient to induce hypertension.

The administration of norepinephrine or nitroglycerin produces a greater response in hypertensive patients but its duration is the same as in normal subjects. This observation led Conway[44] to conclude that the increased reactivity might result from structural changes in the arterial wall. Furthermore, some of the increased resistance in hypertensives was not overcome by nitrite, indicating that the vessels could not dilate as greatly as could those in normal subjects. Gaskell[45] found that abnormally high vascular tone persisted in the vessels of the finger after digital nerve block in patients with persistent hypertension. This tone was attributed to an "abnormal force" exerted by the vascular smooth muscle not under the immediate control of the nervous system.

Hypertrophy in the medial layers of the arterial walls is a prominent feature in the resistance vessels of patients with hypertension. Such hypertrophy might result from repetitive or continuous exposure to elevated internal pressure or from intermittent increases in sympathetic constrictor nerve activity. Folkow et al.[46] postulated that thickening of the arterial walls would reduce the vascular lumen and also significantly increase the degree of vascular constriction induced by a specific degree of smooth muscle shortening. They demonstrated that the resistance through "maximally" distended forearm vessels was higher in hypertensive than in normal subjects. Furthermore, a 30 per cent shortening of the smooth muscle could theoretically increase the resistance as much as two times.

VASCULAR SWELLING. Tobian and Binion[47] found an increased concentration of water and sodium in the renal artery and psoas muscle in humans with hypertension and in the aortic walls of hypertensive rats. Swelling of the arteriolar walls was regarded as a potential cause of increased peripheral resistance since a 13 per cent swelling of the arteriolar wall was computed to increase flow resistance by 54 per cent. A retention of salt and water might represent a change in the electrolyte metabolism in such patients, and low-salt diets might then alleviate hypertension by reducing the fluid content of the vascular walls. Edema of the vascular walls would be roughly equivalent to medial hypertrophy.

UNIDENTIFIED VASOCONSTRICTOR SUBSTANCES. Finally, vasoconstrictor substances yet to be identified might be primarily responsible for the production of essential hypertension. Such substances should have more or less equal effects on such vascular beds as those in the brain and skin and the splanchnic bed, with a slightly more intense effect on renal vessels and a slightly less intense effect on vessels of the skeletal musculature.

SUMMARY

Elevated systemic arterial pressure is a clinical sign which is common to a wide variety of disease states. The many potential mechanisms for the production of sustained high blood pressure are generally grouped into four main classes: endocrine (primarily adrenal glands), renal, cardiovascular and neural. Several specific diseases in each category are characteristically associated with elevated systemic arterial pressure. All these causal mechanisms combined will account for only about 5 to 10 per cent of all patients with high arterial blood pressure. The remaining 90 to 95 per cent of these patients have "essential" hypertension or elevated arterial pressure of unknown origin. Among these patients, the blood pressure rises at different rates. In a small percentage, the blood pressure rises abruptly ("malignant hypertension"); death usually supervenes within a year from severe heart failure, advanced kidney disease or cerebral vascular accident.

The cause of essential and malignant hypertension is not known. Attempts to explain this condition in terms of recognized mechanisms which elevate the blood pressure have been unsuccessful. The distribution of blood flow in the presence of this hypertension is very nearly normal even though the total peripheral resistance is increased. This distribution means that the degree of increased resistance must be more or less equal in all major vascular beds. None of the vasomotor control mechanisms discussed in Chapter 4 produces such widespread, uniform constrictor responses. It thus seems reasonable to seek other mechanisms affecting the various vascular beds which might be responsible for a progressive increase in blood pressure.

First, the presence of elevated arterial blood pressure apparently tends to be self-perpetuating in that it tends to persist after the initiating cause is removed. This persistence may be due to the development of sclerotic vascular lesions in the renal vessels (nephrosclerosis) in the presence of systemic hypertension. Furthermore, the pressoreceptor mechanisms can be shown to be reset to higher levels when the blood pressure is elevated for even a few hours. Thus, the neural control mechanisms may actually tend to sustain a hypertension rather than to induce compensatory reactions to restore the pressure to the control levels. The carotid sinus area is exceptionally susceptible to the development of atherosclerosis. The stiffening of the walls would tend to reduce the sensitivity of the stretch receptors in them, and reflexly induce vasoconstriction in the peripheral vascular system.

Generalized vasoconstriction in the various vascular beds might result from structural changes in the resistance vessels. For example, the smooth muscle in the media apparently hypertrophies in these vessels. If this condition develops in response to repeated vasoconstrictor impulses or to repeated episodes of transient elevation of systemic arterial pressure, a sustained increase in peripheral resistance will occur. Also, the same degree of shortening of the smooth muscle will produce greater constriction of the vessels owing to the greater thicknesses of their walls. Edema of the vascular walls due to increased concentrations of sodium and water in them has been demonstrated in hypertensive patients. This edema would have the same functional effect as hypertrophy of the smooth muscles in the media. Finally, currently unidentified vasoconstrictor substances may be discovered and may turn out to be the primary cause of the progressive rise in systemic arterial pressure observed in this large group of patients.

REFERENCES

1. HAMILTON, W. F., and DOW, P. An experimental study of the standing waves in the pulse propagated through the aorta. *Amer. J. Physiol.*, 125:48–59, 1939.
2. ALEXANDER, R. S. The genesis of the aortic standing wave. *Circulat. Res.*, 1:145–151, 1953.
3. PETERSON, L. H., and GERST, P. H. Significance of reflected waves within the arterial system. *Fed. Proc.*, 15:144–145, 1956.
4. WARNER, H. R. A study of the mechanism of pressure wave distortion by arterial walls using an electrical analog. *Circulat. Res.*, 5:79–84, 1957.
5. ATTINGER, E. O. Pulsatile blood flow. *Proc. of International Symposium on Pulsatile Blood Flow*, April 11-13, 1963. New York, Blakiston Division. McGraw-Hill Book Company, 1964.
6. KOROTKOFF, N. S. A contribution to the problem of methods for the determination of blood pressure. Pp. 126–133 in *Classics in Arterial Hypertension*, A. Rushin, Ed., Springfield, Charles C Thomas, 1956.
7. McCUTCHEON, E. P., and RUSHMER, R. F. Korotkoff Sounds. *Circulat. Res.*, 20:149–160, 1967.
8. THOMSON, A. E., and DOUPE, J. Causes of error in auscultatory blood pressure measurements. *Rev. Canad. Biol.*, 8:337, 1949.
9. WENDKOS, M. H., and ROSSMAN, P. L. The normal blood pressure in the lower extremity. *Amer. Heart J.*, 26:623–630, 1943.
10. GREEN, H. D. Circulatory system: methods. Pp. 208–222 in *Medical Physics*, O. Glasser, Ed. Chicago, Year Book Publishers, 1950.
11. LILLY, J. C. The electrical capacitance diaphragm manometer. *Rev. Sci. Instrum.*, 13:34–37, 1942.
12. ELLIS, E. J., GAUER, O. H., and WOOD, E. H. An intracardiac manometer: its evaluation and application. *Circulation*, 3:390–398, 1951.

13. FRY, D. L. Physiologic recording by modern instruments with particular reference to pressure recording. *Physiol. Rev.* 40:752–788, 1960.
14. WOOD, E. H., LEUSEN, I. R., WARNER, H. R., and WRIGHT, J. L. Measurement of pressures in man by cardiac catheters. *Circulat. Rev.*, 2:294–303, 1954.
15. SCHAPER, W. K. A., LEWI, P., and JAGENEAU, A. H. M. The determinants of the rate of change of the left ventricular pressure (dp/dt). *Archiv für Kreislaufforschung.* 46:27–41, 1965.
16. HEYMANS, C., DELAUNOIS, A. L., and VAN DEN HEUVEL-HEYMANS, G. Tension and distensibility of carotid sinus wall, pressoceptors and blood pressure regulation. *Circulat. Res.*, 1:3–7, 1953.
17. BRONK, D. W., and STELLA, G. The response to steady pressures of single end organs in the isolated carotid sinus. *Amer. J. Physiol.*, 110:708–714, 1935.
18. LANDGREN, S. On the excitation mechanism of the carotid baroceptors. *Acta physiol. scand.*, 26:1–34, 1952.
19. LANDGREN, S., NEIL, E., and ZOTTERMAN, Y. The response of the carotid baroceptors to the local administration of drugs. *Acta phsyiol. scand.*, 25:24–37, 1952.
20. LEUSEN, I., DEMEESTER, G., and BOUCKAERT, J. J. La regulation de la pression arterielle apres hemorragie. *Acta cardiol.*, 11:556–566, 1956.
21. HEYMANS, C., and NEIL, E. *Reflexogenic Areas of the Cardiovascular System.* Boston, Little, Brown & Co., 1958, 271 pp.
22. CARLSTEN, A., FOLKOW, B., GRIMBY, G., HEMBERGER, C. A., and THULESIUS, O. Cardiovascular effects of direct stimulation of the carotid sinus nerve in man. *Acta physiol. scand.*, 44:138–145, 1958.
23. DALY, I. DEB., and DALY, M. DEB. Observations on the changes in resistance of the pulmonary vascular bed in response to stimulation of the carotid sinus baroreceptors in the dog. *J. Physiol.*, 137:427–435, 1957.
24. AVIADO, D. M., JR., and SCHMIDT, C. F. Reflexes from stretch receptors in blood vessels, heart and lungs. *Physiol. Rev.*, 35:247–300, 1955.
25. AVIADO, D. M., JR., and SCHMIDT, C. F. Cardiovascular and respiratory reflexes from the left side of the heart. *Amer. J. Physiol.*, 196:726–730, 1959.
26. PATHAK, C. L. Alternative mechanism of cardiac acceleration in Bainbridge's infusion experiments. *Amer. J. Physiol.*, 197:441–444, 1959.
27. PAINTAL, A. S. The conduction velocities of respiratory and cardiovascular afferent fibres in the vagus nerve. *J. Physiol.*, 121:341–359, 1953.
28. RUSHMER, R. F., VanCITTERS, R. L., and

FRANKLIN, D. Definition and classification of shock. In *Shock: Pathogenesis and Therapy, An International Symposium.* Berlin, Springer Verlag, 1962.

29. RUSHMER, R. F. Shock: a semantic enigma. *Circulation,* 26:445–459, 1962.

30. CLARKSON, B., THOMPSON, D., HORWITH, M., and LUCKEY, E. H. Cyclical edema and shock due to increased capillary permeability. *Amer. J. Med.,* 29:193–216, 1960.

31. OSSIPOV, B. K. On the pathogenetic therapy of shock. In *Shock: Pathogenesis and Therapy: An International Symposium.* Berlin, Springer Verlag, 1962.

32. KOVÁCH, A. G. B., and TAKÁCS, L. Responsiveness of the vegetative nervous system in shock. *Acta Physiol., Acad. Sci., Hung.,* 3:91–101, 1952.

33. MASTER, A. M., GARFIELD, C. L., and WALTERS, M. B. *Normal Blood Pressure and Hypertension.* Philadelphia, Lea & Febiger, 1952, 144 pp.

34. SMIRK, F. H. *High Arterial Pressure.* Oxford, Blackwell Scientific Publications, 1957.

35. PICKERING, G. W. *The Nature of Essential Hypertension.* London, J. and A. Churchill Ltd., 1961.

36. PAGE, I. H. Hypertension, an important disease of regulation. *Advances in Chemistry Series,* 45:50–66, 1964.

37. MILLS, L. C. Clinical observations on the general effects of steroids and the adrenal cortex on blood pressure and relationship to hypertension. Pp. 232–242 in *Hypertension: The First Hahnemann Symposium on Hypertensive Disease.* J. Moyer, Ed. Philadelphia, W. B. Saunders Co., 1959.

38. MOSER, M., and GOLDMAN, A. *Hypertensive Vascular Disease: Diagnosis and Treatment.* Philadelphia, J. B. Lippincott Co., 1967.

39. MENEELY, G. M. The effect of salt and other electrolytes in hypertension. Pp. 250–261 in *Hypertension: The First Hahnemann Symposium on Hypertensive Disease.* J. Moyer, Ed. Philadelphia, W. B. Saunders Co., 1959.

40. SKELTON, F. R. A study of the natural history of adrenal-regeneration hypertension. *Circulat. Res.,* 7:107–117, 1959.

41. KUBICEK, W. G., KOTTKE, F. J., LAKER, D. J., and VISSCHER, M. B. Adaptation in the pressor-receptor reflex mechanisms in experimental neurogenic hypertension. *Amer. J. Physiol.,* 175:380–382, 1953.

42. McCUBBIN, J. W., GREEN, J. H., and PAGE, I. H. Baroceptor function in chronic renal hypertension. *Circulat. Res.,* 4:205–210, 1956.

43. ADAMS, W. E. *The Comparative Morphology of the Carotid Body and Carotid Sinus.* Springfield, Ill., Charles C Thomas, 1958, 272 pp.

44. CONWAY, J. Vascular reactivity in experimental hypertension measured after hexamethonium. *Circulation,* 17:807–810, 1958.

45. GASKELL, P., and DOISY, A. Persistence of abnormally high vascular tone in vessels of the fingers after digital nerve block in patients with chronic high blood pressure. *Circulat. Res.,* 7:1006–1010, 1959.

46. FOLKOW, B., GRIMBY, G., and THULESIUS, O. Adaptive structural changes of the vascular walls in hypertension and their relation to the control of the peripheral resistance. *Acta physiol. scand.,* 44:255–272, 1958.

47. TOBIAN, L., JR., and BINION, J. T. Tissue cations and water in arterial hypertension. *Circulation,* 5:754–758, 1952.

CHAPTER 6

EFFECTS OF POSTURE

I. CIRCULATORY RESPONSE TO ARISING

The cardiovascular system is generally studied in supine subjects or animals. Circulatory dynamics are most stable while the individual is lying down because many of the arteries and veins are horizontally oriented at or near heart level. When one stands upright, many of the arteries and veins are oriented vertically and large hydrostatic pressures are produced by the long, uninterrupted columns of blood. The arterial, capillary and venous pressures are markedly elevated in the dependent extremities, and the circulatory system must promptly make appropriate compensatory adaptation.[1, 2] If these compensatory mechanisms are insufficient or retarded, orthostatic hypotension results. Fainting reactions are frequently produced in erect subjects by stimuli that would have virtually no effect on the supine individual. Recognition that much of man's effective existence is spent in the erect position makes it appropriate to consider the cardiovascular adjustments required in this position.

MEASUREMENT OF VENOUS PRESSURES

A vertical column of fluid in a manometer and an accurate ruler are the only tools needed for measuring steady pressures. It is well to remember that even the most intricate pressure measuring devices require calibration by such simple pressure indicators. Thus, the fluid manometer is the basic instrument for pressure recording.

PERIPHERAL VENOUS PRESSURE

The venous pressure can be measured by a needle connected through a three-way stopcock to a vertical manometer. From the syringe, sterile saline is expressed into the manometer to a level above the expected venous pressure (Fig. 6–1A). The valve on the stopcock is then turned so the vertical tube becomes continuous with the needle. The saline runs into the vein until the vertical height of the column of saline is in equilibrium with the venous pressure at the point of the needle.

Alternatively, the phlebomanometer of Burch and Winsor[3] is well suited to measurement of pressure in both large and small peripheral veins (Fig. 6–1B). In this apparatus, a small needle is fastened to a capillary tube which is connected by a rubber tube

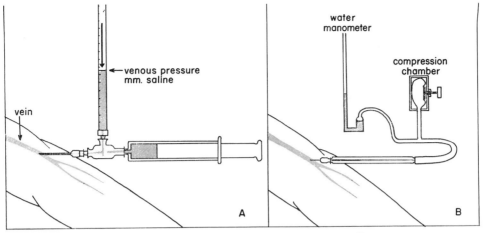

FIGURE 6-1   MEASUREMENT OF PERIPHERAL VENOUS PRESSURE

A, Venous pressure can be measured by a simple vertical manometer filled with saline and connected to a needle which has been thrust into a vein. The fluid column in the vertical tube descends until its pressure is in equilibrium with venous pressure at the point of measurement.

B, The phlebomanometer of Burch and Winsor[3] consists of a small hypodermic needle fastened to a glass capillary partially filled with sterile fluid. The remainder of the system except the water manometer is filled with air. The manometer registers the pressure in the system as adjusted by twisting the screw on the compression chamber until the fluid in the glass capillary is stationary. The pressure in the water manometer then indicates venous pressure when corrected for capillary and hydrostatic pressures in the needle and observation tubing.

to a small air chamber, the capacity of which can be adjusted to elevate the pressure in the system. A water manometer indicates the air pressure within the tubes. Sterile saline is drawn into the capillary tube until the meniscus lies at a reference line. When the needle is inserted into a vein, the meniscus will move farther along the capillary tube if the venous pressure exceeds the pressure within the phlebomanometer. By elevation of the pressure in the system, the meniscus can be brought to a standstill at the reference line when the pressure in the manometer equals the venous pressure. A correction (about 20 mm. H_2O) must be made for the capillarity of the needle and observation tube. A more compact version of this instrument has been described by Sodeman.[4] The advent of sensitive

electronic pressure monitoring systems has greatly increased the ease and continuity of venous pressure measurement. A variety of pressure transducers is now available commercially and permit continuous recording of pressures from veins, large and small, from virtually all parts of the body. The nature and performance characteristics of such gauges have been described in some detail by Fry[5] and by Frank.[6] Techniques of venous catheterization have been described in detail by Thompson and McIntosh.[7]

The Significance of Venous Pressure. The veins originate at the capillaries and terminate at the heart. Thus, venous pressure has important bearing on the function of both the capillaries and the heart. The pressure in the smallest peripheral veins is a basis for deducing the minimal pressure in the capillaries of the region, since the capillary pressure must exceed venous pressure. The effective pressure in the large intrathoracic veins reflects the diastolic filling pressure of the ventricles.

Right atrial pressure ranges just above or below atmospheric pressure but the pressure in extrathoracic veins is 2 to 5 cm. H_2O higher. A rather sudden drop in pressure often occurs as the veins penetrate the thoracic walls, where the extravascular pressure becomes subatmospheric. Branches of the superior vena cava in normal erect subjects are collapsed from the point of entrance into the thorax to a level a few centimeters above the right atrium. The sudden drop in pressure indicates local constriction at or near the point at which the veins pass through the thoracic musculature. In any case, the venous pressure in the arms does not normally reflect right ventricular diastolic pressure. However, if central venous pressure rises, e.g., in congestive failure, the difference between intrathoracic and extrathoracic venous pressure disappears, and the brachial venous pressure becomes a fairly reliable indicator of central venous pressure.

The Phlebostatic Level. To obtain comparable values in different individuals or in a series of measurements, the venous pressure is frequently measured at the level of the right atrium. For this purpose, Burch and Winsor[3] described a reference line (the phlebostatic axis) which passes transversely through the thorax midway between the anterior and posterior surfaces of the trunk at the level of the fourth interspace at the sternum (Fig. 6–2A). The phlebostatic level is a horizontal plane at the level of the phlebostatic axis. Venous pressures anywhere in the body can be meas-

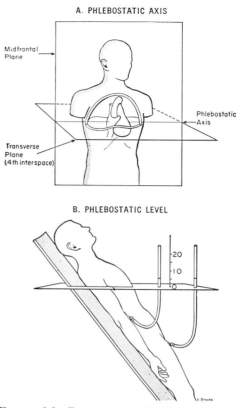

A. PHLEBOSTATIC AXIS

Midfrontal Plane

Phlebostatic Axis

Transverse Plane (4th interspace)

B. PHLEBOSTATIC LEVEL

FIGURE 6-2 BASELINE FOR CENTRAL VENOUS PRESSURE

A, The phlebostatic axis is defined as the line of junction between two planes: a midfrontal plane and a plane at right angles passing through the junction of the fourth rib with the sternum. The phlebostatic axis passes through or near the mid-portion of the right atrial chamber.

B, The phlebostatic level is used as the zero reference for venous pressures measured in different locations with the body in various positions. The phlebostatic level is a horizontal plane passing through the phlebostatic axis.

ured as the vertical height of a fluid column above this plane (Fig. 6–2B).

EXTRAVASCULAR PRESSURES

Water manometers are generally employed for measuring tissue pressures in various sites. For example, pressures in the skin, subcutaneous

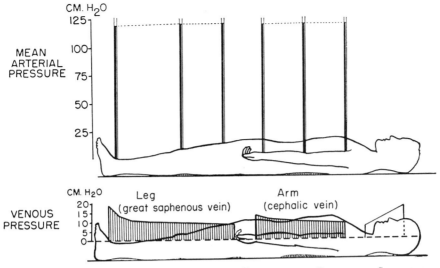

FIGURE 6-3   MEAN ARTERIAL AND VENOUS PRESSURES IN RECLINING SUBJECTS

A, The mean arterial pressure diminishes but slightly from the arch of the aorta to the arterial branches, e.g., the radial. This pressure gradient is responsible for the flow of blood through the system.

B, The peripheral venous pressure also has a very gradual diminution in pressure from the periphery toward the heart. In the smaller venous branches the pressure gradient is considerably steeper. (After Ochsner et al.[8])

tissue and muscle have generally been recorded with apparatus resembling the phlebomanometer (Fig. 6–1B). Cerebrospinal fluid pressure is usually measured with simple vertical manometers of the type illustrated in Figure 6–1A.

VASCULAR PRESSURES IN RECLINING SUBJECTS

When the long axis of the body is horizontal, the long columns of blood are at or near heart level. The mean pressure throughout the entire systemic arterial tree is fairly uniform except for the slight pressure gradients incident to the frictional energy loss during flow through these tubes (Fig. 6–3). The mean arterial pressure diminishes only a few millimeters of mercury during flow of the blood from the aorta to arterial branches the size of the radial artery at the wrist.

In the same way, the venous pressure declines only slightly between the smallest venous branches in the extremities and the large central venous channels. The pressure in peripheral veins of various calibers was measured at various points over the body surface by Ochsner et al.[8]; their data are schematically illustrated in Figure 6–3B. Note that the pressure in the smallest peripheral veins averaged about 17 mm. Hg in the lower extremity and that capillary pressure must exceed the pressures in the corresponding veins.

PRESSURES PRODUCED BY HYDROSTATIC COLUMNS

The pressure in a rigid tube containing a continuous column of stationary fluid is determined by the ver-

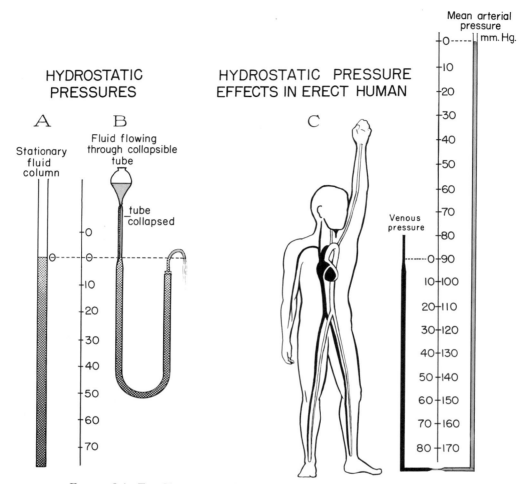

FIGURE 6-4   THE NATURE AND SIGNIFICANCE OF HYDROSTATIC PRESSURES

A, The pressure in a column of fluid is dependent upon its specific gravity and the vertical distance from the point of measurement to the meniscus.

B, A collapsible tube is distended only so long as the internal pressure exceeds the external pressure. These two pressures are exactly equal in the portion of the tube which is collapsed.

C, In the erect position, the arterial and venous pressures are both increased by some 85 mm. Hg at the ankle. With the arm held above the head, the arterial pressure at the wrist is about 40 mm. Hg and the effective venous pressure is zero down to a level just above the heart.

tical distance from the point of measurement to the top of the fluid (Fig. 6–4). At lower levels within the tube, the pressure in the fluid progressively increases owing to the action of gravity on the column of fluid above each point of measurement. Strictly speaking, the meniscus of the fluid represents an interface between the fluid

medium and the atmosphere, so the total pressure equals the hydrostatic pressure in the fluid column plus the ambient atmospheric pressure. In the present discussion the hydrostatic pressure will be considered in relation to the specific gravity of the fluid and the vertical distance from the point of measurement to the level at which fluid pressure equals the pressure immediately outside the tube.

The venous system consists of a series of collapsible tubes, so there is no interface between the venous blood and the external environment of the vein. If at any point along the vein, the pressure within it equals the external tissue pressure, the vessel collapses at that level. If a thin-walled tube containing no air is arranged as indicated in Figure 6–4B, the fluid from the reservoir will flow through the tube in response to a pressure gradient. The tube collapses at a level just above that of the outflow tube. Below this level, the internal pressure exceeds the external pressure, and the tube is distended by hydrostatic pressures which increase progressively toward the lower portion of the system. Above the zero level, the pressure within the collapsed tube is equal to the external pressure. Technically, a free-falling body has no weight because all the potential energy is converted into kinetic energy (movement) or lost as friction (heat). Thus, even though there is fluid flowing through the collapsed portion of the tube, the lateral pressure exactly equals the external pressure. If a normal man assumes a semi-reclining position with his head and trunk oriented about 30 to 45 degrees from the horizontal plane, the lower portion of the jugular vein is distended, but at some point along its course the vein becomes collapsed because venous pressure equals tissue pressure. This represents the level of zero effective venous pressure.

When a normal man is standing, the level of zero effective venous pressure is within the thorax (Fig. 6–4C). If there is a continuous column of blood extending from the foot to heart level, the pressure in an ankle vein should be about 85 mm. Hg (125 cm. H_2O). It has been demonstrated ex-

perimentally that this is approximately true so long as the subject remains relaxed and motionless. Similarly, if the mean arterial blood pressure at heart level is 90 mm. Hg the arterial blood pressure at the ankle should be increased by a corresponding amount, i.e., to about 175 mm. Hg, neglecting the slight frictional losses during flow indicated in Figure 6–3. Since the arterial and venous pressures in dependent extremities are increased to the same extent by hydrostatic pressure, the energy lost during circulation through dependent parts is no greater than that lost when the same vascular bed is at heart level. The pressure differences between arteries and veins at the ankle are essentially the same as those at heart level. The frictional energy loss along a tube is not increased when it is formed into a U tube. For example, the pressure head is the same for tubes A and B in Figure 6–5 and the flow from each tube is essentially identical. Forming a tube into a dependent loop does not increase the amount of energy required to propel fluid through the tube. Thus, the erect position does not require an increased energy output by the heart, but capillary pressure increases tremendously in the dependent parts of the body.

CEREBRAL CIRCULATION

Whenever a man is erect, the pressure within the skull drops well below atmospheric pressure while the pressure in the lower spinal canal is well above this value. It has long been recognized that cerebrospinal fluid protects the cerebrospinal vascular bed. The cerebrospinal fluid pressure and the cerebral venous pressure vary together because these fluids are confined within a relatively rigid chamber

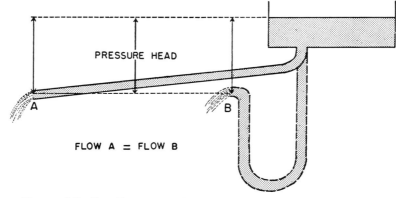

FIGURE 6-5   THE EFFECTS OF DEPENDENCY ON THE FLOW OF FLUID

This simple model illustrates the point that assuming the erect position per se places no additional burden upon the heart. Since the frictional energy loss is essentially the same, the same energy release (pressure head) provides equal flow from *A* and *B*.

(Fig. 6–6). The intravenous and extravenous pressure must be precisely equal at all levels of the cerebrospinal cavity regardless of its position or orientation.

Since the hydrostatic columns in the arteries, capillaries and veins are precisely balanced by equal changes in extravascular hydrostatic pressure,[9] the cerebrospinal circulation exhibits a stability not exceeded in any other tissue of the body. The pressure gradient from the arteries to the veins is precisely equal across all capillary beds. The only mechanism for altering flow through any part of the enclosed circulation is by means of local vasoconstriction or vasodilation. However, the cerebral circulation is remarkably unresponsive to the usual neural, humoral or chemical mechanisms (see Chapter 4). The blood flow through the cerebrospinal vessels is extremely constant, a condition compatible with the more or less uniform oxygen requirements of the central nervous system. The effective capillary pressure is also very similar at all levels within the cerebrospinal canal, and the fluid balance postulated by

Starling (see Fig. 1–15) is probably in effect in all capillary networks. Net filtration probably does not occur in cerebral capillaries other than those of the choroid plexus, which has the specialized function of producing cerebrospinal fluid. In fact, many substances in the blood are greatly impeded in their movement into the cerebrospinal fluid, a fact ascribed to the so-called "blood-brain barrier."

The circulatory pattern and extravascular support within the eye are quite analogous to those of the cerebrospinal cavity. The ciliary body is a structure specialized to produce capillary filtrate (aqueous humour). A similar kind of external support of the vascular beds probably obtains within the medullary cavity of bones.

COUNTER PRESSURES IN PERIPHERAL CIRCULATION

It is obvious that a capillary pressure exceeding a pressure of 85 mm. Hg in an ankle vein must also greatly exceed the maximum colloid osmotic pressure of the plasma proteins (about 30 mm. Hg). If the effective capillary

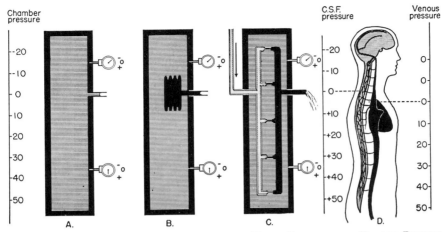

FIGURE 6-6   THE RELATION OF CEREBROSPINAL FLUID PRESSURE TO VENOUS PRESSURE

In a rigid container filled with fluid, the pressure at the level of the horizontal tube equals atmospheric pressure. Below this level the pressure progressively increases owing to the hydrostatic column of fluid. Above the reference level, the pressure progressively diminishes below atmospheric pressure. This situation is unaltered by the presence of a distensible barrier between the contents of the chamber and the outlet tube. If fluid flows into the chamber through rigid tubes and out through collapsible tubes, the pressure within the collapsible tubes is precisely equal to the pressure outside the tube at any level within the rigid system. By the same token, the venous pressure determines the cerebrospinal fluid pressure within the cerebrospinal cavity.

pressure throughout the vascular networks of a region significantly exceeds the maximal colloid osmotic pressure, fluid will filter from all parts of the capillary system, resorption will be impossible and accumulation of fluid in the tissue spaces (edema) can result. It is important to consider the extent to which this kind of situation is alleviated in various regions of the body by such mechanisms as (a) the balancing of intravascular pressures by extravascular or tissue pressure, (b) the reduction of the hydrostatic columns in veins by "pumping" action and (c) the return of unabsorbed capillary filtrate to the circulation by way of the lymphatic system.

INTRAMUSCULAR TISSUE PRESSURE

In reclining subjects the intramuscular pressure ranges from 2 to 5 cm.

H_2O in muscles with loose fascial investment,[10] e.g., biceps brachii and gastrocnemius. Slightly higher values have been obtained from anterior tibial and soleus muscles, which are invested with a tight fascial sheath. After the subject has been tilted into the erect position, intramuscular pressures rise abruptly a few centimeters of water and then gradually increase to values of 20 or 30 cm. H_2O in muscles with tight fascial covering. Maximal pressures developed during voluntary muscular contraction are rarely reported to be over 50 cm. H_2O, although the venous pressure in the legs exceeds this amount. In muscles without tight fascial sheaths the increase in pressure is relatively slight during maximal voluntary contraction. For example, pressure in the rectus femoris could not be raised above 20 cm. H_2O by maximal effort.[10] Although the recorded values for intramuscular

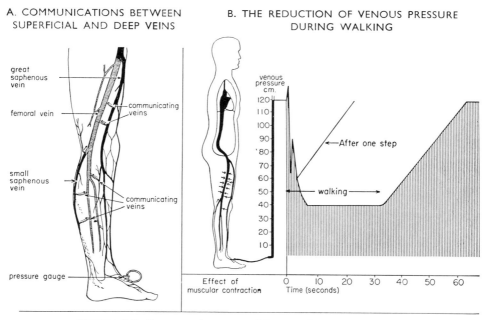

A. COMMUNICATIONS BETWEEN
SUPERFICIAL AND DEEP VEINS

B. THE REDUCTION OF VENOUS PRESSURE
DURING WALKING

FIGURE 6-7   PUMPING ACTION OF MUSCLES DURING WALKING

A, Venous blood may ascend the leg along both deep and superficial channels, which are in communication at many points. To reduce the venous pressure at the ankle, each vertical column of blood draining the area must be interrupted at some point in the leg.

B, After taking one step the venous pressure in a dorsal vein of the foot is markedly reduced and then gradually ascends to the control level; repetitive steps keep the venous pressure depressed (after Pollack and Wood[13]).

pressure are surprisingly low, muscular contraction has important cardiovascular significance. A relationship between low intramuscular pressure and syncope has been demonstrated by Mayerson and Burch.[11] Even more impressive is the fact that voluntary muscular contraction can apparently force blood under a cuff inflated to levels of 90 mm. Hg.[12] By some unknown means, contraction of skeletal muscle in the legs is sufficient to compress the veins of the legs even when their internal pressure is very high. This is the basis of a muscular pumping mechanism by which the venous pressure in dependent extremities may be significantly lowered during ordinary walking or shifting of position.

Muscular Pumping Mechanisms. The veins of the extremities are equipped with many valves located at strategic positions along their course. So long as blood flows continuously throughout the peripheral venous system, the valves along all the venous channels are open and the columns of blood are not interrupted at any point. Under these conditions, the pressure in the veins at the dorsum of the foot is equal to that in a vertical column of blood extending from the point of measurement to heart level (Fig. 6–4). If the subject takes one step (Fig. 6–7), the venous pressure at the ankle drops to a level equivalent to that in a column of fluid extending to the knee and then gradually returns to the previous level at a rate determined by the volume flow of blood through the limb.[13] There are alternate pathways by which blood from the foot may ascend the leg. If any single uninterrupted column of blood from ankle to heart persisted after the step, the venous pressure at the dorsum of the foot would not be altered. Thus, muscular contraction must produce complete or partial emptying of both the deep and superficial veins within the leg or thigh. As the muscles relax, columns of blood are supported by closed intravenous valves. According to Höjensgard and Stürup,[14] the pressure in the deep and superficial leg veins may be reduced simultaneously during walking. The superficial veins must empty into the deep veins of the thigh so that all the veins above the knee are decompressed. This could be accomplished by complete emptying of veins or by segmenting the columns of blood so that each valve in the thigh is closed and supports a column of blood which does not extend to the valve above. As blood flows through the capillaries into the veins, the partially collapsed deep and superficial veins gradually refill, elevating the pressure at the dorsum of the foot back to the initial levels. Repetitive movements of the lower extremities, as in walking, maintain the venous pressures at the lower level (Fig. 6–7) if each successive step occurs before the venous columns in the thighs are refilled.

This muscular pumping mechanism has important functional connotations: (a) It drastically lowers the venous and capillary pressures, reducing the effective capillary filtration pressures. (b) It reduces the volume of blood contained within the veins of the leg and to this extent these veins act as a reservoir which releases stored blood during muscular exercise (see later). (c) It momentarily acceler-

ates the return of venous blood from the legs at the onset of walking or running. After the pumping mechanism is established, the rate of venous return again depends upon the rate of blood flow through the capillaries into the veins. When venous blood flows upward from the leg into the abdomen, the pressure in the veins of the thigh must exceed the pressure in the abdominal portion of the inferior vena cava, which has no valves. In general, the veins within the abdomen are filled with uninterrupted columns of blood under a pressure equivalent to that of a vertical column extending slightly above heart level. A critical analysis of the pumping mechanisms in the leg by Stegall[15] disclosed that muscle contraction of the legs can contribute significantly to the propulsion of the blood during running. The abdominal pressure was found to be elevated by about 22 mm. Hg during exertion, apparently to splint the trunk and pelvis. The contracting leg muscles must elevate venous pressure sufficiently to overcome elevated abdominal pressure and propel blood upward against hydrostatic pressure to the heart. Measured by ultrasonic Doppler flow detector, blood was accelerated in both the deep and superficial veins during contraction of the leg muscles (Fig. 6–8A). Measurements of venous pressures by catheters from the right atrium down the vena cava to the ankle revealed an increase in venous pressure above the popliteal veins and a decrease in venous pressure at the ankle (Fig. 6–8B). The power developed by the leg muscles in pumping blood upward to the heart was computed utilizing data on muscle blood flow from the literature and the pressure drops indicated in Figure 6–8B. The surprising result was an estimate that at least 30 per cent of the

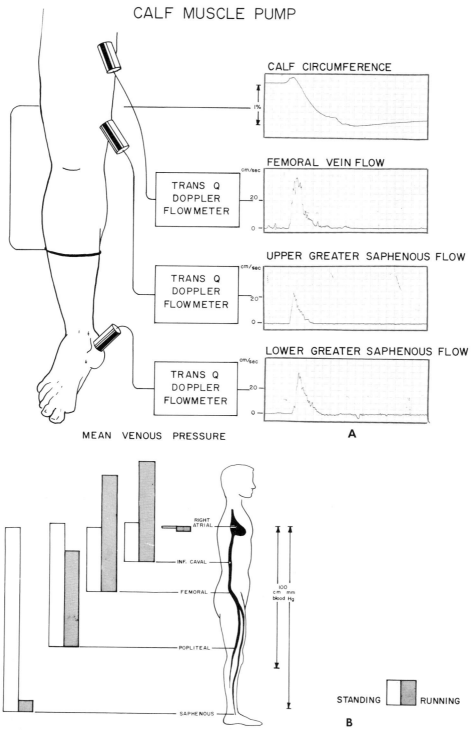

FIGURE 6-8 MUSCULAR PUMPING MECHANISMS

A, Upper calf circumference and venous flow velocity with a brief ankle flexion. Paper speed 25 mm./sec.

B, Mean venous pressures at rest and during running in one subject. The figure is scaled as shown. The bottom of each bar represents atmospheric pressure at the level shown; bar height is proportional to the mean pressure obtained during running. (From *Circulat. Res.* 19:182.)

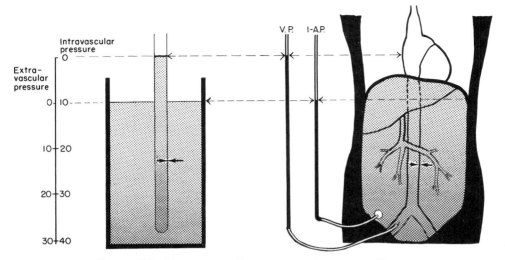

FIGURE 6-9   TRANSMURAL PRESSURES OF ABDOMINAL VEINS

If a collapsible tube is filled with fluid and suspended in a tank of water, the walls must support only the difference in pressure between the inside and the outside. In the case illustrated, the walls of the tube support no more than 10 cm. H₂O pressure at any level in the tube. The abdomen contains movable organs with a specific gravity similar to that of blood. For this reason the transmural pressure of intra-abdominal veins is less than 10 cm. H₂O at any level in the abdominal cavity.

total systemic circulatory work during running must be done by pumping action of the musculature in the legs.

INTRA-ABDOMINAL PRESSURE

The abdominal cavity is filled with organs having a specific gravity approximating that of blood. The hydrostatic pressure of a vertical column of abdominal organs is similar (Fig. 6–9) to that which would be produced if the abdomen were filled with fluid.[16] At rest the venous pressure apparently exceeds the intra-abdominal pressure by only 5 to 10 cm. H₂O at any level within the abdomen in either the supine or the erect position. However, the diaphragm and the abdominal walls may simultaneously exert tension during deep inspiration or straining, so that the overall intra-abdominal pressure exceeds venous pressure in

the thorax and compresses the abdominal veins. Blood is forced onward into the veins of the thorax because retrograde flow out of the abdominal cavity is prevented by closure of venous valves. Since the diaphragm can exert no force in the upward direction, intrathoracic pressure never exceeds intra-abdominal pressure.

INTRATHORACIC PRESSURE

The collapsed volume of the lungs is much smaller than the capacity of the thoracic cage. Since the lungs are stretched or distended to fill their allotted space, the elastic tissue is under stretch even at the end of a forced expiration. This elastic tension of the pulmonary tissue is expressed as a subatmospheric intrathoracic pressure which exerts a distending force on the structures within the chest. An elastic tube filled with fluid is further distended if the tube is confined within a chamber containing a subatmospheric pressure. The level of zero transmural pressure occurs at the point where the internal fluid pressure is balanced by the extravascular pressure. The central venous pressure measured with a catheter ranges slightly above or slightly below the atmospheric pressure. The transmural pressure of the veins and atria, however, is greater than the recorded values because of the subatmospheric pressure in the thorax. If the negative intrathoracic pressure is applied to the top of an external fluid column connected to an intrathoracic vein (Fig. 6–10), the top of the fluid column is elevated by the "suction" of the subatmospheric intrathoracic pressure. The "effective" venous pressure within the chest is indicated by such a manometer. The distending influence of the subatmospheric intrathoracic pressure tends to increase the transmural pressures throughout the thoracic cavity. It augments the central

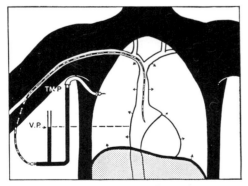

FIGURE 6-10   TRANSMURAL PRESSURE IN THE
                        THORAX

The central venous pressure recorded with a catheter approximates atmospheric pressure. The transmural pressure of the intrathoracic vessels is actually represented by the combined effects of intrathoracic and intravascular pressures. The intrathoracic pressure exerts a distending influence on vasculature within the thorax.

venous pressure in distending the large veins and the heart, reducing, to this extent, the lower end of the pressure gradient from the periphery to the right ventricle.

The intrathoracic pressure fluctuates during normal respiratory activity, averaging about −5.4 cm. H_2O (−4 mm. Hg) at the end of a normal expiration. Inspiration further distends the lungs, lowering the pressure to about −10.8 cm. H_2O (−8 mm. Hg). Increased respiratory excursions produce correspondingly greater fluctuations in the intrathoracic pressure. Changes in intrathoracic and intra-abdominal pressure associated with diaphragmatic movements provide a pumping mechanism that facilitates transfer of blood into the thorax.

THE ABDOMINOTHORACIC PUMPING MECHANISM

During inspiration, the contracting diaphragm descends and the intrathoracic pressure is lowered by increased stretch of the inflated lungs. Simultaneously, the abdominal organs are displaced downward and forward; this displacement tends to stretch the anterior abdominal wall and increases the overall intra-abdominal pressure. Thus, during inspiration, the gradient in pressure between the abdomen and the thorax is increased and the flow of blood into the thoracic veins is accelerated (Fig. 6–11). In addition, the shortening of the inferior vena cava reduces its capacity, contributing to the blood flow into the thorax.[17] The increased intra-abdominal pressure temporarily impedes flow from the periphery into the abdomen; flow is accelerated after the intra-abdominal pressure is lowered during the subsequent expiratory movement.

Exhalation releases tension within the inflated lungs, and the intrathoracic

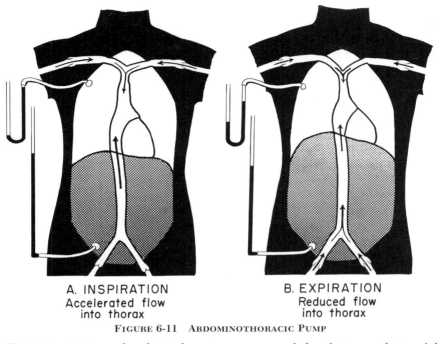

A. INSPIRATION
Accelerated flow
into thorax

B. EXPIRATION
Reduced flow
into thorax

FIGURE 6-11   ABDOMINOTHORACIC PUMP

A, During inspiration, reduced intrathoracic pressure coupled with increased intra-abdominal pressure accelerates the flow of blood from the abdominal veins into the thorax.

B, During expiration, flow into the thorax is retarded by simultaneous increase in intrathoracic pressure and reduction in intra-abdominal pressure.

pressure rises toward atmospheric pressure. Intra-abdominal pressure is reduced as the diaphragm relaxes and ascends. The inferior vena cava becomes elongated and accommodates more blood.[17] Thus, blood flow from abdomen to thorax is accelerated during inspiration and slowed during expiration. If expiration is continued beyond the normal range by active contraction of the abdominal muscles, the diaphragm is stretched as it is elevated beyond the position of rest so that intra-abdominal pressure is increased more than intrathoracic pressure rises. Since the diaphragm applies force only toward the abdominal cavity, and elastic tension in the lungs is continuously present, intra-abdominal pressure always exceeds intrathoracic pressure. By this mechanism, a favor-

able pressure gradient from abdomen to thorax is always maintained under normal conditions.

CONTROL OF CENTRAL VENOUS PRESSURE

The pressure in the intrathoracic portions of the superior and inferior venae cavae is of great importance because the transmural pressure in these veins represents the distending pressure of the heart. A positive effective filling pressure must be maintained in these veins at all times regardless of the position of the body, the magnitude of the blood volume, the redistribution of blood in dilated capillary beds or the accumulation of blood in distended dependent veins. Otherwise, filling of the heart would be deficient during the diastolic intervals. On the other hand, excessive pressure in these veins would raise the gradient in pressure in both the venous and the lymphatic systems, which would promote accumulation of fluid in the tissues. The maintenance of central venous pressure between these two critical levels requires that the venous system compensate for variations in total blood volume and changes in its distribution. The right ventricular pressure during diastole represents the minimal pressure in the systemic venous system, since it is the point of outflow from the entire system. At rest in the horizontal position, the right ventricular pressure varies between +2 and −2 mm. Hg during diastole. Angiocardiographic studies[18] have revealed that, in the supine position, both the superior and inferior venae cavae are distended with blood. In the erect position, the inferior vena cava is distended, but the superior vena cava is partially collapsed just above the level of the right atrium. The point of collapse of the veins represents the level at which the effective venous pressure (intravascular pressure minus extravascular pressure) is essentially zero. If the pressure in the inferior vena cava fell until the point of collapse was just below the right atrium, the effective filling pressure of the right ventricle would be zero. Thus, a decrease in venous pressure of only a few centimeters of water in the right atrium would represent a serious impairment of right ventricular filling. This contingency is prevented by continuous and precise adjustments in the venous reservoir system to maintain the central venous pressure at levels only slightly above that of the right atrium regardless of the body's position.

The mechanism which controls the central venous pressure is best de-scribed by a schematic diagram (Fig. 6–12). Consider a distensible tube filled with water until there is a slight positive internal pressure when it is horizontal. In the vertical position, the fluid level in the tube would descend because the hydrostatic pressure would produce greater distention of the dependent portions. The fluid level could be restored to the previous height only by compression of some portion of the tube (Fig. 6–12). Exactly the same considerations apply whether the fluid is stationary or is flowing through the tube (see Fig. 6–4). The central venous pressure is only slightly above atmospheric pressure in normal reclining subjects. When the individual assumes a vertical position, the hydrostatic pressures produce a distention of the dependent veins which may accumulate relatively large quantities of blood (more than 500 cc.). Unless some portions of the venous vascular bed were compressed, effective central venous pressure would probably fall below that of the heart. A major portion of this blood may come from the lungs. However, external compression of veins by skeletal muscles in the legs, and probably by contraction of large venous channels and other venous reservoirs, restores the central venous pressure so that it is just above the pressure in the right atrium. The exact mechanisms controlling this important adjustment have not yet been elucidated.

The probability that central venous pressure is precisely controlled was strengthened by exposing animals to positive and negative radial acceleration on a large centrifuge.[9] Under forces as great as five times the force of gravity (5 g) the pressures in "dependent regions" became very high, but the level at which venous pressure remained essentially unchanged was at or near heart level whether these

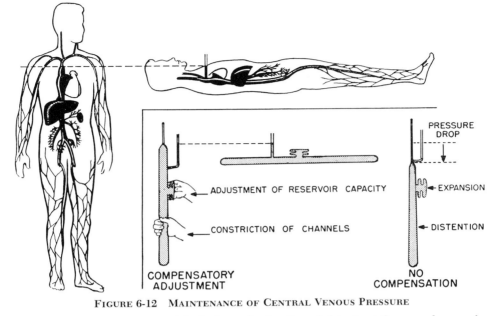

FIGURE 6-12 MAINTENANCE OF CENTRAL VENOUS PRESSURE

The veins in various regions of the body tend to be distended to about the same degree when a subject is recumbent. In the erect position the hydrostatic columns of blood produce distention of the vessels below the heart and collapse of veins above the heart. Since most of the venous reservoir capacity is below heart level, the central venous pressure theoretically could fall below heart level unless compensatory adjustments were promptly instituted. These compensatory mechanisms are illustrated schematically as a constriction of venous channels and regulation of reservoir capacity.

forces were directed toward the head or toward the lower parts of the body. Since the capacity of the veins below the diaphragm greatly exceeds that of those above the diaphragm, the large hydrostatic pressures would tend to cause massive accumulations of blood in dependent regions when the forces acted from head to feet. Control of central venous pressure must certainly involve regulation of the capacity of the venous reservoirs.

THE EFFECTS OF POSTURE ON VENTRICULAR SIZE

In earlier times the ventricular chambers were thought to be nearly empty at the end of each systole. This impression probably stemmed from observation of hearts exposed by thoracotomy, which induces marked shrinkage of the heart (see Fig. 3–9). Measurements under more normal conditions consistently indicate that relatively large volumes of blood remain within the ventricular chambers at the end of a normal ventricular systole. In fact, the ventricles apparently eject only about half of the end diastolic volume.[19, 20] In normal human subjects and in patients with heart disease resting quietly in the supine position the heart functions at or near its maximum dimensions.[21, 22] In resting recumbent dogs, the left ventricle tends to attain near maximum dimensions as recorded by gauges of diameter, length and circumference.

The rapid increase in the left ventricular diameter of a dog during a

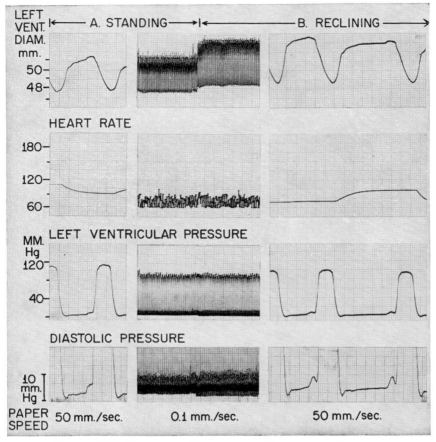

FIGURE 6-13 EFFECTS OF RECLINING ON VENTRICULAR FUNCTION

The changes in left ventricular diameter, heart rate and ventricular pressures as a healthy dog, standing with his trunk horizontal, spontaneously reclines. Note that the diastolic distention increased in spite of a slight drop in mean atrial pressure. The increased stroke deflections in the diameter record indicate an increase in stroke volume which has been amply confirmed by aortic flowmeters. These changes are in accordance with the Frank-Starling mechanism.

change from the standing (with trunk horizontal) to the reclining position is illustrated in Figure 6–13. The transition from sitting (or standing) to the recumbent position was accompanied by a progressive increase in diastolic dimensions over a series of cardiac cycles in which the stroke deflection increased and the systolic pressure was elevated (Fig. 6–14A, B). Thus, the increase in diastolic size was accompanied by an increase in energy

release, in accordance with the Frank-Starling mechanism.[22] The diastolic diameter expanded to a maximum as evidenced by the fact that it reached a plateau early in diastole and atrial contraction produced little or no additional distention.

After the dog was anesthetized and thoracotomized, the heart was observed as it distended to its "maximum" dimensions when the animal succumbed to asphyxia. The diastolic

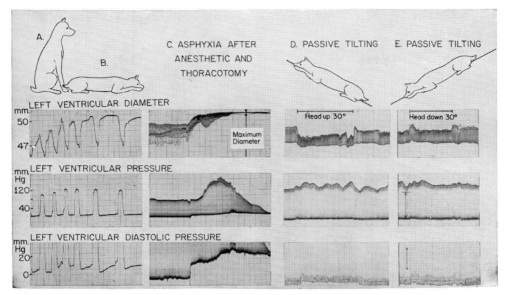

FIGURE 6-14   MAXIMAL DIASTOLIC DISTENTION DURING RECUMBENCY

A, As indicated in Figure 6-13, the left ventricular diameter promptly increases during the next few cycles after a dog assumes the reclining position.

B, After anesthesia, thoracotomy and asphyxia, the left ventricle distended under direct vision. The ventricular diameter after this extreme distention was essentially the same as in the recumbent position in *A*, indicating that under these conditions left ventricular distention may be "maximal" for that ventricle.

C, Changes in ventricular diameter with changes in posture are not due to the effort because they occur during passive tilting with the head up but to a much lesser extent with the head down.

diameter recorded during the distention produced by asphyxia was essentially the same as that recorded previously while the dog was relaxed (Fig. 6–14*B*).

The reduction in ventricular size was not due to the exertion involved in standing since both the diastolic diameter and the stroke deflection were reduced when the head was passively tilted up 30 degrees (Fig. 6–14*C*). However, vertical orientation of the trunk per se is not an essential factor in the reduction in heart size and stroke volume because the trunk is horizontal during both reclining and standing in the dog. Furthermore, the heart size promptly diminishes to about the same extent if the animal merely lifts his head in response to an

unexpected noise. In other words, the cardiac chambers function at or near their maximum dimensions in the relaxed recumbent dog and their size is promptly reduced in all other circumstances observed.

A reduction in stroke volume on arising has been consistently observed in normal human subjects;[23] the average heart rate is slightly accelerated, but the net effect is a diminution in cardiac output. The same observation was made on intact dogs in which aortic flow was measured continuously by means of an indwelling ultrasonic flowmeter.[24] A reduction in cardiac output when the erect position is assumed indicates that the total flow through the peripheral circulation has been curtailed, presumably by vasoconstriction in some peripheral vascular bed.

THE CONCEPT OF VENOUS RETURN

The stroke volume of the heart-lung preparation was generally increased by elevating the venous reservoir. This experimental technique formed the basis for the concept that a prominent factor in the initiation of increased cardiac output was an increase in "venous return" in many cardiovascular responses. A precise definition for the term "venous return" is difficult to derive since it has been employed in many different ways so that it has, at one time or another, included increased volume flow into the ventricles, increased velocity of flow in the central veins, increased central venous pressure, increased filling pressure in the ventricles and so forth. However, there might be general agreement that stroke volume and cardiac output are increased by greater venous return when the central venous pressure, the volume flow into the ventricles, the diastolic ventricular volume, the stroke volume and the cardiac output are all increased. On the basis of these criteria, the increase in stroke volume and cardiac output occurring when an erect man or dog lies down is a most clear-cut example of the results of an increased venous return. Similarly, the reduced stroke volume and cardiac output accompanying standing could be described in terms of reduced venous return. An exaggerated form of this response is seen when positive radial acceleration with centrifugal forces of three to five times the force of gravity (3 to 5 g) are applied. Under these conditions, the ventricles become progressively smaller until they appear to empty maximally during each systole. Evidence of changes in venous return in the initiation of circulatory responses cannot be easily recognized in other spontaneous circulatory adjustments by normal animals or man.

THE EFFECTS OF STANDING ON PERIPHERAL FLOW DISTRIBUTION

When a normal person arises from the recumbent to the erect position, less blood flows through the splanchnic bed and the dependent extremities (Fig. 6–15). For example, the estimated blood flow through the liver decreased on the average from 1713 cc. to 1070 cc. per minute in a group of human subjects.[25] The blood flow through the hand promptly diminishes and then rises somewhat to reach a mean level just below that recorded in the reclining subject. The blood flow through the legs decreases significantly, and the oxygen content of femoral venous blood is reduced, indicating that a much greater proportion of the oxygen reserve is utilized. A most pronounced reduction in flow through renal and superior mesenteric arteries occurred when the dogs in Figure 4–14 stood on their hind legs with the trunk held erect. According to recent evidence, the arteriovenous oxygen difference in blood passing through the leg increases about two-fold without a demonstrable increase in oxygen consumption, and oxygen extraction is augmented by this amount even if the leg bears no weight.

Teleologic explanations for vasoconstriction in the dependent leg are not difficult to imagine. In the erect position, the long columns of blood elevate the pressure in both the arteries and veins of the legs. An increase in the internal pressure within the arteries, arterioles, capillaries and

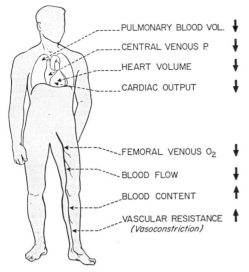

FIGURE 6-15   SOME EFFECTS OF ARISING

Changes in blood distribution and blood flow when a man stands are summarized schematically. Blood content diminishes in the lungs and heart and increases in the legs. Blood flow through the legs and cardiac output both diminish. The oxygen extraction from the blood flowing through the legs is necessarily more complete.

venules by 50 to 90 mm. Hg would tend to produce distention of all these vessels, producing a passive vasodilation throughout these vascular beds unless this tendency were opposed by active vasoconstriction. Vasoconstriction might also serve to diminish the rate at which fluid filters through the dependent capillary beds. If an erect subject moves his legs, as in walking, venous pressure in the lower legs drops to much lower levels owing to the pumping action of the muscles (Fig. 6–7). Under these conditions, the pressure gradient from the arteries to the veins may suddenly increase from about 90 mm. Hg to about 140 mm. Hg. This increase would cause considerably augmented flow through the dependent vascular beds. The consequent accelerated outflow from the

arterial system, coupled with the reduced stroke volume (Figs. 6–13 and 6–14), might produce a precipitous fall in systemic arterial blood pressure unless a peripheral vasoconstriction were promptly induced. The principal sign of a severe reduction in systemic arterial pressure attendant upon standing is a loss of consciousness.

THE TIME SEQUENCE OF POSTURAL RESPONSES

The directional changes illustreated in Figure 6–15 fail to convey the need for very prompt circulatory compensation to avoid precipitous fall in systemic arterial pressure. The vertical orientation greatly increases the hydrostatic pressure in dependent blood vessels which should cause distention and a lowered peripheral resistance at the same time that cardiac output is reduced. The central blood volume and heart volumes are diminishing, and the cardiac output is reduced by some 20 to 30 per cent. Diminished cardiac output accompanying reduced peripheral resistance should result in sharply falling arterial pressure unless reflex vasoconstriction occurs at the same time. In normal individuals actual measurements of systemic arterial pressure reveal no significant change even at the very onset of passive tilting from horizontal to erect positions on a tilt table where muscular pumping action of the legs is minimal or absent. To study the time relations of the integrated response to passive tilt to 60 degrees, Stegall and I recorded the overall reactions in a group of six normal subjects as illustrated in Figure 6–16. The course of changes in venous pressure and volume in the extremities (Fig. 6–16A) demonstrates a prompt but slight reduction in arm volume (10 to 30 ml.) and a sustained drop in

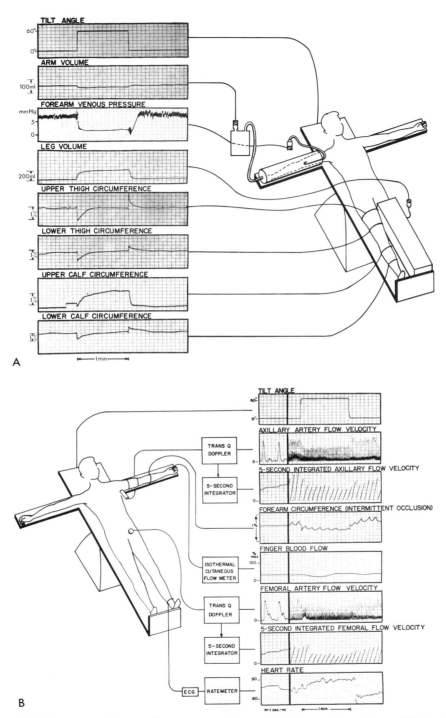

Figure 6-16   CHANGES IN VENOUS PRESSURE AND VOLUME AND BLOOD FLOW DURING PASSIVE TILT

A, Changes in venous pressure, arm and leg volumes and leg circumference at four levels during a passive tilt upright to 60 degrees. The initial downward spike in the circumference records represents easily visible sagging of tissues; the swelling of the leg follows the artifact.

B, Changes in axillary and femoral flow velocity recorded by ultrasonic Doppler flow sensors, forearm circumference changes with intermittent venous occlusion, finger blood flow and heart rate during passive tilting to 60 degrees like that illustrated in part *A.*

forearm venous pressure while the leg volume (by plethysmography) increased very rapidly by some 200 ml. in 10 to 15 seconds and another 50 ml. at the end of a minute. The circumference of the leg at four levels displayed an initial artifact due to visible sagging of tissues on all records. The increase in circumference due to swelling began immediately after the artifact. The upper calf showed the greatest change in circumference. Computations from the circumference gauges indicated that about 130 ml. accumulated in the thigh and some 80 ml. in the calf, accounting for 80 to 90 per cent of the swelling observed by plethysmography. The remaining 10 to 20 per cent must have gone to the foot. On return to the horizontal position, the blood rapidly leaves the legs, reaching pretilt levels within 15 to 20 seconds. The blood pressure recorded by sphygmomanometer repeatedly remained within a few mm. Hg of the pretilt values throughout.

The changes in blood flow during tilting are presented in Figure 6–16B. The instantaneous flow velocity in the axillary and femoral arteries (recorded by ultrasonic Doppler flow sensor) diminished very promptly, and the integrated flow velocity (related to volume flow per 5 seconds) also fell by one-third or one-half within about 10 to 15 seconds, indicating extremely prompt vasoconstriction in both arm and leg. The reduction in blood flow was confirmed by venous occlusion plethysmography using a circumference gauge, showing a reduction in estimated flow from 4.4 to 2.2 m./min./100 ml. of forearm. An isothermal skin blood flow sensor on the finger also showed an initial reduction in apparent blood flow during the first part of the tilt. The heart rate rose gradually after upright tilting from about 75 to about 90 beats/min. On the return to

horizontal, the heart rate dropped abruptly to a level below the control within one or two beats.

The net result of the changes observed in Figure 6–16A and B represents evidence of extremely rapid and effective compensation for the downward displacement of blood by a prompt vasoconstriction and reduction in peripheral blood flow to maintain arterial pressure very near the control levels. Under a wide variety of conditions, the compensatory vasoconstriction is either delayed or insufficient in amount, the arterial pressure falls and the individual experiences giddiness or fainting. This is the fundamental functional disturbance of the so-called orthostatic hypotension discussed in Part II of this chapter.

SUMMARY

In the standing adult of average height, the arterial and venous pressures recorded at the ankle are both as much as 85 mm. Hg higher than the pressures in the reclining subject. The pressure difference between the arteries and veins remains unchanged. The cardiac output has been reported to be diminished when the subjects are relaxed in the upright position rather than when they are supine. The major circulatory change produced by the hydrostatic columns is an increase in the capillary pressure in the dependent extremities and displacement of blood into dependent extremities.

Changes in the position of the body have no functional effect on the vasculature within the cerebrospinal cavity and the eye, and probably not on those in bone, because the extravascular pressure precisely balances the venous pressure.

Contraction of the leg muscles during walking brings into play the so-called "muscular pumping action" which has three effects: (*a*) At the beginning of muscular contraction, blood is displaced from the veins of the legs owing to external compression. (*b*) The pressure in the veins and capillaries in the lower extremities tends to be maintained at lower levels during active walking. (*c*) The arteriovenous pressure difference is increased so that blood flow through the capillaries into the veins would be increased if the state of arteriolar constriction remained unchanged. The quantity of blood flowing through the veins depends upon the rate of flow through the capillaries.

The external pressure provided by the hydrostatic column of abdominal organs tends to balance the hydrostatic pressures in the veins of the abdomen. By this mechanism, the vast splanch-nic venous bed is largely protected from being distended by the increased venous pressures developed in the erect position. The subatmospheric pressure within the thorax provides a favorable pressure gradient from abdomen to thorax. Contraction of the diaphragm can act only to increase intra-abdominal pressure and reduce intrathoracic pressure.

The effective or transmural pressure in the thoracic veins, atria and ventricles is greater than that recorded externally because the subatmospheric pressure acts as a distending force. The filling pressure of the right ventricle is normally maintained at very low and constant levels by adjustments in the capacity of the venous reservoir system to compensate for variations in the distribution of blood and in the total blood volume.

II. POSTURAL HYPOTENSION

Diminished systemic arterial pressure, often accompanied by dizziness, sweating, visual disturbances and even loss of consciousness, is occasionally produced by sudden assumption of the erect posture after an individual has been relaxed while seated or lying down. The principal effects of arising from the recumbent to the standing position result from the hydrostatic pressures of vertically oriented columns of blood. The arterial and venous pressures increase in the dependent regions of the body. In regions above the heart, the veins collapse and the venous pressure becomes approximately equal to the surrounding tissue pressure. The arterial pressure in these regions diminishes by an amount equivalent to the height of the column of blood above the level of the heart. The cerebral circulation, however, is protected against the effects of the reduction in arterial pressure because the gravitational influences on hydrostatic columns affect equally the intravascular and extravascular pressures within the rigid cerebrospinal canal. During standing the arterial pressure at the base of the skull[15] (about 30 cm. above the heart) is about 25 mm. Hg less than the arterial pressure at heart level. The pressure of the cerebrospinal fluid within the skull is also about 25 mm. Hg less than the systemic venous pressure at heart level (i.e., is approximately 25 mm. Hg below atmospheric pressure). Since the arterial, capillary, venous and extravascular pressures within the skull are all reduced by the same amount (25 mm. Hg), the perfusion pressure from the arteries to the veins is not reduced when the erect position is assumed.

The cerebral blood flow is affected by a reduction in the systemic arterial pressure that acts to reduce the perfusion pressure, i.e., the pressure gradient from the cerebral arteries to the veins.

The cerebral circulation is unresponsive to virtually all mechanisms normally exerting control over peripheral blood flow. Lacking effective compensatory mechanisms, the cerebral perfusion diminishes with any significant drop in systemic arterial pressure.

SYNCOPE (FAINTING)

Fainting is characterized by an abrupt fall in blood pressure, bradycardia, pallor, dizziness, dimming or loss of vision and unconsciousness.[12, 26] These changes may be induced by many and varied conditions including emotional reactions (e.g., the sight of blood), standing quietly for long periods, hemorrhage and pain—particularly the diffuse, poorly localized pain carried by visceral afferent fibers.[26] Fainting reactions can be elicited experimentally by passively tilting the subject into the erect position during withdrawal of blood by venesection or trapping of blood in the legs with cuffs, after administration of various dilator drugs or during application of painful stimuli.

Because fainting most commonly develops in erect individuals and is promptly alleviated by falling or lying down, many investigators once attributed it to reduced cardiac output resulting from a combination of the bradycardia with pooling of blood in the dependent veins. Since then, evidence obtained in a variety of ways suggests that such a combination is not necessarily concurrent with fainting. Prevention of the bradycardia with

atropine does not affect the fall in blood pressure. By means of cardiac catheterization, a reduction in both right atrial pressure and cardiac output was observed after passive tilting and during venesection while the arterial blood pressure was well maintained. At the abrupt onset of the fainting reaction the blood pressure drops precipitously to lower levels (i.e., 60/40) with no drop in cardiac output.

Barcroft[12] accidentally discovered that during fainting reactions the blood flow through skeletal muscle increases greatly owing to both release of vasoconstrictor tone and activation of vasodilator fibers serving skeletal muscles. He compared the blood flows in the forearms of subjects with and without sympathetic nerve block during induced fainting reactions and found a flow through the innervated muscles exceeding that through the denervated muscles. These observations led to the concept of sympathetic vasodilator fibers serving skeletal muscles. Although the blood flow through the liver diminishes abruptly at the onset of a fainting reaction, the concurrent fall in blood pressure is disproportionately great. This observation suggests the occurrence of some vasodilation in the splanchnic bed as well as in the skeletal muscle.[26] Resistance to blood flow through the kidney may also be reduced. The loss of consciousness is apparently caused by diminished cerebral blood flow, as evidenced by a marked reduction in the amount of venous blood flowing from the brain.

HYPERSENSITIVE CAROTID SINUS

External pressure on the carotid sinus may activate the pressoreceptor reflex which normally compensates for an abrupt rise in systemic arterial blood pressure. The heart rate slows, and the peripheral vessels dilate as though to correct an increased arterial pressure. Thus, the systemic arterial pressure is abruptly but inappropriately reduced, and the individual experiences lightheadedness or even unconsciousness.

In 1933 Weiss and Baker[27] described 15 patients complaining of dizziness and fainting apparently related to unusual sensitivity of the carotid sinus mechanism. Some of these patients developed cardiac standstill for 2 to 12 seconds when pressure was exerted on their necks by tight collars, during shaving or even by the turning of their heads in a particular manner. Digital pressure over the sinus region readily produced the attacks. In six of these patients there was a definite aneurysmal dilation of one or both carotid sinuses, and in three a small tumor pressed on the sinus. In the remaining six patients no gross lesion was noted.

Four main types of syncope can be produced by compression of the carotid sinus: (a) transient cardiac standstill, (b) precipitous fall in blood pressure with slowing of the heart rate, (c) precipitous fall in blood pressure without bradycardia and (d) cerebral syncope now regarded as a form of epilepsy rather than as cardiovascular collapse.

Circulatory collapse accompanied by a precipitous fall in blood pressure, bradycardia, profuse sweating and pallor can be induced in many erect normal subjects by mechanical stimulation of the brachial arterial wall with a hypodermic needle.[28] Stimulation of visceral afferent fibers in general and pain fibers in particular produces depressor responses in most normal subjects and frequently produces syncopal

reactions. The vasodilation in peripheral vascular beds during syncopal reactions or in response to hyperactive carotid sinus reflexes represents an inappropriate response in the circulatory system which has accommodated to the erect position.

Systemic arterial pressure is most apt to drop during a sudden transition from lying down to standing up. The normal response to this change is a prompt vasoconstriction in the dependent parts, accompanied by a reduction in stroke volume and cardiac output. If the peripheral vasoconstriction is not prompt enough or not great enough, the individual is likely to faint. Thus, patients who have been bedridden for days or weeks may suffer from dizziness or faintness the first few times they stand. This is commonly attributed to a reduced sympathetic constrictor "tone" or to "sluggish" sympathetic responses. A person is much more prone to exhibit a transient drop in systemic arterial pressure on arising if his blood pressure is chronically low.

SYSTEMIC ARTERIAL HYPOTENSION

In any large group of normal individuals the values for systemic arterial pressure conform to the frequency distribution shown in Figure 5–18. Among people with blood pressures below the "normal range" are many who experience transient dizziness, loss of vision or even occasional unconsciousness if they stand up too abruptly, particularly first thing in the morning. These symptoms can be alleviated by arising more gradually or by sleeping on a bed tilted slightly with the head elevated. Such individuals are also prone to develop these symptoms on arising suddenly after kneeling, squatting or stooping. These people have "orthostatic hypotension" primarily because their sympathic constrictor activity is always limited and the response to arising is too slow or too slight. For example, Stead and Ebert[29] reported that the blood vessels of the hands did not constrict normally during a fall in blood pressure when such subjects were in an upright position. The heart rate remained unchanged or increased moderately. The signs and symptoms developed when the systolic pressure was 50 mm. Hg or less. The absence of normal vasoconstriction in response to a fall in arterial pressure was indicated by the following observations: (a) the diastolic pressure dropped markedly when the subject stood up, (b) the blood flow in the hand was higher than that in normal subjects for a given decrease in arterial pressure and (c) trapping blood in the extremities produced a greater reduction in arterial pressure in these patients than normal subjects. Thus, the reflex vasoconstriction which normally accompanies standing does not occur in patients with postural hypotension.

The same sort of symptoms are experienced following surgical excision of the sympathetic chains as a treatment for severe arterial hypertension.

POSTURAL HYPOTENSION FOLLOWING SYMPATHECTOMY

If postural hypotension and syncope result from an inadequate sympathetic constrictor response, elimination of the sympathetic outflow should produce a similar reaction which is more severe. Cutting of the sympathetic fibers running to various organs releases the vasoconstrictor "tone" and increases the blood flow through most tissues except the brain and kidney. (The effects of sympathectomy on the coronary circulation are equivocal for reasons not discussed in this text.) Since the sympathetic constrictor mechanism is dominant in the maintenance of systemic arterial pressure, elimination of this system produces a prompt and severe reduction in arterial blood pressure. However, the increased peripheral blood flow produced by the diminished peripheral resistance does not persist even if the entire sympathetic chains are removed bilaterally. In experimental animals, the peripheral resistance begins to rise again within one or two days and attains preoperative levels within a week or two. This restoration of the blood pressure is an expression of the increased reactivity of the peripheral vessels to catechol amines and other vasoconstrictor substances. This so-called denervation sensitivity has not been satisfactorily explained. Since the arterial blood pressure returns to preoperative levels even after extirpation of the adrenal medullae, the exact mechanism for the return of vascular tone remains a most perplexing problem.

Sympathectomy as a treatment for hypertension has been less than satisfactory because the arterial blood pressure returns to approximately the preoperative levels in about 80 per cent of patients within two years. Immediately after sympathectomy, all patients suffer from hypotension on arising. This orthostatic hypotension persists in very severe form for days or weeks but gradually subsides spontaneously in most instances. Within a few months these patients are able to function quite normally without their sympathetic outflow. In recent years, sympathetic blocking agents have become available for therapy of hypertension. These drugs act to reduce the

Table 6–1.   TYPES OF POSTURAL HYPOTENSION

Primarily an Inadequate Cardiac Output

  Carotid sinus syndrome—cardiac or vagal
    inhibitory type
  Adams-Stokes syndrome
    Ventricular asystole
    Ventricular fibrillation
  Paroxysmal tachycardias
  Cardiac tamponade
  Valvular heart disease (aortic and mitral
    stenosis)
  Ball-valve thrombus and pedunculated
    myxoma of heart
  Myocardial injury
    Infection (diphtheria, rheumatic fever)
    Acute coronary insufficiency
    Infarction (cardiogenic shock)
  Massive pulmonary embolism
  Post-tussive syncope (Valsalva maneuver)
  Pregnancy: Decubitus position with large
    gravid uterus

Primarily an Inadequate Peripheral Resistance

  Neurogenic disturbances
    Mediated through the autonomic nervous
      system
      Chronic orthostatic hypotension
      Surgical splanchnicotomy
      Debilitating infections (atypical pneu-
        monia)
    Mediated through the vasomotor centers
      Direct
        Brain tumor
        Cerebral vascular disease
      Indirect
        Vasodepressor syncope
          Carotid   sinus   syndrome—periph-
            eral vasodilator type

  Primary pulmonary hypertension
  Hypotensive drugs (modified after Wilkins)
    Sympatholytic or adrenergic blocking
      agents
      Ganglionic blockers, e.g., tetraethyl-
        ammonium and hexamethonium
      Centrally acting, e.g., dihydrogenated
        ergot alkaloids, *l*-hydrazinophthala-
        zine
      Peripherally acting, e.g., Dibenamine
    Vasodilator agents, e.g., nitrites (periph-
      eral), veratrum (central neurogenic)
    Agents with modes of action as yet uncer-
      tain, e.g., thiocyanates, pyrogens
  Acute fulminating infections
  Allergic reactions

**Primarily an Inadequate Effective Blood Vol-
ume**

  Hemorrhagic and traumatic shock
  Venesection
  Venous congestion of extremities
  Large varicosities and angiomas of lower
    extremities
  Postexertional hypotension

**Mechanisms Mixed or Not Completely Under-
stood**

  Adrenal cortical insufficiency, crisis
  Diabetic coma
  Low salt syndrome
  Anoxia
    Anemia
    Congenital heart disease, right-to-left
      shunt

systemic arterial pressure by blocking the sympathetic outflow. Like surgical sympathectomy they may induce postural hypotension.

SUMMARY

These few examples illustrate the manner in which physiologic mechanisms for the control of systemic arterial pressure may become involved in circulatory collapse. Obviously, reduction in blood pressure could result from combinations of those factors which reduce the heart rate, stroke volume and cardiac output, reduce peripheral resistance or retard or diminish the vasoconstriction which is a normal component of the cardiovascular response to arising. Judson[30] has based a more comprehensive discussion of these mechanisms on the classification presented in Table 6–1.

REFERENCES

1. HELLEBRANDT, F. A., and FRANSEEN, E. B. Physiological study of the vertical stance of man. *Physiol. Rev.*, 23:220–255, 1943.
2. MAYERSON, H. S. Effect of gravity on the

blood pressure of the dog. *Amer. J. Physiol.*, 135:411–418, 1942.

3. BURCH, G. E., and WINSOR, T. The phlebomanometer. A new apparatus for direct measurement of venous pressure in large and small veins. *J.A.M.A.*, 123:91–92, 1943.

4. SODEMAN, W. A. Direct venous pressure determinations by use of a new instrument. *Amer. Heart J.*, 43:687–690, 1952.

5. FRY, E. L. Physiologic recording by modern instruments with particular reference to pressure recording. *Physiol. Rev.*, 40:753–788, 1960.

6. FRANK, E. K. Physiologic pressure transducer. In *Methods in Medical Research*, Vol. 11, R. F. Rushmer, Ed. Chicago, Year Book Medical Publishers, Inc., 1966.

7. THOMPSON, H. K., JR., and McINTOSH, H. D. Cannulation and catheterization procedures. In *Methods in Medical Research*, Vol. 11, R. F. Rushmer, Ed. Chicago, Year Book Medical Publishers, Inc., 1966.

8. OCHSNER, A., JR., COLP, R., JR.,and BURCH, G. E. Normal blood pressure in the superficial venous system of man at rest in the supine position. *Circulation*, 3:674–680, 1951.

9. RUSHMER, R. F., BECKMAN, E. L., and LEE, D. Protection of the cerebral circulation by the cerebrospinal fluid under the influence of radial acceleration. *Amer. J. Physiol.*, 151:355–365, 1947.

10. WELLS, H. S., YOUMANS, J. B., and MILLER, D. G., JR. Tissue pressure (intracutaneous, subcutaneous and intramuscular) as related to venous pressure, capillary filtration, and other factors. *J. Clin. Invest.*, 17:489–499, 1938.

11. MAYERSON, H. S., and BURCH, G. E. Relationships of tissue (subcutaneous and intramuscular) and venous pressures to syncope induced in man by gravity. *Amer. J. Physiol.*, 128:258–269, 1940.

12. BARCROFT, H., and SWAN, H. J. C. *Sympathetic Control of Human Blood Vessels.* London, Edward Arnold, 1953.

13. POLLACK, A. A., and WOOD, E. H. Venous pressure in the saphenous vein at the ankle in man during exercise and changes in posture. *J. Appl. Physiol.*, 1:649–662, 1949.

14. HÖJENSGARD, I. C., and STÜRUP, H. Static and dynamic pressures in superficial and deep veins of the lower extremity in man. *Acta physiol. scand.*, 27:49–67, 1952.

15. STEGALL, H. F. Muscle pumping in the dependent leg. *Circulat. Res.*, 19:180–190, 1966.

16. RUSHMER, R. F. The nature of intraperitoneal and intrarectal pressures. *Amer. J. Physiol.*, 147:242–249, 1946.

17. FREMONT-SMITH, F. The role of elongation and contraction of the inferior vena cava, coincident with respiration, in the return of blood to the heart: report of an observation on men. *J. Mt. Sinai Hosp.*, 9:432–434, 1942.

18. DUOMARCO, J. L., RIMINI, R., and SAPRIZA, J. P. Attempted evaluation of venous pressure by angiocardiography. *Rev. argent. cardiol.*, 17:15–28, 1950.

19. HOLT, J. P. Estimation of the residual volume of the ventricle of the dog's heart by two indicator dilution technics. *Circulat. Res.*, 4:187–195, 1956.

20. SJÖSTRAND, T. Regulatory mechanisms relating to blood volume. *Minnesota Med.*, 37:10–15, 1954.

21. MUSSHOFF, V. K., and REINDELL, H. Zur Röntgenuntersuchung des Herzens in horizontaler und vertikaler Körperstellung. Der Einfluss der Körperstellung auf das Herzvolumen. [Radiographic examination of the heart in erect and lying position. The influence of the body's position on heart volume.] *Deutsch. med. Wchnschr.*, 81:1001–1008, 1956.

22. RUSHMER, R. F. Postural effects on the baselines of ventricular performance. *Circulation*, 20:897–905, 1959.

23. WEISSLER, A. M., LEONARD, J. J., and WARREN, J. W. Effects of posture and atropine on the cardiac output. *J. Clin. Invest.*, 36:1656–1662, 1957.

24. FRANKLIN, D. L., ELLIS, R. M., and RUSHMER, R. F. Aortic blood flow in dogs during treadmill exercise. *J. Appl. Physiol.*, 14:809–812, 1959.

25. CULBERTSON, J. W., WILKINS, R. W., INGELFINGER, F. J., and BRADLEY, S. E. The effect of the upright posture upon hepatic blood flow in normotensive and hypertensive patients. *J. Clin. Invest.*, 30:305–311, 1951.

26. EDHOLM, O. G. Physiological changes during fainting. Pp. 256–270 in *Visceral Circulation, a Ciba Foundation Symposium*. G. E. W. Wolstenholme, Ed. London, J. & A. Churchill Ltd., 1952.

27. WEISS, S., and BAKER, J. P. The carotid sinus reflex in health and disease: its role in the causation of fainting and convulsions. *Medicine*, 12:297–354, 1933.

28. RUSHMER, R. F. Circulatory collapse following mechanical stimulation of arteries. *Amer. J. Physiol.*, 141:722–729, 1944.

29. STEAD, E. A., and EBERT, R. Postural hypotension; a disease of the sympathetic nervous system. *Arch. Int. Med.*, 67:546–562, 1941.

30. JUDSON, W. E. Hypotension; physiologic mechanisms and treatment. *Med. Clin. North Amer.*, 37:1313–1339, 1953.

CHAPTER 7

CARDIOVASCULAR RESPONSES DURING EXERTION

In everyday life, the adjustments in blood flow accompanying increased activity of tissues or organs impose little stress on the capacity of the cardiovascular system. Digestion of food, formation of urine, secretion of enzymes or synthesis of substances in the liver or glands requires little or no increase in cardiac output above its resting level. Heat dissipation by the skin may involve increased blood flow and slightly augmented cardiac output. In contrast, exercise taxes the ability of the cardiovascular system to convey blood to the peripheral vessels and is the principal normal activity to do so. In man, dog and horse, the cardiac output during exertion is directly related to oxygen consumption.[1] The oxygen consumption of a resting man is about 250 cc. per minute, but during sustained exercise a maximum rate of oxygen consumption of 5350 cc. per minute has been recorded, an increase of 21 fold.[2] This represents a sustained increase in energy release from 0.12 horsepower to 2.6 horsepower. Ekblom and Hermansen[3] reported extremely high values in selected athletes attaining cardiac output up to 42 l./min. with stroke volume of 212 ml. at maximum. In the 10 seconds required to run 100 yards, the athlete consumes oxygen at a rate of about 30 liters per minute, equivalent to 14.4 horspower. During this brief period, however, he burns only about 0.5 liter, so that his oxygen debt is about 5 liters. The rate of energy expenditure increases about 120 times as a man goes from rest to maximum exertion. Fenn[2] computed the actual work done while sprinting as corresponding to 3.95 horsepower of actual external work; the efficiency was thus about 21.5 per cent. Based on these observations, the increased oxygen utilization by exercising muscle must be achieved by (1) increased cardiac output, (2) redistribution of blood flow from inactive to active tissues, (3) increased oxygen extraction from the blood and (4) oxygen debt.

INCREASED OXYGEN UTILIZATION DURING EXERTION

The oxygen consumption of the body is normally increased by significant amounts only during muscular exertion. The magnitude of the increased oxygen requirement is closely related to the quantity of external work which is involved in the exertion. The

220

changes in oxygen consumption from a condition of rest in the supine position to the erect position is so slight that cardiac output need not increase and stroke volume generally decreases considerably (see Chapter 6). Leisurely walking on level ground increases oxygen requirements slightly, but this can be readily accommodated by stroke volume at levels approximating those in the supine position. This effect is discussed in more detail in subsequent sections of this chapter. Moderate exercise can be well sustained by normal individuals utilizing the kinds of control mechanisms described in previous chapters. For any particular individual, maximum exercise which can be sustained for several minutes calls into play an integrated series of mechanisms illustrated in Table 7–1.

Oxygen delivery is increased by a combination of increased total blood flow through the tissues and more complete oxygen extraction from each increment of blood flowing through the tissues. Oxygen extraction is represented by the difference in oxygen content of arterial and venous blood. The oxygen content of arterial blood is normally in the range of 200 cc./liter of blood. The oxygen content in venous blood from all the various tissues averages about 150 cc./liter of

Table 7–1. MECHANISMS FOR INCREASED OXYGEN UTILIZATION DURING EXERTION

Stroke volume   Heart rate

Cardiac output   A-V oxygen difference

Oxygen delivery   Oxygen debt

Oxygen utilization

blood. During exercise, the oxygen content of arterial blood is well-sustained, but the oxygen content of venous blood drops to much lower levels in most tissues. In resting muscle and other tissues which do not participate in the increased metabolic requirements, the oxygen uptake is about the same, but the blood flow is generally reduced to some degree by selective vasoconstriction. The resulting redistribution of blood flow shunts blood generally away from relatively inactive tissues (e.g., splanchnic bed, kidneys) and toward the actively metabolizing muscle, but the magnitude of this shift appears to be variable, depending upon the severity of the exertion and on species differences. For example, exercising dogs exhibit little or no reduction in splanchnic or renal blood flow while humans appear to utilize this mechanism to a much greater extent as discussed in subsequent sections.

The increased cardiac output can be achieved by accelerated heart rate, larger stroke volume or a combination of the two. The changes in autonomic discharge to the heart which would result in tachycardia also induce sympathetic effects on the myocardium producing more rapid tension development and fiber shortening. The effects of increased sympathetic discharge to the ventricles was discussed in detail in Chapter 3 (see Figs. 3–17 and 3–18). Another mechanism which could contribute to increased stroke volume is the Frank-Starling mechanism which proscribes increased energy release in elongated myocardial fibers. If the ventricular myocardium were stretched by greater diastolic distention during exertion, increased energy release during systole would be expected. The relative roles of the sympathetic discharge and the Frank-Starling mechanism has been subject to protracted controversy, in large measure because of differences in control conditions, in experimental procedures, severity of exercise, species differences, types of measurements, and interpretation of the same or similar data. This complex and controversial argument cannot be fully resolved, but we can at least avoid augmentation of disagreement by dealing with the exercise response where it can be most comprehensively described: in dogs with chronically implanted devices for continuously measuring changes in pressures, cardiac dimensions and blood flow. Some sources of variability in canine responses are apparent. The role of the central nervous system in initiating cardiovascular responses in exercise has been demonstrated experimentally, contributing greatly to the variability in observed responses. Finally, recognizable differences between cardiovascular adaptation to exercise in man and dogs will be summarized.

LEFT VENTRICULAR RESPONSE TO EXERTION IN HEALTHY DOGS

Recently, the traditional concepts of cardiac control during exertion have been evaluated by means of new techniques for continuous analysis of left ventricular performance in healthy dogs.[4, 5] Changes in the diameter of the left ventricle and the effective pressure in it were recorded directly, and additional variables were derived by electronic analogue computers as indicated in Figure 7–1.

Comprehensive descriptions of cardiac responses during exercise can be gleaned from continuous and simultaneous recording of the critical physical variables of the type illustrated in Figure 2–23. In dogs, fully recovered from the surgical implantation of re-

cording devices for intraventricular pressure, ventricular outflow and dimensions (ventricular diameter or circumference) can be recorded continuously. Using analogue computers, other essential variables can be derived to provide a remarkably complete picture of the sequential changes in ventricular performance reclining, at rest, standing and during treadmill exercise (Fig. 7–1).

The simultaneous records in Figure 7–1 begin with the dog reclining quietly and then display a sequence of responses of the dog when hearing a loud noise, standing, doing treadmill exercise at 3 m.p.h. on a 12 per cent grade, standing, reclining, repeating exercise, reclining, and so forth. Note the startle response to the loud noise which produced a sharp peak in all the records except the ventricular diameter (top record) and the duration of systole (bottom record). A similar overshoot appeared in most of the records at the beginning of exercise, a pattern characteristic of a dog's initial or early experience with treadmill exercise. The initial overshoot is considerably smaller on the second exercise and after two or three more trials, most if not all the variables would promptly rise to a plateau and remain there during the remainder of the exercise without initial overshoot. This phenomenon has been confirmed in careful studies by Ninomiya and Wilson.[6] They found that the initial overshoot had a response time (63.2 per cent) for all cardiac variables of about 9 seconds. The magnitude of the overshoot was largely dependent upon the number of previous exercise periods, diminishing rapidly with repeated trials. The plateau levels established during more nearly steady state were dependent upon the magnitude of the work loads. The initial response of the inexperienced dogs were clearly re-

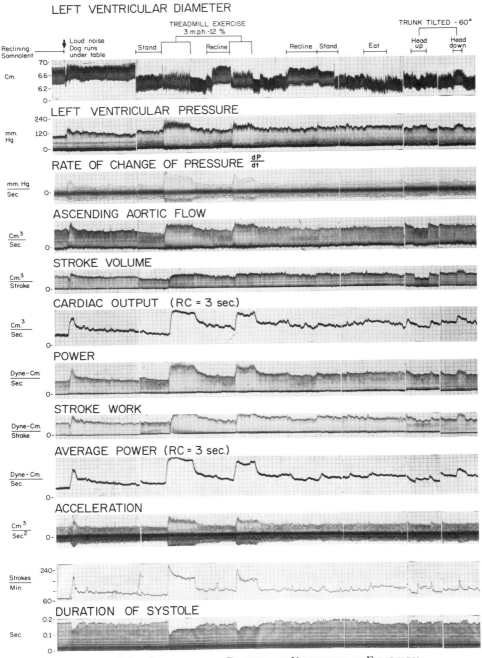

FIGURE 7–1. SPONTANEOUS CHANGES IN VENTRICULAR FUNCTION

The function of the left ventricle, monitored by the techniques illustrated in Figure 2–22, displays marked changes in all significant variables during both postural adaptations and exertion on a treadmill.

lated to the startle response when the treadmill belt started moving without advance warning. It indicates the major contribution of the central nervous system to variability in exercise responses in dogs and probably in man as well.

The magnitude and direction of changes in stroke volume during sustained exercise in dogs remains somewhat equivocal. For example, Wang, Marshall and Shepherd[7] found little or no change in stroke volume at wide ranges of exercise, often less than 5 per cent and the highest reaching 19 per cent. Smulyan et al.[8] reported a reduction in stroke volume at the onset of exertion with a modest increase in stroke volume developing when the heart rate diminished after the initial overshoot. Variability in the responses reported in different animals and by different investigators complicates the problem of providing a "generally accepted" pattern of response.

From more than 200 records of the responses of more than 30 dogs to a standard exercise (running on a treadmill at 3 m.p.h. on a 5 per cent grade), a "typical" ventricular reaction to moderate exertion can be summarized as follows:

1. *Heart rate.* Tachycardia appears promptly, without a lag, and is well sustained throughout the period of exercise.

2. *The left ventricular diameter* tends to change only slightly if the animal is standing at the onset of exertion. Systolic ejection may increase slightly and, on occasion, the diastolic distention may also increase somewhat. In general, the stroke deflections are either unchanged or slightly increased (see also Figs. 7–10 and 7–11).

3. *The left ventricular systolic pressure* is elevated in practically all records.

4. *The left ventricular diastolic pressure* is somewhat variable; the most common changes include a lower pressure during the early rapid filling phase and a higher end diastolic pressure (apparently due to more vigorous atrial contraction) with little change in mean atrial pressure. In some instances the diastolic pressures are definitely reduced.

5. *The instantaneous aortic flow rate* increases, particularly in the early part of systole.

6. *The stroke volume* (integrated instantaneous aortic flow) is unchanged or slightly increased in dogs. In Figure 7–1, the stroke volume increased about as much as was observed in any of the animals studied. In most animals, the stroke volume was increased slightly or not at all at this moderate level of exercise. In dogs exhibiting marked tachycardia, the stroke volume was sometimes reduced during moderate exertion.

7. The peak "power" (rate of doing work) of the ventricle is increased, representing the combined effects of high peak flow and ventricular pressure.

8. *The "stroke work"* increases slightly in dogs, reflecting the increased ventricular systolic pressure combined with the same or slightly augmented stroke volume. The increase in stroke work is undoubtedly greater in man than in the dog. The accumulated stroke "work" ("work" per stroke times heart rate) is definitely greater.

9. *The rate of change of pressure* (dP/dt) is much more rapid during both the rise in systolic pressure and the fall in pressure at the end of systole.

Thus, the principal changes in ventricular performance in dogs during exercise involved a combination of an accelerated heart rate and more dynamic ventricular contraction of the sort produced by increased sympathetic stimulation to the myocardium (see Figs. 3–17 and 3–18). Significant differences between the exercise responses in dogs and in man are described in a subsequent section of this chapter.

Variability in Exercise Responses. Comparison of two successive exercise responses in the same dog and single responses from two other dogs demonstrates fairly similar fundamental patterns, although the details differ. Significant differences in the diastolic diameter, the amplitude of the stroke deflection and the systolic and diastolic pressures are observed. Physiologic variability is a common feature of biologic systems, stemming from individual differences in structure, function, previous state of training and other characteristics. The responses of different animals tend to be more divergent than the responses of the same animal to different bouts of exercise. Successive exercise periods tend to reduce the variability and to produce more stereotyped responses.

The differences in repeated exercise reactions by the same animal can usually be reduced. On a subsequent day, the first exercise may again be associated with an overshoot. Thus, learning or conditioning may play a role in the nature and magnitude of the cardiac responses to exercise.

Some dogs have become so accustomed to the laboratory and so well trained that they will exercise freely on the treadmill for as long as desired without any restraint. When a trained dog is standing quietly on the treadmill, showing him the switch that activates the treadmill may induce a response much like the typical exercise response without any external evidence of muscular movement or tensing (Fig. 7–2). The variability in the ventricular responses of different ani-

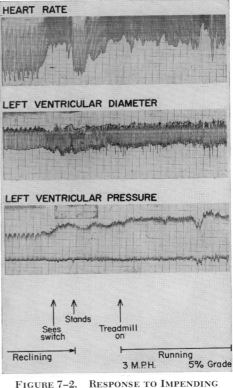

FIGURE 7–2. RESPONSE TO IMPENDING EXERCISE

A dog with extensive experience running on the treadmill was shown the electric switch that activates the treadmill, producing a left ventricular response very similar in kind and magnitude to the subsequent adaptation to running on the treadmill. This example is somewhat more dramatic than is generally seen.

mals, coupled with such evidence of control by higher levels of the nervous system, indicates the interaction of multiple mechanisms. Thus it seems futile to attempt to describe or explain the exercise response in terms of any simple generalization. These observations have required a critical evaluation of a long standing concept that cardiac compensation to exercise characteristically includes marked increase in stroke volume by virtue of the Frank-Starling mechanism.

POSTULATED RESPONSE TO EXERTION BASED ON THE FRANK-STARLING MECHANISM

For many years, the mechanisms for increasing peripheral vascular flow and cardiac output were discussed in terms of increased "venous return" and Starling's law of the heart. In these traditional formulations, the increased cardiac output resulted from two parallel sequences originating with the onset of skeletal muscle contraction (Fig. 7–3).

According to this postulation the cardiac response to exercise should follow the pattern presented schemati-cally in Figure 7–3B. A brief time after exertion begins, the diastolic pressure in the ventricles should in-crease.[9] The diastolic, systolic and stroke volumes should all increase and remain elevated during the exercise. The systemic arterial pressure should fall, exciting the pressoreceptor mech-anisms to induce tachycardia and pe-ripheral vasoconstriction which re-store the blood pressure to normal. This hypothetical sequence of events was generally believed to occur until serious deviations from it were seen during direct measurements on human subjects and intact animals.[10]

In this traditional view five mech-

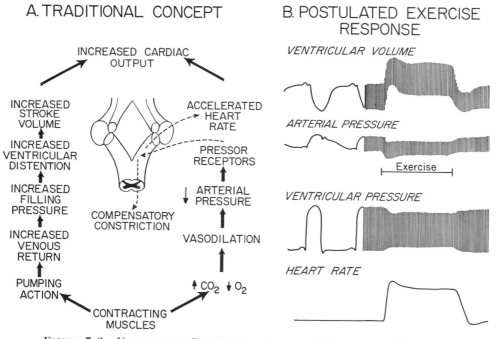

FIGURE 7–3. VENTRICULAR RESPONSE TO EXERCISE (TRADITIONAL CONCEPTS)

A, Schematic representation of the ventricular response, envisioned in terms of the Frank-Starling mechanism. According to this hypothesis, stroke volume would be increased by greater diastolic and systolic distention of the ventricles, reduced systemic arterial pressure, increased ven-tricular diastolic pressure and tachycardia.

B, The sequence of events postulated to explain the increased stroke volume by increased "ve-nous return" and tachycardia in response to diminished systemic arterial pressure through the presso-receptor mechanisms.

anisms were assigned prominent roles in promoting increased cardiac output during exercise: (a) a drop in arterial blood pressure, (b) cardio-acceleration induced reflexly by pressoreceptors, (c) an increase in "venous return," (d) elevated central venous pressure and (e increased diastolic ventricular volume leading to increased stroke volume.

Arterial blood pressure (systolic) is characteristically elevated during exercise with mean pressure remaining relatively unchanged. If a drop in arterial pressure occurs at all, it is so transient at the beginning of exertion that it cannot be consistently demonstrated in man or experimental animals.

Tachycardia often occurs in anticipation of exertion, before muscular contractions begin. During exercise, the elevated arterial blood pressure should slow the heart. What sustains the accelerated heart rate during exertion? Furthermore, cardio-acceleration per se does not increase cardiac output. With constant "venous return" the cardiac output cannot be increased by tachycardia.

"Venous return" is a term which is widely used but rarely defined. It appears to stem from experiments with heart-lung preparations in which an ample venous reservoir of blood could be artificially maintained. The intact circulation, in contrast, is a closed system. A sustained increase in volume flow through the entire circuit has been correspondingly increased. Some authors have used the expression *increased venous return* as though it implied an elevated central venous pressure or increased filling pressure of the ventricles.

Increased ventricular filling pressure. Although an increase in peripheral venous pressure during exercise has been repeatedly demonstrated,

evidence of changes in central venous pressure has been somewhat equivocal.

Changes in ventricular volume. Although the traditional concepts of cardiovascular control appear to call for an increase in diastolic volume whenever the stroke volume is increased, there is considerable evidence that the heart often becomes smaller during exertion.[11, 12]

Critical Evaluation of These Traditional Concepts. The traditional concepts of cardiac adaption to exercise were based for many years on the Frank-Starling mechanism, calling for an increase in central venous pressure, increased ventricular distention and greater stroke volume resulting from increased "venous return" and greater diastolic extension of the myocardium. A drop in systemic arterial pressure was predicted to result from reduced peripheral resistance from net vasodilation as illustrated schematically in Figure 7–3. These concepts stemmed directly from certain experiments with anesthetized animals. The development of techniques for continuous analysis of cardiac function during spontaneous exercise has made it possible to re-evaluate the role of these hypothetical mechanisms by directly comparing the response to treadmill exercise with the responses to the classic experimental procedures in the same dog on the same day.[4]

Increased venous return to the heart clearly corresponds to an elevation of the venous reservoir in the heart-lung preparation (Fig. 3–11). Similar effects are commonly expected to follow intravenous infusion of blood or other fluids. Increasing "venous return" (by rapid or slow infusion of blood, by compression of the abdomen with pneumatic cuffs or by tilting dogs into the head-down position) failed to produce cardiac responses bearing any obvious relation to the normal exercise responses even when the central venous pressure was greatly elevated.[4] Studies on human subjects have demonstrated that increased cardiac output does not result when central venous pressure has been elevated by intravenous infusion of blood. Infusion of fluids containing no blood cells may be followed by an increase in cardiac output to compensate for the relative anemia produced by the dilution of the blood.[13, 14] Thus, there is little positive evidence that an increase in "venous return," in the most common usage of the term, is essential for initiation of an increase in cardiac output when exercise begins.

Reduced peripheral resistance was simulated experimentally by rapidly pumping blood from a femoral artery into a femoral vein exposed under local anesthesia. The systemic arterial pressure declined and this reduction was accompanied by tachycardia. However, the overall response did not resemble the normal exercise response.

Naturally occurring catechol amines, l-epinephrine and norepinephrine, were infused intravenously in doses calculated to be within the physiologic range. In virtually all experiments on dogs, these substances in physiological doses produced bradycardia along with elevation of the systemic arterial pressure. Under these conditions the normal ventricular exercise response cannot be reproduced unless tachycardia is induced artificially. When the right atrium was stimulated with an artificial pacemaker during infusion of catechol amines, normal exercise responses were simulated with a fair degree of precision.

Stimulation of sympathetic nerves distributed to the heart from the stellate ganglia profoundly affected both the heart rate and the dynamic ventricular performance as defined in Chapter 3 (see Figs. 3–17 and 3–18). Prompt and sustained tachycardia can be produced by relatively weak stimulation. The ventricular contraction was much more vigorous, as indicated by a more rapid rise in ventricular pressure, a more rapid ejection, a higher peak pressure, a more rapid fall in pressure and a shorter systole. Stimulation of the same sympathetic fibers through electrodes implanted in a healthy dog produced changes in ventricular performance of the same general type as those commonly observed during spontaneous exercise.[15]

Stimulation in the central nervous system was next undertaken to locate sites from which impulses could reach the heart through the autonomic pathways. Since the hypothalamic region is generally recognized as the locus of important integrating mechanisms governing autonomic activity, the diencephalon was explored by means of stimulating electrodes.[16-18] The success of the search for sites of electrical stimulation which would produce cardiac responses similar to the natural exercise responses is indicated in Figure 7–4.

After a typical treadmill exercise response was recorded, the dog was anesthetized with chloralose and an electrode was positioned in the subthalamus (H_2 fields of Forel). Stimulation there produced changes in cardiac function of the proper type, and the similarity of responses to unipolar and bipolar stimulation indicated that the electrode tip was directly in or very near the source of the nerve impulses producing this change. The electrode shaft was cemented to the skull, and the animal was permitted to recover. Three days later the same locus was stimulated through the implanted electrode while the unanesthetized dog stood quietly. The

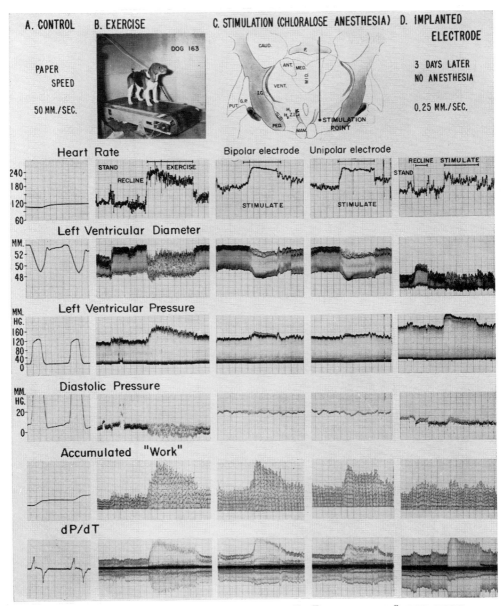

FIGURE 7–4. EXERCISE RESPONSE SIMULATED BY DIENCEPHALIC STIMULATION

A, Control records at fast paper speed (50 mm./sec.).

B, Left ventricular response to exercise on a treadmill at 3 m.p.h. on a 5 per cent grade.

C, On the same day, unipolar and bipolar stimulation in the H_2 fields of Forel under chloralose anesthesia produced changes of the same general type as were recorded during exercise. The electrode was implanted at that site.

D, Three days later, without any anesthesia, stimulation using the implanted electrode reproduced the original left ventricular response to exercise with considerable precision. The principal difference was in the ventricular diastolic pressure change.

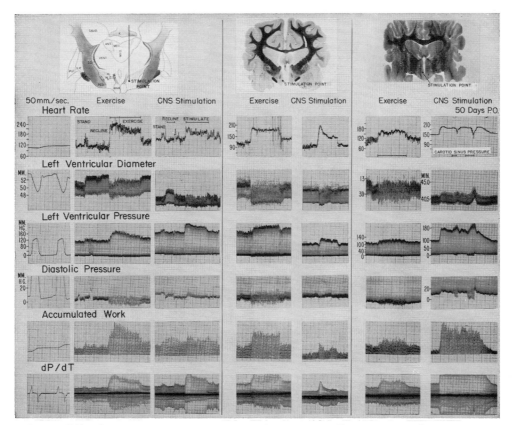

FIGURE 7–5.   COMPARISON OF RESPONSES TO EXERCISE AND DIENCEPHALIC STIMULATION

Diencephalic stimulation in the region of the H_2 fields of Forel and in the periventricular gray matter produces changes in left ventricular function comparable to those produced by spontaneous exercise.

response to stimulation reproduced nearly all details of the exercise response with considerable precision (Fig. 7–4B). The same kind of cardiac responses can be elicited routinely by stimulation of the H_2 fields of Forel or the periventricular gray matter, as evidenced by records from three different dogs (Fig. 7–5).

When the animal is under chloralose anesthesia, electrical stimulation of these areas often results in increased ventilation and distinct running movements as well as the cardiovascular response. Syncurine completely abolished the limb and respiratory move-

ments but did not affect the magnitude of the cardiac response. If the electrode was moved a very short distance up or down, cardiac responses without running movements or running movements without cardiac responses could be elicited. Unfortunately, the activated neural structures are never exactly the same during electrical stimulation and normal activity. For this reason, the role of these diencephalic sites in normal function cannot be assessed with confidence by stimulation alone. Additional evidence obtained by selective destruction of such areas is also necessary.

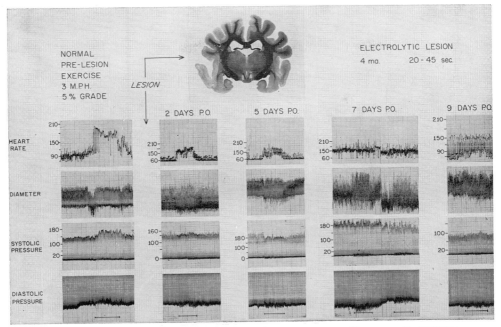

FIGURE 7–6. EFFECT OF DIENCEPHALIC LESIONS ON THE EXERCISE RESPONSE

The response to the standard treadmill exercise was recorded. Small bilaterally symmetrical lesions were placed in the H_2 fields of Forel. Two days later the systolic ventricular pressure rise during exercise was slightly reduced. After five days, the systolic ventricular pressure fell during exercise. Seven days after the lesions, the heart rate did not accelerate. After nine days, the animal performed the standard exercise without any significant changes in the recorded variables. The explanation for this sequence is not obvious, but it suggests that, before the lesions, these discretely localized sites may have played a significant role in the normal response to exercise.

Diencephalic lesions of a very small size were made bilaterally in regions which produced powerful cardiac responses. In one animal with such lesions the ventricular response to exertion decreased progressively during successive treadmill exercises (Fig. 7–6). By the seventh day after the lesions were made, the animal's ventricular performance did not change significantly when he exercised. Obviously, he could run only a short time. He then stopped and let the treadmill slide beneath him. During the period after the diencephalon was damaged, the animal displayed other signs of autonomic disturbance including vomiting, diarrhea, reduced food intake and easy fatigability. In spite of these complications it seems evident that the bilateral lesions destroyed pathways or collections of nerve cells important to normal cardiovascular regulation.

In summary, the changes in ventricular performance during exercise in dogs can be characterized by increased heart rate, increased ejection velocity and acceleration of blood leaving the ventricles, shorter systolic interval with little or no increase in stroke volume (Fig. 7–7). The differences between the recorded exercise responses in dogs and the traditional postulates are illustrated in Figure 3–14.

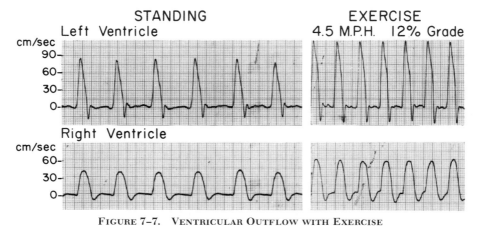

FIGURE 7–7.   VENTRICULAR OUTFLOW WITH EXERCISE

The instantaneous outflow velocity of blood from the right and left ventricles displays steeper upslope to a higher peak velocity during exertion. This signifies greater outflow acceleration of blood. The duration of ejection is reduced so that the stroke volume (area under each stroke deflection) may not be increased to any significant degree.

REDISTRIBUTION OF BLOOD FLOW DURING EXERTION

Contracting skeletal muscles need a greatly increased blood flow, which can be supplied by an increase in cardiac output. The load on the heart can be reduced somewhat by diversion of some flow from relatively inactive tissue to the active muscle. For example, about one fourth of the total cardiac output at rest flows through the kidney, a quantity far greater than necessary to meet that organ's oxygen requirement. A significant proportion of the renal blood flow could be diverted to serve active muscles at the expense of a reduction in the oxygen content of renal venous blood. If this mechanism is operable, the cells in the renal parenchyma must function in an environment of reduced oxygen tension to achieve the greater oxygen extraction. Curtailment of renal blood flow during exercise not only is a very reasonable concept but is supported by evidence from normal human subjects. For example, Bucht et al.[19]

catheterized the renal veins and measured renal clearances to determine the blood flow during mild and moderately severe exercise. When the work was slight, the renal blood flow was unchanged but the cardiac output was somewhat augmented. During more strenuous work the renal blood flow decreased by 20 per cent and the cardiac output was almost doubled.

The blood flow through the splanchnic bed and liver might also be curtailed during exertion. During supine exercise the hepatic blood flow, measured indirectly, was about 400 ml. per minute below a mean resting level of approximately 1500 ml. per minute.[20] The extent to which differences in posture would affect these observations is not known (see later discussion). The blood flow in the arm diminishes 50 per cent in the early minutes of exercise, primarily because circulation through the skin decreases;[21] this reduced flow does not persist throughout the exertion. According to Scheinberg et al.,[22] cerebral blood flow increased in subjects walking on a treadmill.

The distribution of blood flow during exercise most commonly has been studied in human subjects by means of indirect methods applied to one portion of the circulation at a time. Installation of ultrasonic flowmeters at several sites in the canine circulation makes possible continuous, simultaneous monitoring of several patterns of flow at rest, during exercise and under other conditions. When a dog ran on the treadmill, the flow through the

lower abdominal aorta to the hindquarters increased promptly and was sustained throughout the exercise (Fig. 7–8). The instantaneous flow velocity and the integrated flow (flow per stroke) rose, and there were more strokes per minute. In contrast, the blood flow through the renal artery was essentially unchanged, not only in the example presented in Figure 7–8 but also, consistently, in a series of exercise responses by six dogs. The flow through the hepatic artery to the liver and stomach was substantially

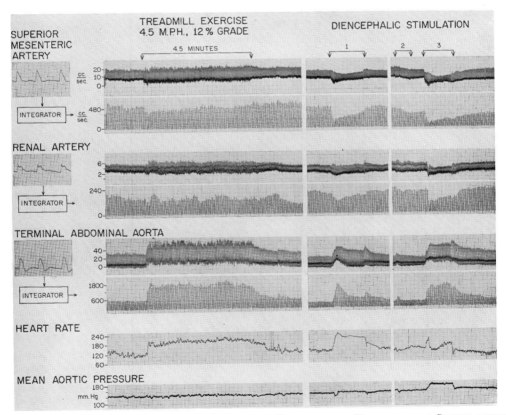

FIGURE 7–8.   BLOOD FLOW DISTRIBUTION DURING EXERTION AND DIENCEPHALIC STIMULATION

During exercise, the flow through the superior mesenteric and renal arteries may change transiently, but the integrated flow is essentially unchanged, while the flow to the hindquarters is greatly increased. A similar change in flow distribution can be induced by stimulation in the same regions that produced the pronounced changes in cardiac function illustrated in Figure 7–5.

reduced, as was the flow through the hepatic portal vein; these observations suggest that the splanchnic flow diminished. The blood flow through the common carotid artery was generally greater than at rest. Since flow through the internal carotid could not be distinguished from that through the external, the flow through soft tissues of the head might have increased without a change in the cerebral vascular bed.

The hypothesis that blood flow to the visceral organs would be reduced during exertion was not confirmed by these experiments. Van Citters and Franklin[23] utilized telemetry to record the blood flow velocity to kidneys and gut in husky dogs pulling sled and driver during cross country races. Although the flow in terminal aorta increased by 9 to 12 fold and coronary flow increased 5 to 6 fold, the mesenteric and renal flows were unchanged during this violent and prolonged exercise.

Electrical stimulation of selected sites in the diencephalon consistently influenced flow distribution directionally as exercise did (Fig. 7–8B). These sites were at or near those which induced corresponding changes in cardiac function, hyperpnea and running movements (see previous discussion). Thus, complete patterns of somatic and visceral adaptation (e.g., exercise) can be induced by selective diencephalic stimulation. It should be emphasized, however, that the motor and visceral components can appear individually after stimulation of slightly different diencephalic loci, so that the motor activity is not the cause of the changes in visceral function. Abrahams and Hilton[24] reported that stimulation of certain hypothalamic sites produced muscle vasodilation in anesthetized cats and defense reactions in conscious cats — pupillary

dilation, hissing, snarling, massive pilo-erection and running about the cage.

Uvnäs[25] noted that, although the vasodilator mechanism induces additional blood flow through muscle, the clearance of radioactive materials from the muscle is somewhat retarded and its oxygen consumption decreases. These observations were interpreted as evidence that the sympathetic vasodilator system tends to open arteriovenous shunts (or arteriovenous capillaries) and to reduce flow through true capillaries. Such a mechanism would at least deliver more blood to the muscles. It could then be distributed to the true capillaries by an opening of the precapillary sphincters during exercise (i.e., opening induced by local metabolic products).

BLOOD FLOW IN MUSCLES DURING EXERTION

At the beginning of exercise the flow of blood through the contracting muscles increases greatly to maintain and restore the supply of energy that is being released as work and wasted as heat. Barcroft and Dornhorst[26] presented evidence that contraction of skeletal muscles actually hinders the flow of blood through them; thus, the vasodilation must be great enough to permit very large flows in the intervals between contractions.

The widely accepted concept that vasodilation in active muscle results directly from the diminution of oxygen tension, decline of pH and accumulation of carbon dioxide and other metabolites appears to be logical and to be evidenced by the extreme vasodilation occurring after temporary obstruction of the arterial supply to an extremity (reactive hyperemia). As mentioned in Chapter 4, the evidence that a lowered oxygen level or an elevated carbon dioxide level is normally an important regulator of blood flow to muscles and certain other tissues is tenuous and indirect. The blood flow through the human calf immediately after exercise does not consistently reflect the severity of the preceding exertion[27] and remains elevated after the oxygen debt has been repaid and the heart rate has returned to normal. Then, too, the venous blood from the legs may contain more oxygen during recovery from either exercise or temporary arterial occlusion than during rest.

Most concepts of the intimate nature of the control exercised by metabolites, hormones or neural mechanisms over the peripheral vasculature are based on very indirect evidence and remain extremely controversial.[28] Evidence can be marshalled to support any one of several widely divergent views, and the solution to the dilemma does not appear close at hand. The specific chemical(s) which produce local vasodilation in active muscle have not been identified with certainty. Kjellmer[29] presented evidence that potassium ions released from within muscle cells during exercise can reach concentrations high enough to account for a major portion of vascular dilation during exertion. Intra-arterially injected potassium appears to simulate vascular responses observed during exercise. It is generally agreed that the sympathetic nerves serving vessels in skeletal muscle are predominantly constrictors. If the constrictor portion of this action is blocked, a vasodilation is elicited by stimulating sympathetic trunks which has been ascribed to a specialized sympathetic vasodilator system (see also Chapter 4).

Sympathetic Vasodilator Fibers to Skeletal Muscle. Nerve fibers are assigned to the sympathetic system on purely anatomic grounds. Although the vast majority of these fibers release a transmitter substance closely resembling norepinephrine, exceptions exist. For example, the fibers innervating the sweat glands of the skin are anatomically sympathetic, but they release acetylcholine as a transmitter substance and thus may be blocked by atropine. In recent years an eminent group of Swedish investigators has presented a great deal of experimental evidence[30-32] which suggests that some sympathetic fibers distributed to skeletal muscles (and possibly to the heart) release acetylcholine as a transmitter substance to induce vasodilation.

The use of the term "vasodilator" in this connection deserves additional consideration. After all accessible sympathetic fibers to the extremities are cut, the smooth muscle in vessels serving skeletal muscle retains a fairly high degree of tone, evidenced by the fact that the blood flow increases five- or six-fold when acetylcholine is administered. This effect is blocked by atropine. Activation of the sympathetic vasodilator fibers can also increase the blood flow above the level sustained under "basal tone." This effect can also be blocked by atropine administered in doses too small to affect the vasodilation caused by inhibition of vasoconstrictor tone. Such dual innervation of vessels in skeletal muscle is generally interpreted as mediating two forms of vascular reaction, the vasoconstrictor activity serving in the control of systemic arterial pressure and the vasodilator activity serving to accelerate muscle blood flow promptly at the onset of muscular exertion.[31]

The pathway of the sympathetic vasodilator system has been traced from the motor cortex[32] to the supraoptic area in the hypothalamus, through the medulla and thence down to spinal levels. Quite naturally, it has been suggested that impulses from higher neural levels traverse these connections to elicit vasodilation in skeletal muscles, "in circumstances when a sudden increase in blood flow in the skeletal muscles is needed in order to create optimal conditions for muscular effort."[33]

POSTURAL EFFECTS ON THE EXERCISE RESPONSE

Over some five years the changes in the ventricular dimensions of healthy dogs were measured hundreds of times by different techniques during various spontaneous adjustments. When the animal had stood quietly on the treadmill during the control period, exercise at 3 m.p.h. on a 5 per cent grade was accompanied by only slight changes in the ventricular dimensions. The diastolic dimensions might increase slightly in some instances and not at all in others. The systolic dimensions might decrease slightly, but, in general, the systolic deflections were not significantly augmented during the moderate exercise employed. The

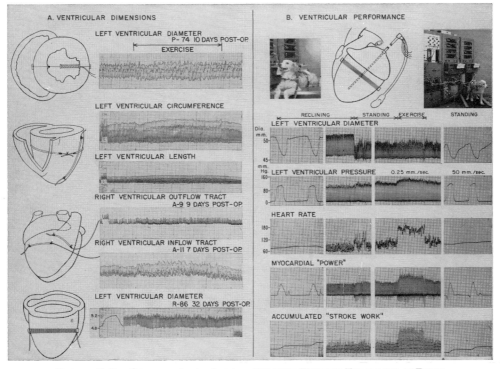

FIGURE 7–9.   CONSTANCY OF STROKE VOLUME DURING EXERTION IN DOGS

A, Direct recordings of changing internal left ventricular diameter, external left ventricular circumference and length, various dimensions of the right ventricular wall and the external left ventricular diameter consistently demonstrated little or no shift in baseline or increase in the amplitude of the deflections. This observation indicates that the total ventricular volume and stroke volume remain essentially unchanged in dogs during moderate exercise from a standing control.

B, When a recumbent dog stands up, the diastolic and systolic dimensions abruptly diminish and the stroke deflections become much smaller (see also 6–13 and 6–14). These changes in ventricular dimensions are much greater than were typically recorded during exertion.

examples in Figure 7–9A represent about the greatest changes in the stroke deflections of the left and right ventricles recorded by each of three different techniques. These observations suggested that the stroke volume did not increase materially when the standing animal began to run. This conclusion was confirmed by measuring the aortic flow directly with the ultrasonic flowmeter. On the other hand, if the dog was reclining quietly during the control period, the diastolic and systolic ventricular dimensions

and the stroke deflections all diminished significantly when he began to exercise (Fig. 7–9B). Clearly the cardiac output was augmented in either case primarily by an increase in heart rate rather than by greater stroke volume.

Tachycardia alone does not effectively increase cardiac output. This fact is shown clearly by the left ventricular response to cardio-acceleration induced by an artificial pacemaker (Fig. 7–10). Stimulating electrodes were implanted in the region of

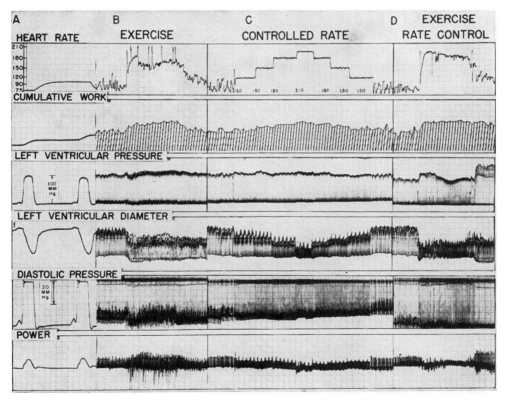

FIGURE 7–10. RELATION OF TACHYCARDIA TO STROKE DEFLECTIONS

A, B, The principal change in left ventricular function during spontaneous exercise is a pronounced acceleration of the heart with little increase in stroke deflections (see also Fig. 7–9).

C, Stepwise increase in heart rate induced by an artificial pacemaker in the same alert dog produced a progressive decline in diastolic and systolic dimensions and stroke deflections.

D, The changes in heart rate during exercise were precisely reproduced from a tape recording activating the artificial pacemaker, and the stroke deflections were greatly diminished as compared with the normal exercise response.

the sino-atrial node during an aseptic operation in which recording devices were also attached to the heart. After recovery the animal was exercised on the treadmill (Fig. 7–10B). The left ventricular dimensions decreased as the animal stood up and began to run. The stroke deflections were now slightly larger than those after exertion, during a standing control period. Stimulation through the electrodes near the sino-atrial node was then begun to increase the heart rate in a stepwise fashion (Fig. 7–10C). This artificial tachycardia was accompanied by a progressive reduction in the diastolic and systolic dimensions and the stroke deflections. Similarly, an artificially induced tachycardia reproducing the rates recorded during exercise resulted in a markedly reduced stroke deflection (Fig. 7–10D). Thus, an

artificial tachycardia does not produce the normal increase in cardiac output because the stroke volume is decreased. The normal exercise response involves no change or a slight increase in the stroke volume.

The nature of the cardiac response to exertion depends to a considerable extent on the state of the animals during the control period. For example, if a dog is lying quietly on the treadmill during a control period and then stands and begins to exercise abruptly, systolic and diastolic left ventricular diameters diminish along with stroke deflections (Fig. 7–11B). On the other hand, if the animal is standing quietly on the treadmill during the control period, the left ventricular diameter is not greatly altered when the exercise begins (Fig. 7–11D).

To summarize, the cardiovascular

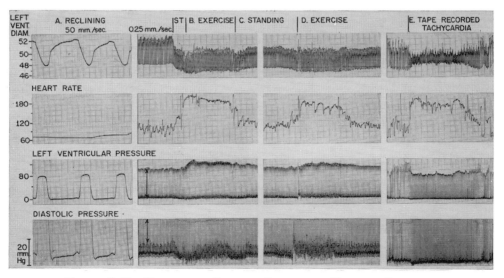

FIGURE 7–11. EFFECTS OF CONTROL POSTURE ON EXERCISE RESPONSE

A, In reclining dogs, the left ventricular diameter is approximately maximal and the stroke deflections are large.

B, If the animal stands and immediately begins to exercise, the ventricular dimensions and stroke deflections appear to diminish promptly in relation to the exercise.

C, D, Exercise begun from a standing control demonstrates that the ventricular dimensions and stroke deflections are not greatly affected by the exercise.

E, Artificial tachycardia produced greatly reduced stroke deflections.

response to physical exertion in dogs can be characterized as follows. If the dog is reclining during the control period, his heart rate will range around 70 beats per minute and his diastolic ventricular dimensions and stroke volume are at or near their maximal levels. When the dog stands, diastolic and systolic dimensions are abruptly reduced and the stroke volume diminishes by as much as 30 per cent. (See also Chapter 6.) Exercise of moderate degree is accompanied by a substantial increase in heart rate and little or no change in stroke volume (generally less than 10 per cent according to Wang, Marshall and Shepherd[34]). Strenuous exercise produces greater tachycardia and wider variability in stroke volume in either intact or sympathectomized dogs.[35] However, dogs without cardiac nerves revealed less tachycardia and larger stroke volumes, particularly during mild exercise.[36] With cardiac nerves intact, the cardiac output is increased primarily by increased heart rate, with stroke volume generally maintained or slightly increased, depending upon the magnitude of the tachycardia, particularly at the onset of exertion. In our experiments, the stroke volume during exertion failed to reach the recumbent values even during the maximum exertion we could induce the animals to sustain.

The blood flow is greatly augmented through arteries serving actively contracting muscles (e.g., terminal aorta). In contrast with traditional concepts, the visceral blood flow (e.g., to kidneys and gastrointestinal tract) was well maintained; indeed it did not diminish even during extremely severe exertion by husky sled dogs pulling heavy loads over long distance.[23] The redistribution of blood away from inactive or visceral tissues was not displayed by these studies as compensation to exertion in dogs.

EXERTIONAL RESPONSES IN MAN

The cardiovascular adaptation to exercise in dogs has been described quantitatively and comprehensively by continuous recordings capable of rapid responses to abrupt changes. Available information regarding cardiovascular adaptations in man are neither so comprehensive nor so dynamic. However, the data at hand suggest many points of similarity between human and canine exercise responses.

The constancy of the stroke volume which had been so consistently observed in the animal experiments (Figs. 7–9 and 7–11) led to a survey of the literature to determine how the stroke volume behaves during exercise by human subjects.[38] In eight different studies, summarized in Figure 7–12, the stroke volume changed only slightly over a wide range of exercise levels, graded for severity on the basis of oxygen consumption. This apparent failure of stroke volume to increase progressively as the work load increased was not consistent with observations by certain investigators, notably Mitchell, Sproule and Chapman.[39] In a personal communication Chapman pointed out that this discrepancy might be partly explained by the fact that the stroke volume during exercise is very little higher than that in the recumbent position. It seems quite possible that the stroke volume in the relaxed recumbent subject is at or near the maximal level ordinarily reached during heavy work. When the individual stands up, his stroke volume, and his heart volume, consistently diminish.[40] Beginning at this smaller baseline, the stroke volume in-

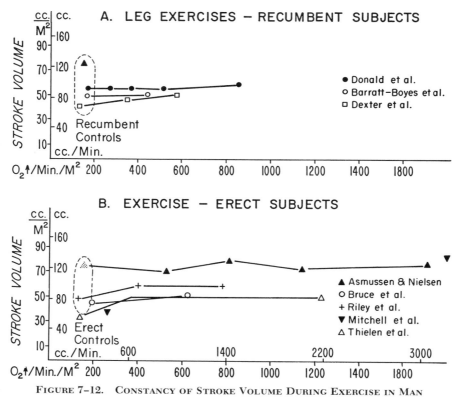

FIGURE 7–12.   CONSTANCY OF STROKE VOLUME DURING EXERCISE IN MAN

A, Human subjects exercising in the recumbent position exhibit little increase in stroke volume over a fairly wide range of exercise as judged by the oxygen consumption.

B, Normal human subjects in the erect position have smaller stroke volumes during the control period, and at the onset of exercise the stroke volume increases to a higher level where it tends to remain over a wide range of oxygen consumption. At the extreme levels of exercise, a further increase in stroke volume is observed (see Fig. 15–2).

creases promptly with even slight exertion, but does not necessarily increase progressively as the external work becomes more intense. Chapman has, however, presented evidence that there is an additional increase in stroke volume under conditions of maximal exertion.[41]

In summary, relaxed men typically appear to have a slow heart rate, large ventricular dimensions and large stroke volume (at or near maximum). Exercise in the supine position produces little or no increase in stroke volume even when the exertion is severe. Athletes tend to have slower heart rates, larger blood volumes,

higher ventricular filling pressures, larger ventricular dimensions and larger stroke volume than sedentary individuals equally relaxed and recumbent. Athletes also tend to respond to supine exercise primarily by tachycardia with little or no increase in stroke volume.[42]

On assuming the erect position, the heart rate increases somewhat and stroke volume declines precipitously by some 30 to 40 per cent.[42] Wang and Shepard[43] demonstrated that even the mildest exercise (alternately lifting the feet two inches off the floor) was sufficient to restore stroke volume to approximately the recumbent control values. Increasing exertion up to rather extreme levels produced only slight increases in stroke volume above either mild exercise or recumbent control levels.

Distribution of blood flow in man. Evidence for a shift of blood flow from inactive or visceral tissues to actively contracting muscle during exercise remains controversial. For example, Brod[44] reported no pronounced change in blood flow to kidney or splanchnic bed with light work. Greater reduction in kidney flow could be much more readily produced by neural mechanisms (such as the suggestion of heavy work, disagreeable situations, mental arithmetic), more or less as startle reactions produce profound renal vasoconstriction in dogs. In contrast, Rowell *et al.*[45] found that hepatic blood flow (estimated using indocyanin green) was reduced by 50 to 70 per cent during prolonged treadmill exercise requiring 48 to 70 per cent of maximum oxygen uptake. With more severe exertion, estimated hepatic blood flow was diminished by as much as 80 per cent or more.

Conditions Under Which Stroke Volume Increases. According to Yandell Henderson,[46] "The athlete's heart is supernormal." Many other investigators have also observed this tendency,[47] although Freedman *et al.*[48] could find no differences attributable to training in the way a trained and an untrained athlete meet the tissues' demands for oxygen. In any event, there seems little doubt that, during exertion, the heart rate accelerates less and the stroke volume is higher in trained athletes than in average subjects. Warner *et al.*[49] demonstrated that, if tachycardia is prevented by artificial control of the heart rate, the cardiac output increases normally during exertion through an increase in stroke volume.

Patients with chronically high cardiac output (resulting from anemia, thyrotoxicosis or an arteriovenous fistula) also tend to have a normal heart rate and an increased stroke volume at rest and to utilize increased stroke volume rather than cardioacceleration during exertion.[50] The cardiac responses of such patients resemble those of trained athletes.

Normal persons who stand during the control period will generally exhibit an increase in stroke volume at the onset of exertion, be it severe or mild. There is little evidence that stroke volume increases progressively with more strenuous work in average normal subjects. Subjects whose apprehensions induce tachycardia and reduced stroke volume during the control period will tend to display greater increases in stroke volume than relaxed subjects will.

SUMMARY

Traditional concepts of the cardiac response during exertion, based primarily on the Frank-Starling mechanism, have been evaluated for human subjects and intact dogs and found wanting. The patterns of ventricular response to exercise could not be duplicated by many different standard experimental methods including increased "venous return," reduced peripheral resistance, intravenous administration of natural autonomic hormones or by artificial tachycardia. Electrical stimulation of specific areas in the diencephalon reproduced ventricular responses similar to those occurring during exercise both with and without anesthesia. Lesions in the regions which produced these responses have been shown to produce profound changes in the responses to treadmill exercise. In both dogs and man, the stroke volume does not necessarily increase with increased severity of exertion as judged by oxygen consumption. The stroke volume is characteristically smaller during standing control measurements than in the recumbent position. During exercise in the erect position, the stroke volume may increase above the values measured during standing control but rarely exceeds the recumbent controls to any great extent. The stroke volume does not necessarily increase from very mild to quite severe exercise in human subjects. A further increase in stroke volume may occur at maximal levels of exertion.

REFERENCES

1. BARGER, A. C., RICHARDS, V., METCALFE, J., and GUNTHER, B. Regulation of the circulation during exercise. *Amer. J. Physiol.*, 184:613–623, 1956.
2. FENN, W. O. Acute and sustained high energy output. Pp. 8–17 in *Symposium on Stress* (16–18 March, 1953). Washington, D. C., Army Medical Service Graduate School, 1953.
3. EKBLOM, B., and HERMANSEN, L. Cardiac output in athletes. *J. Appl. Physiol.*, 25: 619–625, 1968.
4. RUSHMER, R. F., SMITH, O. A., JR., and FRANKLIN, D. Mechanisms of cardiac control in exercise. *Circulat. Res.*, 7:602–627, 1959.
5. FRANKLIN, D. L., VAN CITTERS, R. L., and RUSHMER, R. F. Left ventricular function described in physical terms. *Circulat. Res.*, 11:702–711, 1962.
6. NINOMIYA, I., and WILSON, M. F. Cardiac adaptation at the transition phases of exercise in unanesthetized dogs. *J. Appl. Physiol.*, 21:953–958, 1966.
7. WANG, Y., MARSHALL, R. J., and SHEPHERD, J. T. Stroke volume in the dog during graded exercise. *Circulat. Res.*, 8:558–563, 1960.
8. SMULYAN, H., CUDDY, R. P., VINCENT, W. A., KASHEMSANT, U., and EICH, R. H. Initial hemodynamic responses to mild exercise in trained dogs. *J. Appl. Physiol.*, 20:437–442, 1965.
9. RUSHMER, R. F. Anatomy and physiology of ventricular function. *Physiol. Rev.*, 36: 400–425, 1956.
10. RUSHMER, R. F., and SMITH, O. A., JR. Cardiac control. *Physiol. Rev.*, 39:41–68, 1959.
11. LILJESTRAND, G., LYSHOLM, E., and NYLIN, G. The immediate effect of muscular work on the stroke and heart volume in man. *Scand. Arch. Physiol.*, 80:265–282, 1938.
12. SJÖSTRAND, T. Regulatory mechanisms relating to blood volume. *Minnesota Med.*, 37:10–15, 1954.
13. SUNAHARA, F. A., HATCHER, J. D., BECK, L., and GOWDEY, C. W. Cardiovascular responses in dogs to intravenous infusions of whole blood, plasma, and plasma followed by packed erythrocytes. *Canad. J. Biochem.*, 33:349–360, 1955.
14. FOWLER, N. O., FRANCH, R. H., and BLOOM, W. L. Hemodynamic effects of anemia with and without plasma volume expansion. *Circulat. Res.*, 4:319–324, 1956.
15. ANZOLA, J., and RUSHMER, R. F. Cardiac responses to sympathetic stimulation. *Circulat. Res.*, 4:302–307, 1956.
16. SMITH, O. A., JR., RUSHMER, R. F., and LASHER, E. P. Similarity of cardiovascular responses to exercise and to diencephalic stimulation. *Amer. J. Physiol.*, 198:1139–1142, 1960.
17. RUSHMER, R. F., SMITH, O. A., JR., and LASHER, E. P. Neural mechanisms of cardiac control during exertion. *Physiol. Rev.*, 40(Suppl. 4): 27–34, 1960.
18. SMITH, O. A., JR., JABBUR, S. J., RUSHMER, R. F., and LASHER, E. P. Role of hypothalamic structures in cardiac control. *Physiol. Rev.*, 40 (Suppl. 4):136–145, 1960.
19. BUCHT, H., EK, J., ELIASCH, H., HOLMGREN, A., JOSEPHSON, B., and WERKÖ, L. The effect of exercise in the recumbent position on the renal circulation and sodium excretion in normal individuals. *Acta physiol. scand.*, 28:95–100, 1953.
20. BISHOP, J. M., DONALD, K. W., TAYLOR, S. H., and WORMALD, P. N. Changes in arterial-hepatic venous oxygen content difference during and after supine leg exercise. *J. Physiol.*, 137:309–317, 1957.
21. BISHOP, J. M., DONALD, K. W., TAYLOR, S. H., and WORMALD, P. N. The blood flow in the human arm during supine leg exercise. *J. Physiol.*, 137:294–308, 1957.
22. SCHEINBERG, P., BLACKBURN, L. I., RICH, M., and SASLAW, M. Effects of vigorous physical exercise on cerebral circulation and metabolism. *Amer. J. Med.*, 16:549–554, 1954.
23. VAN CITTERS, R. L., and FRANKLIN, D. L. Cardiovascular responses in Alaska sled dogs during exercise. *Circulat. Res.*, 24: 33–42, 1969.
24. ABRAHAMS, V. C., and HILTON, S. M. Active muscle vasodilatation and its relation to the "flight and fight reactions" in the conscious animal. *J. Physiol.*, 140:16P–17P, 1958.
25. UVNÄS, B. Sympathetic vasodilator system and blood flow. *Physiol. Rev.*, 40 (Suppl. 4):69–80, 1960.

26. BARCROFT, H., and DORNHORST, A. C. The blood flow through the human calf during rhythmic exercise. *J. Physiol.*, 109:402–411, 1949.

27. HALLIDAY, J. A. Blood flow in the human calf after walking. *J. Physiol.*, 149:17P, 1959.

28. FOLKOW, B. Nervous control of the blood vessels. *Physiol. Rev.*, 35:629–663, 1955.

29. KJELLMER, I. The effect of exercise on the vascular level of skeletal muscle. *Acta physiol. scand.*, 62:18–30, 1964.

30. UVNÄS, B. Sympathetic vasodilatory outflow. *Physiol. Rev.*, 34:608–618, 1954.

31. LINDGREN, P., and UVNÄS, B. Vasoconstrictor inhibition and vasodilator activation — two functionally separate vasodilator mechanisms in the skeletal muscles. *Acta physiol. scand.*, 33:108–119, 1955.

32. ELIASSON, S., LINDGREN, P., and UVNÄS, B. Representation in the hypothalamus and the motor cortex in the dog of the sympathetic vasodilator outflow to the skeletal muscles. *Acta physiol. scand.*, 27:18–37, 1952.

33. ELIASSON, S., FOLKOW, B., LINDGREN, P., and UVNÄS, B. Activation of sympathetic vasodilator nerves to the skeletal muscles in the cat by hypothalamic stimulation. *Acta physiol. scand.*, 23:333–351, 1951.

34. WANG, Y., MARSHALL, R. J., and SHEPHERD, J. T. Stroke volume in the dog during graded exercise. *Circulat. Res.*, 8:558–567, 1960.

35. ASHKAR, E., and HAMILTON, W. F. Cardiovascular response to graded exercise in the sympathectomized-vagotomized dog. *Amer. J. Physiol.*, 204:291–296, 1963.

36. DONALD, D. E., and SHEPHERD, J. T. Response to exercise in dogs with cardiac derevation. *Amer. J. Physiol.*, 205:393–400, 1963.

37. FRANKLIN, D. L., ELLIS, R. M., and RUSHMER, R. F. Aortic blood flow in dogs during treadmill exercise. *J. Appl. Physiol.*, 14:809–812, 1959.

38. RUSHMER, R. F. Constancy of stroke volume in ventricular responses to exertion. *Amer. J. Physiol.*, 196:745–750, 1959.

39. MITCHELL, J. H., SPROULE, B. J., and CHAPMAN, C. B. The physiological meaning of the maximal oxygen intake test. *J. Clin. Invest.*, 37:538–547, 1958.

40. LINDERHOLM, H., and STRANDELL, T. Heart volume in the prone and erect positions in certain heart cases. *Acta med. scand.*, 162:247–261, 1958.

41. FISHER, J. M., CHAPMAN, C. B., and SPROULE, B. J. Effect of exercise on stroke volume in human subjects. *Clin. Res.*, 8:73, 1960.

42. BEVEGARD, S., HOLMGREN, A., and JONSSON, B. Circulatory studies in well trained athletes at rest and during heavy exercise with special response to stroke volume and the influence of body position. *Acta physiol. scand.*, 57:26–50, 1963.

43. WANG, Y., MARSHALL, R. J., and SHEPHERD, J. T. The effect of changes in posture and of graded exercise on stroke volume in men. *J. Clin. Invest.*, 39:1051–1061, 1960.

44. BROD, J. Haemodynamic changes in the body during severe muscular exercise and preparation for exercise under physiological and pathological conditions. *Proc. 5th National Cong. Czechoslovak Physiol. Soc.*, June 13, 1961.

45. ROWELL, L. B., KRANING, K. K., EVANS, T. O., KENNEDY, J. W., BLACKMON, J. R., and KUSUMI, F. Splanchnic removal of lactate and pyruvate during prolonged exercise in man. *J. Appl. Physiol.*, 21:1773–1783, 1966.

46. HENDERSON, Y., HAGGARD, H. W., and DOLLEY, F. S. The efficiency of the heart, and the significance of rapid and slow pulse rates. *Amer. J. Physiol.*, 82:512–524, 1927.

47. MUSSHOFF, K. VON, REINDELL, H., and KLEPZIG, H. Stroke volume, arteriovenous difference, cardiac output and physical working capacity and their relationship to heart volume. *Acta cardiol.*, 14:427–452, 1959.

48. FREEDMAN, M. E., SNIDER, G. L., BROSTOFF, P., KIMELBLOT, S., and KATZ, L. N. Effects of training on response of cardiac output to muscular exercise in athletes. *J. Appl. Physiol.*, 8:37–47, 1955.

49. WARNER, H. R., and TORONTO, A. F. Regulation of cardiac output through stroke volume. *Circulat. Res.*, 8:549–552, 1960.

50. BISHOP, J. M., DONALD, K. W., and WADE, O. L. Circulatory dynamics at rest and on exercise in the hyperkinetic states. *Clin. Sci.*, 14:329–360, 1955.

CHAPTER 8

ELECTRICAL ACTIVITY
OF THE HEART

Electrical potentials associated with waves of excitation which spread through the heart can be recorded from electrodes applied to the surface of the body. The electrodes consist of curved metal plates firmly applied to areas of skin which have been coated with electrode paste and gently abraded to reduce skin resistance. Since the largest cardiac potentials recorded from the skin rarely exceed 2 mV., very sensitive recording equipment is needed to register them. Since electrocardiograms represent potentials inscribed on paper moving at a constant speed, the records indicate the rate and sequence of cardiac excitation. Thus, heart rate can be accurately measured and abnormalities of rhythm and conduction can be readily identified. The principles involved in detecting changes in rate, rhythm and sequence of cardiac excitation can be mastered with little effort. Electrocardiography becomes more complicated when changes in the shape of the individual deflections are analyzed. Basic theories used to explain variations in the configuration of electrocardiographic complexes will be given consideration.

The sequence of cardiac excitation and the specialized conduction system of the heart were described in Chapter 2 (see Fig. 2–12). The normal sequence of excitation initiates myocardial contraction, and establishes the mechanical events of the cardiac cycle. If the sequence of cardiac excitation and contraction is not clearly understood, the reader would profit by a review of those sections before proceeding.

I. THE SOURCE OF CARDIAC POTENTIALS

The changes in potentials, recorded as electrocardiograms, resemble electrical phenomena occurring in other excitable tissues such as skeletal muscle, smooth muscle and nerves (see Fig. 2–6). In the resting state there is a difference in potential between the inside and the outside of these cells. This potential difference can be detected by inserting a microelectrode into individual muscle fibers (Fig. 8–1). The difference in potential between the inside and the outside of a resting myocardial fiber ranges

POTENTIALS IN SINGLE MYOCARDIAL FIBERS

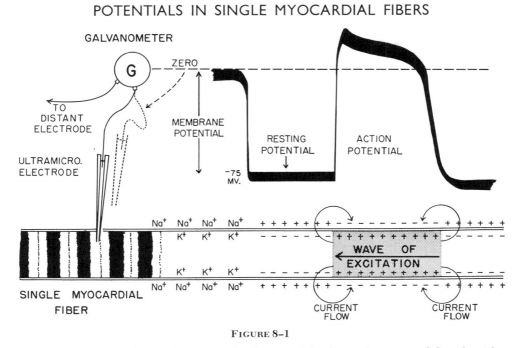

FIGURE 8–1

Potentials between the inside and outside of myocardial cells can be measured directly with an ultramicroscopic electrode consisting of a thin glass tube drawn out to a very fine tip (less than 0.5μ) and filled with a solution of potassium chloride. The potential difference recorded when the electrode is inserted into the cell amounts to about 75 mV. This potential is due to a difference between the concentrations of ions (mainly Na^+ and K^+) inside and outside of the cell, so that the inside of the cell is negative ($-$) in relation to the outside. As a wave of excitation passes over the fiber, an action potential is recorded; the potential rapidly approaches zero and overshoots (reversed polarity of the membrane). The resting potential is restored gradually at first and then very rapidly during the later stages of the repolarization process.

around 75 mV.[1, 2] Its presence has been ascribed to a charged cell "membrane."

THE ORIGIN OF MEMBRANE POTENTIALS

The cell membrane serves as a semipermeable barrier between two very different solutions. Outside the cell, the concentration of sodium is very high and the potassium level is very low. Within the normal resting cell, potassium is the predominant cation and the sodium concentration is very small. To attain a low concentration of sodium within the cells, sodium

ions must be selectively transferred from regions of low concentration across the cell membrane to the extracellular spaces where the concentration is high. Since active transfer of Na^+ requires movement of a charged particle against a concentration gradient, energy must be expended by the oxidative metabolic processes of the cell. As Na^+ is removed from the cell, a potential difference develops across the cell membrane and drives K^+ into the cell until its outward diffusion pressure is balanced by the electrical potential. Thus, the only requirement for the development of a resting potential across a cell membrane is the selective transfer of sodium ions out of the cell.

ACTION POTENTIALS

If the membrane potential is diminished to some critical level in a local area, either spontaneously or by an external electrical stimulus, the permeability of the membrane to sodium and potassium increases suddenly, permitting these ions to pass through the membrane.[3] This process rapidly reduces and then reverses the membrane potential. At the same time, current flowing into the depolarized portion of the membrane passes out through adjacent regions of the cell membrane. This local current flow is sufficient to depolarize these adjacent regions and produce propagation of the impulse down the fiber.[4] In this way, a wave of increased permeability (with its associated changes in membrane potential) spreads rapidly down the myocardial fiber. The fiber is restored to the resting state when membrane permeability to sodium and potassium returns to normal and the unequal ion distribution again becomes manifest.

The rapidly propagating area of increased membrane permeability produces a flow of electrical current and changes in potential which can be recorded from an intracellular electrode (Fig. 8–1). As the wave of excitation passes the electrode at a velocity of about 0.3 m. per second, the membrane potential decreases and reverses very rapidly (the inside of the cell becomes positive with respect to the outside). Thus, an active myocardial cell is not only "depolarized," but actually exhibits an overshoot to a positive potential. The membrane potential returns toward the resting value, slowly at first and then very rapidly.

Action potentials measured from single myocardial cells bear little resemblance to cardiac potentials recorded from the surface of the body. These differences must be resolved by considering the principles underlying the recording of external potentials from masses of myocardial tissue rather than from single cells.

ELECTRICAL MANIFESTATIONS OF POLARIZED MEMBRANES

The changes in the concentrations of Na^+ and K^+ cannot be easily measured during the passage of an action potential. However, the changes in potential caused by the movements of these charged particles can be amplified, recorded and studied. Thus, it is important to consider the electrical manifestations of the distribution of charged particles. To this end, it is necessary to be familiar with a few definitions.[5]

DEFINITIONS

The fundamental quantities in electricity are positive and negative *charges*, which are equal in magnitude and mutually attract each other. Electrical currents are defined in terms of the number of unit charges passing a cross section of conducting medium each second. *Current density* refers to the number of charges passing through a unit area each second. Electrical *potentials* are actually differences in potential between two specific points (e.g., electrode positions). The *potential difference* between two points is defined as the work necessary to carry a unit positive charge between these two points.

Potential differences and current flow in biologic systems occur in volume conductors instead of wires. A

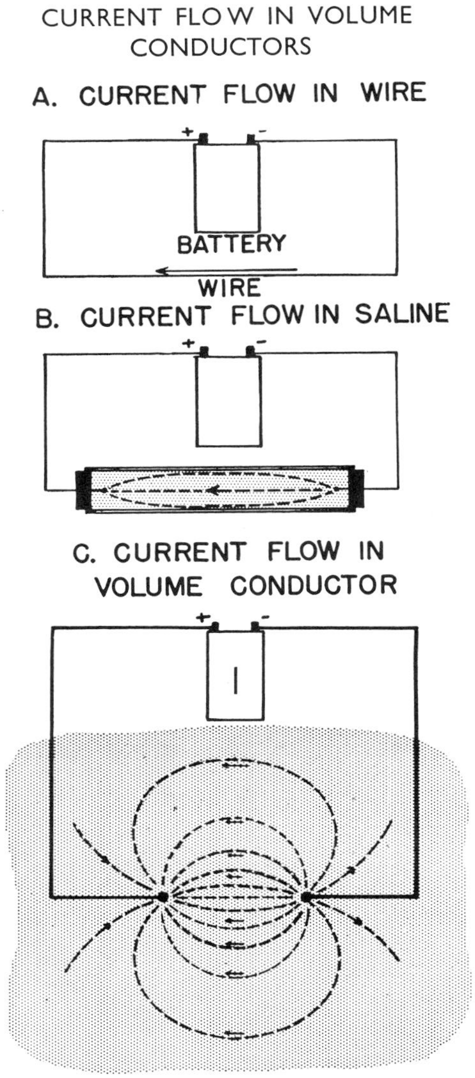

CURRENT FLOW IN VOLUME
CONDUCTORS

A. CURRENT FLOW IN WIRE

B. CURRENT FLOW IN SALINE

C. CURRENT FLOW IN VOLUME CONDUCTOR

FIGURE 8–2

A, Electrical current in a wire is carried by electrons which travel from the negative to the positive terminals of a battery.

B, Electrical currents are carried through solutions by positive and negative ions which move in opposite directions through liquid media.

C, A volume conductor is a medium through which electrical current can flow in three dimensions, as in a large volume of an electrolyte solution. Current density is greatest on a line directly connecting the two electrodes and diminishes along the more circuitous routes.

volume conductor is a medium, such as a large vessel containing an electrolytic solution (Fig. 8–2), which conducts electricity in three dimensions. Since all the body fluids contain electrolytes, the body is a volume conductor. Electrical currents flowing through volume conductors may traverse an infinite number of pathways (Fig. 8–2). If the solution is homogeneous, the current density is greatest along a direct path between the electrodes. Potential differences can be recorded between any two points along a current pathway, either on a wire or in a volume conductor (Fig. 8–3). On the other hand, if recording electrodes are placed at appropriate points on two comparable current pathways, no potential difference is present. The current flow progressively diminishes through the portions of the volume conductor at greater distances from the current source. The

POTENTIALS IN VOLUME CONDUCTORS

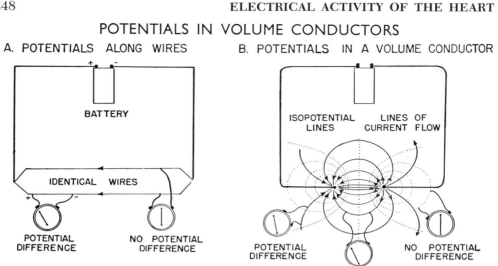

FIGURE 8–3

A, Differences in potential can be recorded along a current pathway, as in a wire. Indeed, the potential difference is the cause of current flow. No potential is recorded from corresponding points on two identical wires and no current flows between these two points.

B, Potential differences can be recorded along the lines of current flow in volume conductors. No potential difference can be recorded along lines which are perpendicular to the lines of current flow (see *A*, above). The dotted lines indicate isopotential lines along which no potential difference can be recorded.

potentials diminish with the square of the distance, schematically illustrated by the greater separation of isopotential lines in Figure 8–4.

At a great distance from the current source, the potential may be nearly zero, so an electrode placed in such a region can be used as a zero reference (indifferent electrode). Since the potential actually becomes zero at an indefinite distance, the indifferent electrode must be at a point where the potentials are too small to be significant. If an indifferent electrode is connected to one side of a galvanometer, the electrode on the other side can be used as an "exploring electrode" to measure the potentials in any portion of the volume conductor. Measurement of potentials with an exploring and an indifferent electrode (termed unipolar recording) is simpler to visualize and to illustrate than bipolar recording, in which both electrodes are in regions of high current density (e.g., the standard limb electrodes in routine electrocardiography).

UNIPOLAR ELECTRODE

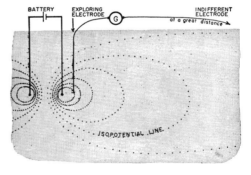

FIGURE 8–4

A galvanometer records the difference in potential between two points. If absolute potential is to be measured, one side of the galvanometer must be connected to an electrode at zero potential. The potentials in a volume conductor diminish with the square of the distance from a current source, as indicated by the progressively increasing separation between isopotential lines. If one of the electrodes is placed at a sufficient distance in the volume conductor, the potentials become negligible for practical purposes. Using this distant (indifferent) electrode as a zero reference, the exploring electrode can be used to determine the "absolute" potentials at any point in the volume conductor. This process is called "unipolar" recording, since only one electrode is affected by the potentials.

POLARIZED MEMBRANES

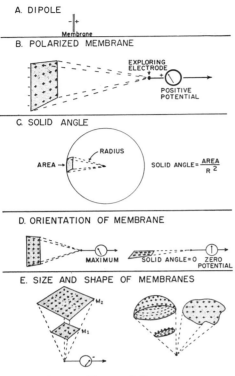

FIGURE 8–5

A, A dipole consists of a positive and a negative charge on opposite sides of a membrane.

B, A membrane with dipoles arranged so that the positive charges are on one surface and negative charges are on the other is called a polarized membrane. A potential from a polarized membrane in a volume conductor can be recorded on a distant electrode. A positive potential is recorded if the positive charges on the membrane face the electrode. The magnitude of the potential depends upon the solid angle subtended by the polarized membrane.

C, A solid angle actually refers to the apparent size of a surface as viewed from a specific position (e.g., the site of an electrode).

D, When a polarized membrane is perpendicular to a line drawn through its center to the electrode it has maximum apparent size when viewed from the electrode position and it produces its maximal potential in this orientation. No potential is recorded if only the edge of the membrane is presented to the electrode because the distances from it to the positive and negative charges of each dipole are exactly equal.

E, The potential recorded from a charge decreases with the square of the distance, but the number of charges on a uniformly charged membrane increases with the square of the dis-

DIPOLES

The difference in potential on the two sides of a membrane can be represented by a positive charge (+) outside the membrane balanced by an equal negative charge (−) on the inside (Fig. 8–1). Each pair of positive and negative charges is called a dipole (Fig. 8–5A). The potential produced by a single dipole is insignificant, but in biologic systems, many pairs of positive and negative charges are arranged on opposite sides of membranes.

MEMBRANE POTENTIALS

When a membrane has positive and negative charges arranged symmetrically as a double layer on opposite sides of it, it is said to be "polarized" (Fig. 8–5B). A large number of charges symmetrically arranged on a membrane combine to produce a potential which can be recorded at some distance. A positive potential will be recorded whenever the electrode is closer to the positive than to the negative charges. In other words, when the positive charges on a membrane face the exploring electrode, a positive potential is recorded by that electrode. If the number of charges per unit area (charge density) is constant, the magnitude of the recorded potential will be determined by three factors: (*a*) the area of the membrane (total number of charges), (*b*) the orientation of the membrane with respect to the electrode and (*c*) the proximity of

tance. Thus, if M_2 is twice as far from the electrode as M_1, the potential recorded from each charge on M_2 is one-quarter as great but there are four times as many charges as on M_1. Thus, each of these membranes would develop the same potential at the electrode. So long as polarized membranes subtend the same solid angle, they will produce equal potentials at the electrode regardless of their size or shape.

the electrode to the membrane. These three variables can be most easily described in terms of the solid angle subtended by the charged membrane (see Fig. 8–5C). The solid angle is greater when the area of the polarized membrane is increased or the radius is diminished according to the formula: Solid angle = Area/Radius² (Fig. 8–5C). The solid angle is maximal when a flat membrane is oriented perpendicular to a line drawn from its center to the electrode (Fig. 8–5D). If the membrane is tilted from this position, the solid angle is diminished, as is the potential recorded by the electrode. No potential is recorded when the distances from the electrode to the positive and negative charges are precisely equal (Fig. 8–5D).

By means of solid angles, the relative magnitude and sign of potentials from polarized membranes of any size, shape, orientation or distance from the electrode can be predicted. For example, the two membranes (M_1 and M_2) illustrated in Figure 8–5E subtend the same solid angle and, individually, each would produce the same potential at an electrode. The basic mechanism by which two membranes with the same solid angle produce equal potentials at an exploring electrode is indicated in Figure 8–5E. On the other hand, the pairs of membranes illustrated in Figure 8–6A subtend the same solid angles, but positive charges on one membrane and negative charges on the other face the electrode. The potentials from these pairs of membranes counteract each other, and no potential can be recorded by the exploring electrode. By the same token, no potential can be recorded by an exploring electrode near a cell which is polarized equally over its entire surface (Fig. 8–6B).

This principle is basic to electrocardiographic interpretation because it applies equally to collections of cells such as the heart.[6] During the intervals when the myocardium is completely polarized or uniformly depolarized, no potentials are recorded by external electrodes and the galvanometer remains at the baseline. Electrocardiographic complexes are inscribed only when part of the myocardium is polarized and the remainder is depolarized (e.g., during excitation or return to the resting state).

When an area on a cell is depolarized, the charges on the membrane are reduced in number or reversed in sign and a potential can then be recorded. In the region outlined by the solid angle in Figure 8–6C, a portion of the membrane facing the electrode is illustrated as completely depolarized and the portion of the membrane immediately behind has negative charges facing the electrode. Current flows from the surrounding polarized membrane into the depolarized zone and, as soon as current flows, a potential can be recorded at the electrode. Under these conditions, the electrode records a negative potential with a magnitude proportional to the solid angle drawn to the junction of the polarized and depolarized areas (Fig. 8–6C). This rather complicated picture can be simplified schematically by substituting a suitably charged membrane conforming to the zone of transition between the polarized and the depolarized membrane. Such a hypothetical membrane precisely reproduces the electrical effects illustrated in the more complicated drawing. Thus, a wave of excitation produces a negative potential when it is moving away from an electrode and a positive potential when it approaches an electrode (Fig. 8–6D). In the same way, a wave of excitation passing through a mass of myocardial tissue can be outlined by a solid angle which indicates the relative magnitude and sign of a potential recorded from an

POLARIZED CELL MEMBRANES

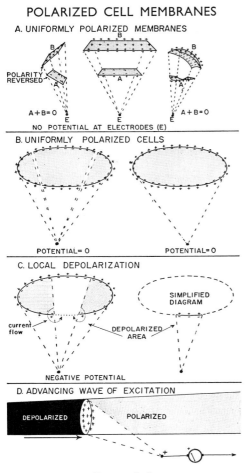

A. UNIFORMLY POLARIZED MEMBRANES

POLARITY REVERSED

A+B=0   A+B=0

NO POTENTIAL AT ELECTRODES (E)

B. UNIFORMLY POLARIZED CELLS

POTENTIAL= 0   POTENTIAL= 0

C. LOCAL DEPOLARIZATION

SIMPLIFIED DIAGRAM

current flow   DEPOLARIZED AREA

NEGATIVE POTENTIAL

D. ADVANCING WAVE OF EXCITATION

DEPOLARIZED   POLARIZED

FIGURE 8–6

electrode at a specific site in relation to the electrical disturbance.

In summary, myocardial cells produce no external potentials so long as they are either completely polarized or completely depolarized, because the equal and opposite charges in each fiber precisely counteract each other. Potentials are recorded only from a transition zone between the polarized and depolarized regions where the charged surfaces are not cancelled. Stated another way, potentials can be recorded only when electrical current flows in response to potential differences (e.g., between polarized and depolarized regions). This is the essence of electrocardiography.

SEQUENCE OF CARDIAC EXCITATION

ATRIAL EXCITATION AND REPOLARIZATION

The wave of excitation normally spreads as a concentric ring from its origin at the sino-atrial node.[7, 8] As atrial depolarization spreads, the area of the excitatory wave first increases

A, The potentials from pairs of uniformly polarized membranes will cancel if they present the same solid angles and the orientation of the charges is reversed. In each of the three examples, the potential at the electrode is zero because the negative charges of one membrane are precisely balanced by the positive charges of its mate.

B, If a uniformly polarized cell is considered in three segments, the principle illustrated in Figure 8–6A applies. In each of the three solid angles, the proximal portion of the membrane has positive charges and the more distant portion has negative charges facing the electrode. Since the near and distant portions of the membrane subtend the same solid angle and the charges are oriented in opposite directions, their effects cancel and the potential at the electrode is zero. Thus, a uniformly polarized (or uniformly depolarized) cell produces no potential which can be recorded by an external electrode. In other words, if the membrane is uniformly polarized, there is no potential difference and no flow of electrical current, and no potential can be recorded.

C, When a region of a polarized cell becomes partially or completely depolarized, electrical currents flow from the polarized regions into the depolarized zone. A potential can then be recorded by a distant electrode; the magnitude of the potential is determined by the solid angle subtended by the depolarized area. On the far side of the cell, negative charges are not balanced by opposite charges in the depolarized region, so the electrode records a negative potential. On the right, a suitably charged membrane conforming to the depolarized area is comparable to the more complicated picture on the left, since the solid angle is the same.

D, The advancing wave of excitation can be visualized as though a suitably charged membrane were placed at the junction between polarized and depolarized regions (as in C, above). Since the outside of the polarized area is positive in relation to the inside, an electrode records a positive potential when a wave of excitation advances toward it and a negative potential when a wave of excitation is moving away.

EXCITATION OF THE ATRIA

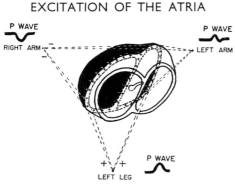

FIGURE 8–7

As a wave of excitation spreads concentrically through the atrial musculature, different patterns are recorded by unipolar electrodes placed on the extremities. For example, the wave of excitation is advancing toward the left leg which therefore responds to the positive charges facing this electrode and inscribes an upward deflection (see Fig. 8–6D). In contrast, the wave of excitation moves away from the right shoulder, so a downward deflection is recorded from the right arm. If the wave of excitation first advances toward the left shoulder and then recedes from this position, a diphasic deflection is recorded from a unipolar electrode on the left arm. In each case the magnitude of the deflection at any instant is determined by the solid angle subtended by the wave of excitation as viewed from the effective electrode position (right and left shoulders and symphysis pubis).

and then diminishes. Viewed from an electrode facing the apex (left leg), the advancing ring of excitation has positive charges facing the recording electrode, and the recorded P wave is an upward deflection (Fig. 8–7). A negative potential is recorded from the electrode at the right shoulder because the wave of excitation is moving away from this point. The wave of excitation travels toward the left shoulder at first, and during the last stages it may pass beyond this position, producing first a positive, then a negative (diphasic) deflection (Fig. 8–7).

The wave of repolarization normally follows the same course as the wave of excitation, but the pol-

arity is reversed.[9] The myocardial fibers in advance of the wave of repolarization are relatively negative (the outside is negative in relation to the inside of the cell), and the repolarized tissue is relatively positive. This condition is the reverse of that existing during depolarization, and can be represented by a charged membrane with negative charges oriented in the direction of the wave's movement. Thus, the wave of repolarization (T_a wave) causes a deflection in the opposite direction to that of the P wave. The T_a wave has longer duration and smaller amplitude than the P wave because repolarization is a slower process. It is generally obscured by the QRS complex, which normally occurs during inscription of the T_a wave.[10]

VENTRICULAR EXCITATION AND REPOLARIZATION

As the wave of excitation passes down the conduction system, the solid angle subtended by this bundle of tissue is very small, and the resultant potentials are not sufficient to produce a deflection. The first recorded potential develops when a significant area of ventricular myocardium has been invaded by a wave of excitation. The configuration of the QRS complex will depend upon the sequence of ventricular excitation and the direction taken by the excitatory waves.[11]

THE QRS COMPLEX. Ventricular excitation can be schematically illustrated by a simplified diagram as in Figure 8–8. The magnitude and sign of the potentials are indicated by solid angles subtended by the margins of the transitional zone between the polarized and depolarized regions. The wave of excitation travels toward the left leg (V_F), producing a positive deflection, and moves away from the

VENTRICULAR EXCITATION

A. VENTRICULAR DEPOLARIZATION (QRS)

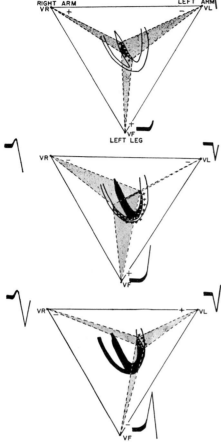

FIGURE 8–8

VENTRICULAR RECOVERY

B. UNIFORM DEPOLARIZATION (ISOELECTRIC S–T)

C. REPOLARIZATION (T WAVE)

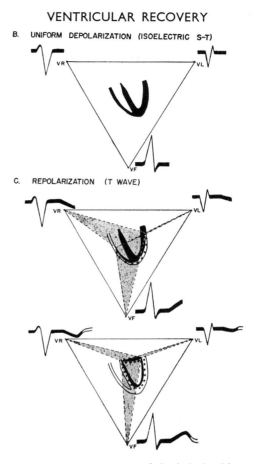

A, The origin of the potentials recorded by unipolar extremity electrodes during ventricular depolarization is illustrated schematically. The initial wave of excitation is presented as originating on the left side of the interventricular septum and moving toward the right ventricle. This area of excitation would produce an upward deflection in both V_R and V_F because the positive charges face these electrodes. A downward deflection would be recorded from V_L because the wave of excitation is moving away from the left shoulder.

At a later stage, the wave of excitation conforms roughly to a cuplike shell of excitation progressing from endocardium to epicardium. Since the wave of excitation is moving toward V_F and away from V_R, the deflections in these two leads are in opposite directions.

If a wave of excitation invades the basilar portion of the left ventricular wall in the final stages, it is moving toward the left shoulder. A downward deflection is inscribed from V_R and V_F and an upward deflection from V_L.

B, When the ventricles are uniformly depolarized no potentials are recorded from any of the external electrodes (see Fig. 8–6*B*).

C, Since depolarized regions are negative with respect to polarized myocardium, a negative deflection is recorded when a wave of repolarization advances toward an electrode. Assuming that repolarization begins on the epicardial surface of the ventricle and progresses inward, a negative deflection would be recorded at V_R since the activity is moving toward the right shoulder. A positive deflection would be recorded at V_R and, in the example illustrated, very little potential would be recorded by V_L because a very small solid angle would be subtended.

The endocardial region of the left ventricle must be the last portion to be repolarized. Here, as in the other examples, the cuplike configuration of the wave of excitation can be represented by a flat, polarized membrane at the junction between polarized and depolarized myocardium at the base of the heart (see Fig. 8–6*C*).

right shoulder as indicated by the negative deflection at V_R. The small solid angle subtended at V_L is associated with a small deflection which may be upward or downward depending upon the exact orientation of the spreading wave. In Figure 8–9 the largest deflections during the entire course of depolarization occur in V_R and V_F, since the solid angles from these electrode positions are greater than that from V_L. The patterns derived from V_L are very susceptible to variations in the orientation of the heart. They are generally diphasic; the downward deflection predominates when the heart is oriented more vertically and the upward deflection is more prominent if the long axis of the heart approaches horizontal.

THE S-T SEGMENT. When ventricular excitation is complete, the degree of membrane polarization is normally uniform throughout the myocardium (Fig. 8–8B). Under these conditions, no potentials are recorded by external electrodes (see Fig. 8–8B), and the galvanometer returns to the baseline, where it remains until the effects of repolarization are manifest in the inscription of the T wave.

THE T WAVE. The normal sequence of ventricular repolarization is unknown. Since a wave of repolarization should produce potentials opposite in sign from those developed during depolarization, the QRS and T waves would deflect in opposite directions if these two processes followed the same course. On the contrary, the QRS and T waves usually deflect in the same direction, so the process of repolarization does not follow the same sequence as depolarization. Experimentally, repolarization can be delayed by applying pressure to the myocardium. Repolarization may be delayed in the subendocardial layers of myocardium owing to high intraventricular pressure affecting the inner layers more than the external layers. On this basis, repolarization is frequently visualized as beginning in the outer layers of myocardium and progressing toward the endocardial surface, in general retracing the path of the wave of excitation. This traditional view will be followed in the present discussion, although it has not been adequately established by direct experimental evidence. The T waves are generally of smaller amplitude and longer duration and have a more rounded contour than the QRS complex because repolarization is a slower process than depolarization. The delay in repolarization is illustrated in the monophasic action potential from a single myocardial fiber (Fig. 8–1) in which the upward deflection (depolarization) occurs much more rapidly than the return to the baseline (repolarization). A schematic representation of the inscription of a T wave from unipolar extremity electrodes is illustrated in Figure 8–8C.

With simplified diagrams as in Figure 8–8C, it is possible to illustrate a mechanism by which ventricular excitation can produce reasonable facsimiles of the deflections recorded from unipolar limb leads.

II. INTERPRETATION OF THE SEQUENCE OF EXCITATION

The electrical activity of the heart is routinely recorded in a standardized manner on graph paper moving at a constant speed. Such electrocardiograms are graphic representations of the sequence of the excitation of the heart. For this reason, any change in this sequence should be readily visible on the records. Even without extensive experience in interpretation of electrocardiograms, changes in the rate or rhythm of the heart beat or in the conduction of the wave of excitation can be analyzed on a purely logical basis. Only a few principles and a few simple rules are required for this type of interpretation. Additional information of great value can be obtained by more detailed analysis of the changes in the shape of the electrocardiographic deflections, which will be considered in Section III of this chapter.

brating potential of 1 mV. produces a vertical deflection of precisely 1 cm. Thin horizontal lines on the paper are 1 mm. apart and represent 0.1 mV., and the thick lines indicate 0.5 mV. The recording paper routinely moves at a constant rate of 25 mm. per second (approximately 1 in. per second). The thin vertical lines demarcate intervals of 0.20 second (1/5 second). Routine electrocardiography includes records obtained by registering potential differences between the extremities as indicated in Figure 8–9.

STANDARDIZATION

The sensitivity of the recording equipment is adjusted until a cali-

THE NORMAL PATTERN OF EXCITATION

On typical electrocardiograms, P waves are followed, after an interval,

THE STANDARD LIMB LEADS

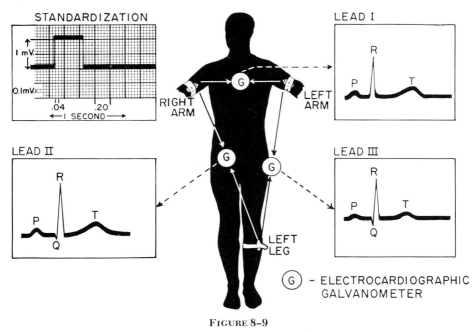

FIGURE 8–9

Electrocardiograms are recorded on paper divided into 1 mm. and 5 mm. squares. Standardization of the electrocardiograph is accomplished by adjusting its sensitivity until a potential of 1 mV. produces a vertical deflection of 1 cm. The paper moves at a standard rate of 25 mm. per second, so 5 mm. along the horizontal axis represents an interval of 0.20 second and 1 mm. indicates 0.04 second.

The standard limb leads are lead I, lead II and lead III. Lead I records the differences in potential between electrodes on the right and left arms. In lead II the galvanometer is connected to electrodes on the right arm and left leg. Lead III refers to connections between the left arm and left leg.

by the electrical signs of ventricular excitation (QRS) and recovery (T). The duration of the various waves and of the intervals between them usually varies within fairly definite ranges in normal individuals. Average values rounded to the nearest 0.04 second are indicated in Figure 8–10. The duration of the P wave ranges around 0.08 second. During the interval between the end of the P wave and the beginning of the ventricular excitation (Q or R wave) the galvanometer remains at the baseline for about 0.08 second because no external potentials are recorded during the A-V nodal delay and the passage of the wave of excitation to the ventricular myocarddium. The QRS interval (0.08 second) represents the time required for waves of excitation to spread through the ventricular walls. The flat segment between the end of the QRS complex

DURATION OF WAVES AND INTERVALS

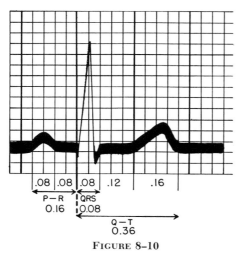

FIGURE 8–10

The average durations of electrocardiographic waves and intervals are rounded to the nearest 0.04 second so they are easier to remember. The P-R interval, QRS interval and Q-T interval are among the most common values measured during routine electrocardiographic interpretation.

and the beginning of the T wave (S-T interval, 0.12 second) represents the period during which the ventricles are more or less uniformly excited, and the T wave occurs during the restoration of the ventricular myocardium to the resting or excitable state.

VARIATIONS IN HEART RATE

The heart rate is determined normally by the frequency with which the sinoatrial node emits excitatory impulses. The frequency at which the S-A node discharges is influenced by activity of nerve fibers from the autonomic nervous system.

MEASUREMENT OF HEART RATE

Since the electrocardiogram contains an accurate representation of the intervals between successive cardiac cycles, atrial and ventricular rates can be easily measured. The simplest method is to determine the number of cycles (and fractions thereof) occurring in 3 seconds and multiply this number by 20 to give the number of cycles in one minute (60 seconds) (Fig. 8–11). At the normal paper speed (25 mm. per second), 1 second is represented by five large squares; 3 seconds by fifteen large squares (3 in.). The QRS complexes, easily identified because of the rapid deflections, are tallied over a 3 in. distance. If exactly four ventricular cycles occur during 3 seconds, the ventricular rate is 80 per minute (see Fig. 8–11). If the P waves can be identified, the same process can be used to determine the atrial rate. P waves can usually be differentiated from T waves, which always follow QRS complexes at a fairly characteristic interval (see Fig. 8–10).

MEASUREMENT OF VENTRICULAR RATE

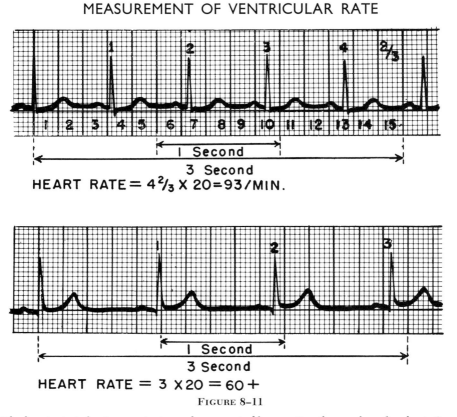

FIGURE 8-11

The heart rate in beats per minute can be computed by counting the number of cycles in 3 seconds and multiplying this value by 20 ($3 \times 20 = 60$ seconds). At standard paper speed, 3 seconds is represented by 15 large squares. In the first example, there are 4⅔ cycles in 3 seconds so the heart rate is about 93 per minute. In the second example, there are slightly more than 3 cycles in 3 seconds so the heart rate is a little over 60 per minute.

ABNORMALITIES OF HEART RATE

Variations in the intensity of the sustained vagal tone have greater influence on the S-A node than does altered sympathetic activity. The slow heart rates found in certain athletes and during sleep, and the tachycardia found in fever, emotion and exercise, are attributed largely to variations in vagal tone. Respiratory activity also may produce variations in vagal tone leading to phasic changes in heart rate with acceleration near the end of inspiration and slowing at the end of expiration. This condition (*sinus arrhythmia*) is frequently encountered in normal individuals, particularly when the heart rate is relatively slow.

A heart rate faster than some arbitrary value (e.g., 100 beats per minute) is termed *sinus tachycardia* if the impulses originate in the S-A node. By the same token, a heart rate of sinus origin below some value (e.g., 60 beats per minute) is called *sinus bradycardia*. Intense vagal stimulation (e.g., from carotid sinus pressure) may transiently interrupt impulse formation by the S-A node. If such *sinoatrial arrest* is sufficiently prolonged, some other site in the heart may begin to discharge conducted impulses. The fact that excitation of the heart can be initiated at many sites in myocardium or conduction system is the basic cause of cardiac arrhythmias.

ABNORMAL RHYTHMS

Since abnormal rhythms of the heart usually result from variations in the site and frequency of impulse formation, the nature of pacemaker activity deserves special consideration.[12]

PACEMAKER ACTIVITY IN MYOCARDIAL FIBERS

The functional differences between smooth muscle, skeletal muscle and myocardium lie in the mechanisms for excitation and control. Under appropriate conditions, all forms of muscle may exhibit myogenic excitation originating within the muscle itself.

If the heart of a chick embryo is sectioned between the common atrium and ventricle, these two segments of myocardium may continue to contract rhythmically but the rate of ventricular contraction is slower than that of the atrium.[13] Similarly, excised myocardial tissue from mammalian hearts may contract repeatedly and, again, the inherent rhythmicity of atrial tissue exceeds that of ventricular myocardium. Every portion of the myocardium and conduction system can assume the role of pacemaker and initiate impulses conducted to contiguous regions. At any moment, the pacemaker of the heart abides in the region with the fastest inherent rate of impulse formation, which is nor-

mally the sino-atrial node. If impulses from the atria are blocked at the atrioventricular node, the atria continue to contract at their characteristic rate and another pacemaker in the ventricles emits impulses at a slower rate (30 to 60 beats per minute). When the pacemaker is situated in the ventricles, impulses may be conducted in a retrograde direction to the atria or they may be blocked at the A-V node.

The functional and electrocardiographic characteristics of arrhythmias are dependent upon four factors: (*a*) Many portions of the myocardium and conduction system are capable of originating waves of excitation. (*b*) Functionally the heart consists of two double shells of myocardial fibers (atria and ventricles) joined by the common bundle of Purkinje fibers (Fig. 8–12). (*c*) Owing to the syncytial arrangement of myocardial fibers, these waves of excitation spread to all contiguous myocardial cells. (*d*) The wave of excitation pursues an abnormal course through some parts of the myocardium.

PREMATURE CONTRACTIONS

The inherent capacity of all the myocardial fibers to rhythmically generate conducted impulses is not apparent so long as the *sino-atrial* node retains its position as pacemaker. However, impulses are generated in regions other than the S-A node fairly often in both normal individuals and patients with organic heart disease. Changes occurring in regions of increased irritability (ectopic foci) have been the subject of considerable speculation with little or no direct experimental evidence. It is fairly well established that myocardial fibers returning to their resting state after a cardiac contraction pass through

TYPES OF PREMATURE CONTRACTIONS

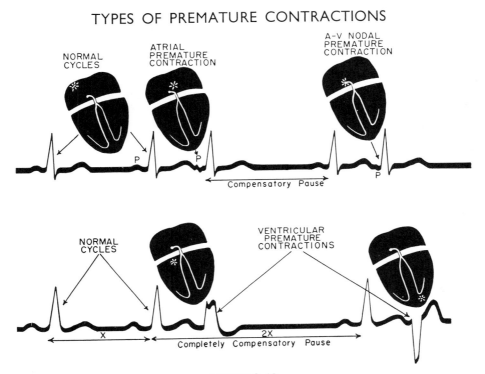

FIGURE 8–12

Premature contractions can originate at ectopic foci in any portion of the atria or ventricles. A few examples are illustrated schematically.

Atrial premature contractions begin with a deformed P wave shortly after the T wave of the preceding normal cycle. The P-R interval is usually shortened but the QRS complex is characteristically unchanged in configuration. The interval between the premature contraction and the next normal cycle is somewhat prolonged (compensatory pause).

Premature contractions originating at the A-V node are similar to atrial premature contractions except that the P wave is largely buried within the QRS complex since the atria and ventricles are excited more or less simultaneously.

Ventricular premature contractions are characterized by markedly deformed and prolonged QRS complexes with no definite S-T segment and with the T wave deflected in a direction opposite to the major deflection of the QRS. P waves are not visible.

a stage of increased excitability which appears to correspond to a similar state during the negative after-potential in nerve fibers.[14] Conducted impulses originating at various sites in the ventricles tend to occur just after the T wave and the abnormal contractions follow closely behind the preceding beat. Such premature contractions per se have little or no clinical significance because they occur in so many normal persons. Frequent premature contractions from multiple sites often occur with various types of heart disease. The general location of the ectopic focus giving rise to these premature contractions can usually be determined electrocardiographically.

ATRIAL* PREMATURE CONTRACTIONS

If an irritable focus in the atrium generates a conducted impulse very soon after the preceding contraction, the wave of excitation spreads out concentrically from this new site (Fig. 8–12). The course of this wave is different from that of an impulse arising in the sino-atrial node and, therefore, the shape of the P wave is altered. The time required for the atrial wave of excitation to engulf the atrioventricular node is different, so the P-R interval also varies from that of the preceding normal beat. The QRS and T waves are generally unchanged because the excitatory impulse follows a normal course from the A-V node through the ventricular myocardium and repolarization of the

---

*The word *auricle* has been widely used as though it were a synonym for *atrium*. Anatomically, *auricle* refers to an atrial appendage and is not appropriate for indicating the main atrial chamber. To avoid inconsistency, the correct term will be used in spite of traditional usage in such familiar conditions as "auricular" premature contractions, "auricular" fibrillation, etc.

ventricles is usually not affected. However, in some cases, slight changes in the configuration of QRS and T waves are produced, probably because the impulse follows the previous excitation so closely that some portion of the conduction system has not fully recovered. This is called *aberrant ventricular conduction*. The abnormal wave of excitation in the atrium envelops the S-A node, which cannot discharge another impulse until it has passed through its complete recovery cycle. Thus, the interval between an atrial premature contraction and the next normal beat is prolonged (compensatory pause in Fig. 8–12). The salient features of atrial premature contractions are: altered configuration of the P wave which closely follows the T wave of the preceding normal contraction, altered P-R interval (usually diminished), normal or nearly normal QRS and T complexes and a compensatory pause. The extent of the changes in P wave configuration and in the P-R interval varies with location of the ectopic focus in relation to the S-A node. If the wave of excitation originates from the region of the A-V node, the P waves are inverted and the P-R interval is very brief (Fig. 8–12).

A-V NODAL PREMATURE CONTRACTIONS

Premature contractions may be initiated from an irritable focus in or near the atrioventricular node. The wave of excitation passes immediately down the Purkinje system to the ventricles, so a QRS complex closely follows the preceding normal T wave (Fig. 8–12). Usually, conduction into the atria is blocked and no P waves appear. Occasionally a P wave begins just before the onset of QRS or is buried in the QRS complex, indicating retrograde conduction into the atrial musculature. Usually the ventricular excitation occurs in its normal sequence and the form of the QRS complex is similar to the patterns displayed during normal cycles. In the absence of retrograde conduction into the atria, the rhythm of the S-A node is undisturbed and the interval between the normal cycles preceding and following the premature contraction is equal to that of·two normal cycles. In other words, the short interval before the premature contraction is precisely balanced by the greater delay following the abnormal beat (completely compensatory pause). The characteristic signs of A-V nodal premature contractions are normal or relatively normal QRS complexes appearing just after the preceding T wave, with P waves absent, buried in the QRS complex or beginning just before the premature QRS.

VENTRICULAR PREMATURE CONTRACTIONS

If a focus within the ventricular musculature discharges prematurely, the course of the wave of excitation and the sequence of ventricular depolarization are abnormal and the configuration of the QRS complex is correspondingly distorted. Since such ectopic foci can develop anywhere in the ventricles, an infinite variety of complexes may result.

The typical electrocardiographic picture consists of slurred, prolonged QRS complexes, beginning without a P wave just after the termination of the preceding normal cycle. Repolarization occurs in an abnormal sequence and the T waves are also deformed, tending to deflect in a direction opposite to the major QRS deflection (Fig. 8–12). When an ectopic focus is located near the base of the heart, at some distance from the conduction system, the general course of the wave of excitation extends from base to apex, and the major QRS deflections are upward in all standard limb leads as in a normal cycle. If, in contrast, a premature ventricular contraction originates near the apex, excitation spreads from the apex toward the base of the heart and the major QRS deflections are downward in all standard limb leads (Fig. 8–12). A completely compensatory pause follows the typical premature ventricular contraction, just as in the A-V nodal ectopic beats.

Premature ventricular contractions, recurring regularly after every normal cycle, may persist for extended periods of time. These premature contractions are termed *coupled* beats and the resulting rhythm is called *bigeminy* because two pacemakers alternate in discharging excitatory impulses to the ventricular myocardium. In a few patients with slow heart rates, premature ventricular contractions are regularly interposed between normal beats without a compensatory pause. These ectopic beats are called *interpolated* premature ventricular contractions.

PAROXYSMAL TACHYCARDIA

A burst of three or four ectopic impulses is generally classed as multiple premature contractions. However, an ectopic focus may discharge a long series of premature contractions in rapid succession at rates higher than 140 per minute (Fig. 8–13). Such sustained ectopic pacemaker activity lasting minutes or days is called paroxysmal tachycardia. This arbitrary distinction between premature contractions and paroxysmal tachycardia indicates the close functional relation between them. Ectopic foci producing either isolated pre-

TYPES OF PAROXYSMAL TACHYCARDIA

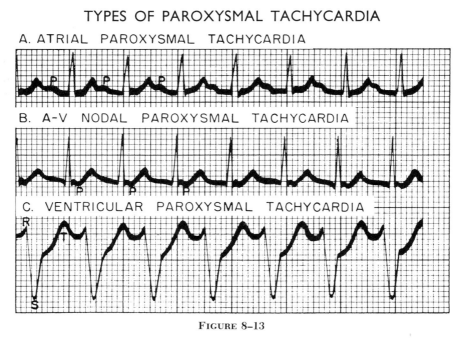

A. ATRIAL PAROXYSMAL TACHYCARDIA

B. A-V NODAL PAROXYSMAL TACHYCARDIA

C. VENTRICULAR PAROXYSMAL TACHYCARDIA

FIGURE 8–13

The fact that paroxysmal tachycardia actually represents a series of premature contractions is clearly indicated by comparing atrial, A-V nodal and ventricular paroxysmal tachycardia with corresponding isolated premature contractions in Figure 8–12.

mature contractions or paroxysms of tachycardia may develop anywhere in the heart. In a typical attack of paroxysmal tachycardia, the heart rate is abruptly elevated to levels of 140 to 240 beats per minute, most commonly around 160 per minute. Once attained, this rapid rate is exceedingly regular, and is essentially unaffected by respiratory activity, exercise, or other controlling mechanisms until the attack is abruptly terminated.

Clinical diagnosis of paroxysmal tachycardia depends upon a history of a very fast, extremely regular heart rate which begins abruptly and does not change until it suddenly reverts to normal. Paroxysmal tachycardia originating from sites in the atria or A-V node is often terminated promptly by inducing intense vagal discharge (pressure on the carotid sinus, deep inspiration with mild Valsalva maneuver, induced vomiting, pressure on the eyeballs, etc.). These procedures

generally have no effect on an ectopic pacemaker in the ventricular walls; this fact suggests that parasympathetic distribution to the ventricular myocardium is scanty or absent. Successful therapy by carotid sinus pressure or other procedures producing vagal discharge represents a diagnostic test for atrial or A-V nodal tachycardia. It may be difficult to differentiate atrial and nodal paroxysmal tachycardia because P waves may be obscured by T waves when the cycle length is short. This poses no practical problem, since the functional significance and therapy of these two conditions are similar. The prolonged and bizarre QRS complexes which occur with ventricular paroxysmal tachycardia simplify its recognition (Fig. 8–13).

ATRIAL FLUTTER

Very rapid regular atrial excitation can be caused experimentally by inducing a wave of excitation which continuously follows a circular pathway in the atrial musculature around some obstruction (e.g., around the roots of the superior and inferior venae cavae). This "circus movement" can be produced by damaging the atrial myocardium between the superior and inferior venae cavae and electrically stimulating the atrium to induce a wave of excitation which circles the obstruction at a rate determined only by the conduction velocity of the myocardium and the circumference of the circle.[15] From this circular pathway, excitation spreads to the remainder of the atrium and to the A-V node (Fig. 8–14B). Thus, the atria are excited at rates of 150 to 350 times per minute. Apparently the A-V node cannot respond to repetitive excita-

tion at these high rates and transmits alternate impulses (2:1 block), every third impulse (3:1 block) or every fourth impulse (4:1 block), depending upon its recovery time. The concept that the atrial flutter observed in patients was due to a circus movement in the atria held sway for many years but a large body of subsequent evidence indicates that atrial flutter is due to rapid, repetitive excitation from a single ectopic focus (Fig. 8–14A). This conclusion, discussed in detail by Scherf and Schott,[16] implies that atrial flutter must be considered comparable to paroxysmal tachycardia except that the atrial waves of excitation occur at a rate which is faster than the A-V node can transmit impulses. The electrocardiographic signs of atrial flutter can be predicted from either of

ATRIAL FLUTTER

A. ECTOPIC ATRIAL FOCUS

B. CIRCUS MOVEMENT

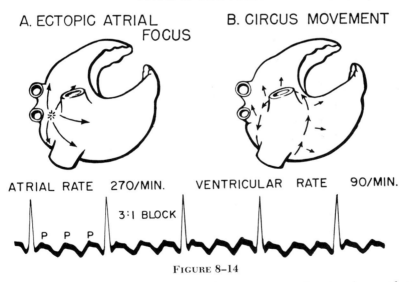

ATRIAL RATE 270/MIN.   VENTRICULAR RATE 90/MIN.

3:1 BLOCK

P P P

FIGURE 8–14

Atrial flutter is characterized by repetitive atrial excitation occurring at such a rapid rate that all waves of excitation are not transmitted through the A-V node into the ventricles. Thus, there may be two P waves for each QRS complex (2:1 block), three P waves to one QRS (3:1 block) or even 4:1 block.

A, According to one theory, the rapid atrial rate results from the rapid firing of an ectopic focus in the atrial musculature, similar to atrial paroxysmal tachycardia except for the failure of the A-V node to transmit all the impulses.

B, According to another theory, atrial flutter occurs when a wave of excitation encircles the roots of the superior and inferior vena cava at a rate determined by the conduction velocity of the myocardium. Waves of excitation spread from the circular pathway to the remainder of the atrial musculature. Circus movements of this type can be produced experimentally (see text).

these descriptions even though the etiology of the condition remains controversial. The ventricular rate is usually regular although a shift from one degree of block to another may occur. The major difficulty in interpreting the records stems from the fact that the P waves tend to be superimposed upon the T waves. If this fact is not recognized, half of the P waves may be overlooked and erroneous conclusions drawn. P waves hidden in T waves or in other complexes can generally be detected by carefully inspecting the record at a point just halfway between the clearly defined P waves. A pair of calipers adjusted until the distance between the points is just half the distance between obvious P waves is often helpful in the procedure.

The functional significance of atrial flutter depends ultimately upon the ventricular heart rate. If the A-V node transmits alternate atrial impulses (2:1 A-V block), the ventricular rate is very rapid (e.g., 150 beats per minute). Under these conditions, the diastolic filling interval for the ventricles is seriously curtailed and the resulting condition closely resembles paroxysmal atrial tachycardia (see above). If 3:1 or 4:1 block persists during various levels of activity, the heart rate remains relatively fixed at levels of 70 to 100 beats per minute at rest and the cardiac reserve is curtailed during exertion because tachycardia does not occur.

ATRIAL FIBRILLATION

If more than one wave of excitation were moving over the atrium at all times, coordinated atrial contraction could not occur and individual P waves could not be identified on electrocardiograms. Instead, the P waves would be replaced by irregular oscillations of the baseline: "fibrillation" waves. A similar situation would result if multiple ectopic atrial foci were discharging asynchronously at rates. Here again, a number of postulates have been advanced (Fig. 8–15) but the ultimate answer must await further evidence. In any event, waves of excitation arrive at the A-V node at random intervals. Only a portion of these excitatory waves are transmitted to the ventricles. Some excitatory waves are too weak or diffuse to invade the A-V node and others arrive during its refractory period. By this mechanism, the ventricular rate is absolutely irregular since the A-V node receives its excitation in a completely random sequence. The complete lack of ventricular rhythm can be readily perceived by palpation of the radial pulse or auscultation over the precordium. The electrocardiographic signs of atrial fibrillation are illustrated in Figure 8–15.

The principal functional disturbance produced by atrial fibrillation is the elimination of effective atrial contractions. Multiple waves of excitation traversing the atrial muculature produce uncoordinated contraction waves which change the shape of the chamber but produce no concerted evacuation of blood into the ventricles. Loss of atrial contribution to ventricular filling may not be very important at rest. However, the reserve capacity of the heart may be significantly restricted by elimination of atrial contraction at the proper interval before ventricular contraction and by uncontrolled irregular rhythms. The extent to which stroke volume is limited by atrial fibrillation is not known but it could be very important. Furthermore, neural control of ventricular rate is lost and the cardiac reserve is diminished by the lack of compensatory tachycardia.

A. SINGLE ECTOPIC FOCUS   B. MULTIPLE ECTOPIC FOCI   C. MULTIPLE CIRCUS WAVES

(Aberrant Conduction)   (Asynchronous Discharge)

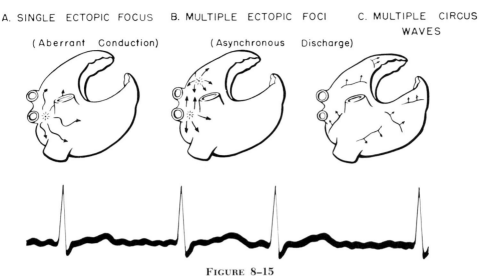

FIGURE 8–15

Atrial fibrillation is characterized by a totally irregular ventricular rhythm. The A-V node transmits impulses in a completely random fashion, apparently because impulses arrive in its vicinity at varying intervals. At least three explanations for this condition can be advanced:

A, A single ectopic focus may discharge impulses so rapidly that portions of the atrial muscle are refractory. Thus, the waves of excitation are broken up and follow aberrant pathways irregularly over the atrial musculature.

B, Multiple ectopic foci, discharging asynchronously at high rates, would produce an apparently random distribution of excitatory processes traveling through the atrial walls.

C, Multiple waves of excitation could follow random courses through the atrial myocardium, following pathways where the myocardium has returned to the excitable state. This concept is an extension of the circus movement theory for atrial flutter.

VENTRICULAR FIBRILLATION

A random distribution of excitatory waves traversing the ventricular musculature would preclude a coordinated contraction in the ventricle just as it does in the atrium. Thus, ventricular fibrillation can be survived for only brief periods and is a common immediate cause of death. Thus, electrocardiographic records of spontaneous ventricular fibrillation are rarely obtained. They consist of broad irregular waves of varying amplitude and configuration. Transient bouts of ventricular fibrillation are occasionally responsible for periodic fainting reactions.

CLINICAL SIGNIFICANCE OF ARRHYTHMIAS

The preceding discussion of arrhythmias does not represent a comprehensive coverage of the subject but illustrates the type of logic which leads to their identification. The presence of arrhythmia does not necessarily indicate heart disease. Premature contractions and paroxysmal tachycardia occur in hearts in which no pathologic changes are demonstrable in subsequent postmortem examinations. On the other hand, they are more frequently found in patients with organic disease. Certain arrhythmias are more likely to be associated with particular types of heart disease. For example, atrial fibrillation is frequently encountered in patients with hyperthyroidism or with left atrial dilatation from stenosis of the mitral valve. Premature contractions often originate in portions of the myocardium in which the blood supply is insufficient (e.g., from obstruction of coronary arteries). In any case, abnormal rhythms must be evaluated along with all other available evidence to arrive at a judgment concerning the cardiac status of the patient.

ABNORMAL CONDUCTION

Since the atrium contains no specialized conduction system, waves of excitation are rarely delayed during their spread over the atrial musculature. A very common site of delayed conduction occurs at the transition between the atrial myocardium and the atrioventricular node. Indeed, some A-V nodal delay occurs normally and is frequently prolonged by inflammatory and toxic effects on the heart.

DISTURBANCES OF ATRIOVENTRICULAR CONDUCTION

Theoretically, delay in the excitation of the A-V node might be detected by measuring the interval between the end of the P wave and the beginning of the ventricular complex (QRS). However, variability in the duration of the P wave limits the accuracy of this measurement. Instead, the time elapsing between the beginning of the P wave and the beginning of ventricular excitation (Q or R wave) is measured. This interval (P-R) includes the A-V nodal delay and is routinely used to detect its prolongation (Figs. 8–10 and 8–16).

The P-R interval averages about 0.16 second, but varies with age and with heart rate. This interval includes the time required to excite the atria, the A-V nodal delay and the time occupied by conduction along the common bundle and the bundle branches to the ventricular myocar-

dium. The upper limits of normal for the P-R interval vary from 0.20 second in an adult with an average heart rate (72 per minute) to 0.125 second in an infant with a fast heart rate (e.g., 160 per minute). It is convenient to remember that the upper limit of normal in adults is 0.20 second; in adolescents between the ages of 14 and 17 years, the P-R interval should remain below 0.18 second, and in children under 14 years, below 0.16 second.

PROLONGED P-R INTERVAL (FIRST DEGREE A-V BLOCK)

The P-R interval should be measured on the lead in which a prominent Q wave occurs and the P wave is well formed. If the Q wave is absent, the lead with the longest QRS interval should be used. In most cases, these criteria are best met in lead II. When the measured P-R interval exceeds the upper limits of normal, an electrocardiographic diagnosis of prolonged P-R interval or first degree A-V block is indicated (Fig. 8–16A). Since a number of different conditions may produce prolongation of the P-R interval, this electrocardiographic sign does not imply either an etiologic or an anatomic diagnosis of the conditions which produced it. However, prolonged P-R intervals occur quite frequently during acute rheumatic fever.

Functional Significance of Prolonged P-R Interval. The P-R interval is prolonged most frequently in the course of inflammatory disease processes involving the entire myocardium (e.g., acute rheumatic fever). This being the case, the principal functional disturbances are due to the underlying disease process which caused the delayed A-V nodal conduction. In addition, a prolonged interval between atrial and ventricular

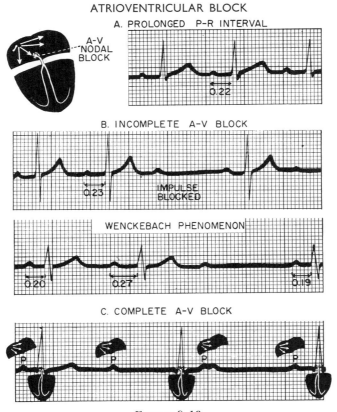

FIGURE 8–16

A, Prolongation of the P-R interval implies increased delay in conduction between the atrial myocardium and the A-V node (A-V nodal delay). This condition is called merely *prolongation of P-R* or sometimes *first degree A-V block.*

B, When A-V nodal conduction has been impaired, an atrial wave of excitation may occasionally fail to invade the A-V node and no QRS complex follows the normal P wave. This is called *partial A-V block.* Occasionally the P-R interval becomes progressively longer and longer with each successive cycle until an impulse is blocked at the A-V node (*Wenckebach phenomenon*).

C, Complete A-V block implies that none of the normal atrial waves of excitation pass the A-V node to enter the ventricles. Under these conditions, another pacemaker becomes established in the ventricle which usually generates impulses at a slower rate. The ventricular pacemaker is often situated at or near the A-V node, as indicated above, and the QRS complexes remain normal. If the QRS complexes are slurred and deformed, as occurs with ventricular premature contractions (Fig. 8–12), the ventricular pacemaker is somewhere in the ventricular myocardium. The atrial and ventricular rates are completely independent.

systole may deleteriously affect closure of the mitral and tricuspid valves. During atrial contraction, blood is driven into the already distended ventricular chambers and the atrioventricular valves move toward the position of closure. If ventricular systole is delayed, the valves gape wide again and some of the blood ejected by atrial systole probably flows back into the atria. When ventricular systole begins, the valves are separated and additional regurgitation occurs before the valves are closed and sealed. The effectiveness of atrial contraction in producing ventricular filling is also reduced in other forms of A-V block (see below).

PARTIAL A-V BLOCK (SECOND DEGREE A-V BLOCK)

More severe degrees of A-V block may produce occasional or regularly recurring dropped ventricular beats. For example, in some patients, the P-R interval becomes progressively longer in a sequence of cycles until a point is reached at which a P wave is not followed by a QRS complex (Wenckebach phenomenon). In this particular cycle, the spreading wave of atrial excitation is blocked at the A-V node and fails to reach the ventricles. In other cases, an occasional ventricular complex is missing without a change in the P-R interval (Fig. 8–16B).

COMPLETE A-V BLOCK

If all atrial waves of excitation fail to pass the A-V node, a pacemaker in the ventricle must be established. The inherent rhythmicity in the ventricular conduction system or myocardium, generally ranging from 40 to 60 impulses per minute, is characteristically much slower than that of the A-V node or the atrial musculature. Under these conditions, the atria and ventricles are excited by independent pacemakers discharging at very different rates. The P waves occur regularly and with a frequency almost double that of the QRS complexes, but the two chambers are sufficiently out of phase that the P-R intervals are continuously variable and have no meaning. If the ventricular excitation originates near the A-V node, the course of excitatory impulses to the ventricular muscle is along the normal pathways and the QRS complex is essentially normal in duration and configuration. On the other hand, excitation spreading from an ectopic pacemaker somewhere in the ventricular myocardium will, of necessity, follow an abnormal and more devious course, producing al-

terations in both the configuration and the duration of the QRS interval.

DISTURBANCES OF VENTRICULAR CONDUCTION

Rapid conduction of the excitatory impulse over the Purkinje system provides almost simultaneous distribution of waves of excitation to the endocardial surfaces of both ventricles. Since excitation normally reaches all parts of the ventricular wall within a very brief interval, the potentials develop rapidly and end promptly, producing QRS complexes of short duration and deflections which are sharp and clean. If the excitation of any large portion of the ventricle is delayed, the duration of the QRS complex is increased and the configuration is altered by slurred, notched, multiphasic or prolonged deflections in various leads (Fig. 8–17). Despite the fact that an almost endless variety of QRS configurations can be produced by different alterations in ventricular conduction, an electrocardiographic

ABNORMAL INTRAVENTRICULAR CONDUCTION

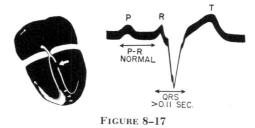

FIGURE 8–17

Blocked or delayed conduction in major branches of the Purkinje system produces asynchronous excitation of the ventricular walls. Since the wave of excitation follows a normal course from the S-A node through the A-V node, the P waves and the P-R interval are normal. Delayed excitation of a major portion of the ventricular walls produces prolonged, bizarre QRS complexes. The types and significance of ventricular conduction disturbances are considered further in the next section.

diagnosis of intraventricular conduction disturbance (intraventricular block) can be made whenever the QRS interval exceeds certain arbitrary values.

The QRS interval is measured from the point at which the first deflection (Q or R wave) leaves the baseline, to the termination of the complex. It should be measured in the standard limb lead in which it is longest. An average value for QRS interval in adults is about 0.08 second. The maximal normal QRS interval is approximately 0.10 second in adults, 0.09 second in children from 5 to 14 years of age and 0.08 second in children under 5 years of age. Although the electrocardiographic diagnosis of defective intraventricular conduction is readily made, its clinical significance requires analysis of the type and location of the disturbance. The nature and extent of abnormal ventricular conduction can be assessed only by an analysis of the configuration of the QRS complexes in various leads.

THE DURATION OF ELECTRICAL SYSTOLE (Q-T INTERVAL)

The interval occupied by the QRS-T complex represents the time required for excitation and repolarization of the ventricular myocardium. The so-called Q-T interval is measured from the beginning of the QRS complex (Q or R wave) to the end of the T wave (Fig. 8–10). As the Q-T interval varies somewhat with heart rate, age and sex, it is generally necessary to refer to a table to determine if a particular value is within normal limits or exceeds the upper limit of normal.

SUMMARY

Electrocardiographic signs of abnormal heart rate, rhythm and conduc-

tion were summarized briefly to illustrate the kind of logic which can be applied to an analysis of electrocardiograms. Electrocardiographic interpretation was introduced in this way to demonstrate that information can be gleaned from electrocardiographic tracings on logical grounds. It is not considered appropriate to attempt an exhaustive discussion in a text of this sort. Additional details should be sought in standard textbooks of electrocardiography. With a little experience, following a simple routine will disclose most of the common types of abnormal heart rates, arrhythmias and conduction disturbances.

PROCEDURE FOR DETECTING ABNORMALITIES OF HEART RATE, RHYTHM AND CONDUCTION

Analysis of electrocardiograms should begin with the following steps:

1. Determine ventricular rate and atrial rate
2. Examine the record for variations in rhythm
3. Examine the complexes to detect changes in configuration
4. Measure P-R interval
5. Measure QRS interval

Determining the ventricular rate is the first step in analyzing an electrocardiogram. If a P wave precedes each QRS complex by a constant interval, the atrial rate is the same as the ventricular rate. The P-R interval is measured in several complexes. If this value is relatively constant and within the range of normal, the rhythm is probably of sinus origin. In adults, heart rates below 60 can be termed sinus bradycardia and those above 100 are labeled sinus tachycardia. If the heart rate is absolutely constant at levels above 140 at rest and the QRS complex is normal, the diagnosis is atrial paroxysmal tachycardia when P waves precede the QRS complexes by a normal interval. If P waves cannot be distinguished, the term supraventricular (atrial or A-V nodal) paroxysmal tachycardia is applied. Premature contractions are identified while scanning the records by noting two cycles in rapid succession followed by a slightly prolonged interval or compensatory pause. A P-R interval in excess of the maximal normal values presented in Table 1 means a first degree A-V block or increased A-V nodal delay. Regularly recurring cycles consisting of a P wave without a QRS-T complex signify partial A-V block (second degree A-V block). A continuously variable P-R interval suggests complete A-V block.

The QRS interval is measured as indicated in Figure 8–10, and if this value exceeds 0.10 second in adults with normal heart rates, an interventricular conduction disturbance is present. When P waves precede the prolonged QRS complexes by normal intervals, conduction within the ventricles is delayed or blocked. If P waves are absent and the ventricular rate is very regular at rates in excess of 140 per minute at rest, and if the QRS complexes are prolonged and bizarre, the diagnosis is ventricular paroxysmal tachycardia. Very slow ventricular rates (less than 60), with P waves absent or buried in a prolonged, bizarre QRS complex, imply sinus block with an ectopic pacemaker in the ventricles.

If the process of cardiac excitation can be clearly visualized and the P, QRS and T waves can be identified on the records, most of the common disturbances of rhythm and conduction can be recognized with little effort. More complete analysis, particularly as it involves interpretation of the changes in shape of the various waves, can best be approached with an understanding of the basic principles of electrocardiographic theory.

III. INTERPRETING DIFFERENCES IN WAVE FORM OF ELECTROCARDIOGRAPHIC COMPLEXES

The shape of the various electrocardiographic deflections is altered by many different factors including: the position of the recording electrodes on the body surface, the orientation of the heart within the thorax, the thickness of the walls of the heart, the course of the excitation through the myocardium, the rate of depolarization and repolarization, and the extent of polarization and depolarization. The changes in wave form due to the electrode position and to the orientation of the heart in the thorax must be distinguished from changes in these patterns produced by various disease states. Certain changes observed on electrocardiograms are frequently associated with specific abnormal functional states of the myocardium (e.g., myocardial ischemia, myocardial infarction and the effects of varying electrolyte concentrations and drugs). The altered electrical activity of the heart under these conditions can be assessed by two very different approaches: (a) empirically or (b) by theoretical analysis. Empirical interpretation involves matching certain electrocardiographic patterns with specific disease states. Such correlations require considerable experience

CENTRAL TERMINAL OF WILSON

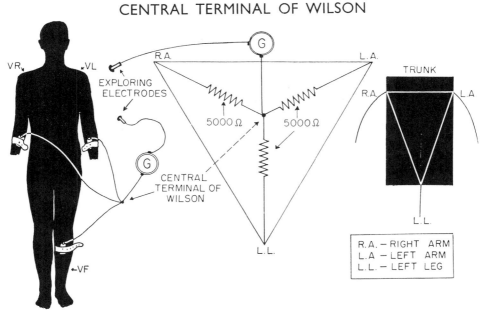

FIGURE 8–18

Accurate unipolar recording of cardiac potentials requires an indifferent electrode which is unaffected by potentials developed by the heart. If electrodes on all three extremity leads are connected through 5000 ohm resistors to a single terminal (the central terminal of Wilson), the potentials at the extremities almost completely cancel out to provide a fairly reliable indifferent electrode. The heart is not exactly equidistant from each electrode, since it is situated toward one end of a roughly rectangular volume conductor, but the resulting errors have not proved too serious for practical purposes.

since they involve learning and applying a vast quantity of detailed information collected over the years. Comprehensive coverage of this material cannot be achieved in a text of this scope. Instead, the theory underlying the production, distribution and recording of potentials from the heart is used to describe factors which may affect the form of electrocardiographic complexes.

THE EFFECTS OF ELECTRODE POSITION OF ELECTROCARDIOGRAPHIC PATTERNS

The potentials developed in a volume conductor were described in terms of a unipolar exploring electrode and an indifferent electrode so distant from the source of potentials as to be unaffected. The most distal portions of the arms and legs are not sufficiently distant to be truly indifferent because electrocardiograms can be readily recorded by placing electrodes on the wrists or ankles. Thus, there is no point in or on the body which could serve as an indifferent electrode. With the body immersed in a large tank of salt water the indifferent electrode can be placed at a great distance from the heart, but this is impractical. However, if wires from three electrodes, equidistant from each other and from the heart, are joined at a single terminal, the potentials developed at the electrodes tend to cancel each other (Fig. 8–18). This principle has been utilized in the cen-

DERIVATION OF STANDARD LIMB LEADS

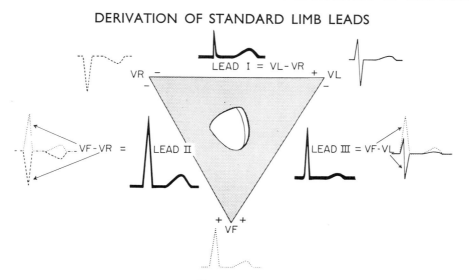

FIGURE 8–19

Each standard limb lead represents the difference in potential between two extremities. Since the unipolar limb leads record the potentials at the individual extremities, subtracting the potential recorded at the right arm (V_R) from the potentials at the left arm (V_L) should produce the patterns recorded from lead I. The process is more easily visualized in deriving lead II complexes by subtracting V_R (dashed line) from V_F (dotted line). An upward deflection is inscribed in lead II when V_F is positive with respect to V_L (note positive and negative signs on the Einthoven triangle). This schematic drawing indicates the complex origin of the standard limb leads as compared to the unipolar extremity leads.

tral terminal of Wilson,[17, 18] to provide an acceptable indifferent electrode for unipolar recording.

Wilson's central terminal is connected to one side of the galvanometer and an exploring electrode to the other (Fig. 8–18). If the exploring electrode is placed on the surface of the body at the right shoulder (V_R), left shoulder (V_L) and left leg (V_F), the wave of excitation passing through the heart can be "viewed" from different angles (see Fig. 8–8). These electrode positions are called the unipolar limb leads, and can be employed to illustrate the potentials developing during cardiac excitation and recovery, i.e., ventricular excitation.

STANDARD LIMB LEADS

When electrodes are applied to two extremities and connected to a galvanometer, the records indicate continuously the difference in potential between the two electrode positions. The standard limb leads can be recorded by measuring the potential difference between each pair of unipolar records, as in Figure 8–19. In accordance with the polarity indicated on Einthoven's triangle (+ and − signs), the complex at the negative end of the lead line is subtracted from the complex at the positive end. It is apparent that the standard limb leads are more complicated than unipolar leads, since the potentials fluctuate at both electrodes and the final record represents the difference in potential at each instant in time. Because it is difficult to visualize the result of subtracting one solid angle from another, this method is not widely used to describe the origin of the potentials recorded on standard limb leads. Instead, an electrical axis is usually employed for this purpose.

THE ELECTRICAL AXIS OF THE HEART

Although the amplitude and polarity of potentials recorded from unipolar electrodes can be predicted by knowing the solid angle subtended by an area of uniform charge density, the process cannot be reversed. In other words, the portions of the heart undergoing depolarization cannot be determined from externally recorded potentials such as the electrocardiogram. Areas of depolarization in an infinite variety of combinations can theoretically produce the electrocardiographic pattern recorded from any particular electrode position. For this reason, electrical activity in the heart is often represented by vectors which indicate the magnitude and mean direction of excitation without specifying the location of the activity. An arrow can be erected in the center of an area of spreading activity (see Fig. 8–20C) to indicate the mean direction of progression (the mean orientation of the charges), with the length of the arrow proportional to the solid angle (the magnitude of the recorded potential). Vectors can be derived from the electrocardiographic records obtained with the standard limb leads. Such vectors indicate the mean direction and magnitude of potentials developed within the heart as projected upon a frontal plane. However, they do not identify the specific regions of the heart being invaded by waves of excitation.

Instantaneous Electrical Axes. An electrical axis or vector can be determined for any instant during the cardiac cycle from simultaneously recorded standard limb leads (e.g., leads I and III). The method requires use of the Einthoven triangle, which is based on the concept that the heart

INSTANTANEOUS ELECTRICAL AXES

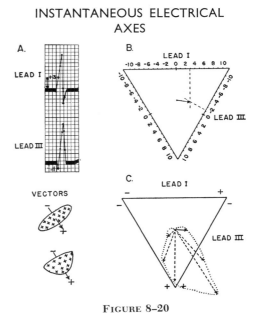

FIGURE 8–20

A, An instantaneous electrical axis can be derived from two standard limb leads recorded simultaneously. Simultaneous points on the two complexes are slected (e.g., 0.02 second after the beginning of the QRS complex). At this instant, the galvanometer had deflected upward 3 mm. in lead I.

B, From a point +3 units on the lead I line of Einthoven's triangle a perpendicular line is erected. Similarly, at this same instant, the deflection was 1 mm. below the bottom of the baseline in lead III. A perpendicular line is erected at −1 unit on the lead III line. An arrow drawn from the center of the triangle to the intersection of the perpendicular lines is the instantaneous electrical axis.

C, Such vectors indicate the mean direction in which the wave of excitation is advancing at a particular instant. If vectors are derived at intervals of 0.02 second during the remainder of the QRS complex (black dots on the QRS complexes), a series of instantaneous electrical axes can be derived. This series of vectors indicates the changing orientation and magnitude of potentials developing during ventricular excitation and is called a *vectorcardiogram.*

lies in a large, uniform volume conductor at the center of an equilateral triangle with the limb electrodes at the apices. In spite of the rectangular configuration of the trunk (Fig. 8–18) and the lack of homogeneity of the body, these assumptions are more completely realized than would appear at first glance. The positive and negative signs on Einthoven's triangle (Fig. 8–20) indicate that the limb electrodes are connected to the recording galvanometer in such a way that an upward deflection is recorded under the following conditions in each lead:

Lead   I: When the left arm is positive in relation to the right arm.

Lead   II: When the left leg is positive in relation to the right arm.

Lead III: When the left leg is positive in relation to the left arm.

The method of determining an instantaneous electrical axis at a particular moment in time is illustrated in Figure 8–20. The instantaneous axis indicates the mean direction in which the wave of excitation is traveling at a particular instant, and its length represents the relative magnitude of the externally recorded potentials developed at that time (Fig. 8–20B). If instantaneous electrical axes are determined at short intervals during the remainder of ventricular excitation, the series of instantaneous vectors change in length and orientation during the cardiac cycle (Fig. 8–20C). A series of instantaneous electrical axes constitutes a *vectorcardiogram*.

VECTORCARDIOGRAMS

A line connecting the points of the instantaneous vectors describes a loop. Loops of this type can be inscribed on the face of a cathode ray oscilloscope, thus continuously indicating the instantaneous electrical axis from moment to moment. The instantaneous electrical axes illustrated in Figure 8–20C actually represents three-dimensional vectors as projected on a frontal plane. Since the

original potentials actually develop in three dimensions, a more complete picture of the shifting patterns of potentials can be derived from three-dimensional vectors: stereovectorcardiography.

Although stereovectorcardiography has added little to our basic knowledge of electrocardiography, the graphic representation of vectors helps to visualize the process of ventricular excitation (see Fig. 8–21B). An average or mean electrical axis has proved useful in electrocardiographic interpretation even though it is not nearly as accurate or complete as a vectorcardiogram or a series of instantaneous vectors.

MEAN ELECTRICAL AXIS

Theoretically, a mean electrical axis should be the resultant of instantaneous vectors such as those illustrated in Figure 8–20C. The routine method of determining the mean electrical axis is a compromise based on the questionable assumption that the height of the Q, R and S deflections is proportional to the area under them. The net upward or downward deflection is determined for the typical QRS complex in two of the three standard leads (e.g., leads I and III). As indicated in Figure 8–21, the mean electrical axis is determined in much the same way as an instantaneous electrical axis (see Fig. 8–20). Note that in Figure 8–21 the mean electrical axis approximates the resultant of all the instantaneous axes illustrated in Figure 8–20C. Although the mean electrical axis is intended to represent the mean value for the instantaneous axes, serious discrepancies often occur, particularly in the presence of ventricular conduction disturbances.

The direction of the mean electrical axis is expressed in degrees on a

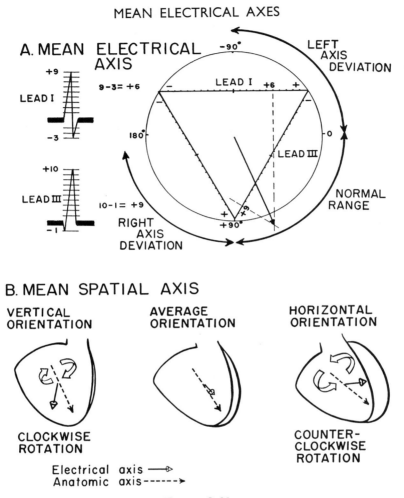

MEAN ELECTRICAL AXES

A. MEAN ELECTRICAL AXIS

B. MEAN SPATIAL AXIS

VERTICAL ORIENTATION

AVERAGE ORIENTATION

HORIZONTAL ORIENTATION

CLOCKWISE ROTATION

COUNTER-CLOCKWISE ROTATION

Electrical axis ⟶
Anatomic axis ------➤

FIGURE 8–21

A, The mean electrical axis is computed from two of the three standard limb leads (e.g., leads I and III). The sum of the downward deflections is subtracted from the sum of the upward deflections. For example, the vertical height of the R wave above the baseline is measured in millimeters (+9 mm. in lead I). The total amplitude of the downward deflections (−3 mm. in lead I) is added algebraically to the height of the R wave (+9) and leaves a net value of +6. At a point 6 units toward the plus sign on the lead I line of the triangle, a perpendicular is erected. The net amplitude of upward and downward deflections in lead III is +9 (+10 − 1). A perpendicular erected 9 units toward the plus sign on lead III is extended to intersect the perpendicular from lead I. An arrow drawn from the center of the triangle to the intersection of these two perpendicular lines is the *mean electrical axis*.

B, The mean electrical axis oriented in three dimensions (spatial vector) is directed rather strongly posteriorly. For this reason, rotation of the heart around a longitudinal axis produces large changes in the orientation of the mean electrical axis as projected on a frontal plane. This is the principal mechanism by which changes in the orientation of the heart produce changes in both the mean electrical axis and the configuration of patterns from the various electrocardiographic leads.

circle drawn from the center of the equilateral triangle. In most normal subjects the mean electrical axis lies in the range from 0 to +90 degrees (+100 degrees according to some authors). A mean electrical axis greater than +90 degrees is termed right axis deviation, while a shift of the electrical acis into the negative range is called left axis deviation. A large downward deflection in lead III and a tall R wave in lead I produces left axis deviation. A number of factors influence the orientation of the mean electrical axis, including the position of the heart within the thorax, the rotation of the ventricles around their longitudinal axis (Fig. 8–21B), the thickness of the ventricular walls (e.g., hypertrophy), and the rate and sequence of ventricular conduction. For example, left axis shift occurs when the heart is horizontally oriented, as in short, stocky individuals with high diaphragms. Vertical orientation of the heart tends to shift the mean electrical axis toward the right (Fig. 8–21B). So long as the heart is normal, these axis shifts are generally confined to the normal range. More extreme axis deviation may result from predominant enlargement of one ventricle (e.g., left ventricular preponderance produces left axis deviation).

UNIPOLAR PRECORDIAL LEADS

The anterior and posterior aspects of the heart can be explored by means of electrodes applied directly to the surface of the thorax (Fig. 8–22). This is important because the limb leads respond primarily to potentials developed on the lateral, superior and inferior regions of the heart. Electrical activity on the anterior and posterior surfaces subtends very small solid angles from the limb electrodes and

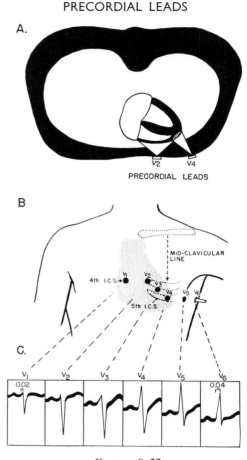

PRECORDIAL LEADS

FIGURE 8–22

A, Electrodes placed at prescribed positions on the precordium are influenced to a greater extent by the myocardium directly beneath than by more distant regions. For this reason they are termed "semi-direct" precordial leads. A local region of depolarization at the apex would have a greater effect on V_4 than on V_2, illustrating the utilization of these leads for detecting altered potentials from local areas under the electrodes.

B, Unipolar precordial electrodes are routinely placed on six positions. V_1 is in the fourth intercostal space (I.C.S.) at the right sternal edge. V_2 is in the fourth I.C.S. just to the left of the sternum. V_4 is in the fifth I.C.S. in the midclavicular line with V_3 midway between V_2 and V_4. On a horizontal line drawn from V_4, V_5 is located at the anterior axillary line and V_6 at the midaxillary line.

C, Electrocardiographic patterns recorded from the six precordial electrode positions are schematically presented. In V_4 the amplitude of R and S are approximately equal. This is termed the *transitional zone*, which is believed to lie over the interventricular septum.

produces relatively small potentials. For these reasons, records of cardiac potentials from unipolar electrodes, positioned at specific points on the thoracic wall over the heart, have become a part of the routine electrocardiographic examination. The myocardium immediately under these precordial electrodes contributes more to the recorded deflections than do myocardial walls farther away. A small area of altered polarization in the proximal zone subtends a relatively large solid angle (see V_4 in Fig. 8–22A), and appears as a large deflection from that particular electrode. The central region of the solid angle has the greatest influence on the recorded potentials. Around the periphery of the solid angle, the membranes approximate a radius of the solid angle and contribute very little to the recorded potentials.

Changes in the functional state of small myocardial areas can be detected by an electrode placed sufficiently near the defect (e.g., local myocardial ischemia). Unfortunately, unipolar electrodes can be placed close to the myocardium only over the precordium. In some cases it is desirable to explore additional areas on the surface of the thorax. For example, unipolar electrodes placed on the back provide an appreciable degree of localization over the posterior surface of the heart, even though these points are farther from the electrodes. An electrode in the lower esophagus has a fairly high degree of specificity for certain regions on the posterior aspect of the atria and ventricles. Small areas of myocardial destruction caused by occlusion of coronary arteries may produce characteristic signs at these various electrode positions when no indication appears on records from the more distant standard limb leads. Electrocardiographic changes during myocardial infarction are discussed below.

The precordial leads are also used to assess the orientation of the heart within the thorax and the presence of ventricular enlargement. These applications require an understanding of two characteristics of the precordial electrocardiograms: (a) the intrinsicoid deflection and (b) the transitional zone. (See Figs. 8–24, 8–25)

THE ELECTROCARDIOGRAPHIC POSITION OF THE HEART

The orientation of the heart within the thorax has important bearing on the interpretation of electrocardiograms. For example, electrocardiographic patterns which suggest enlargement of the left ventricle can result solely from a horizontal orientation of the heart. However, the electrocardiographic indications of cardiac orientation do not correspond to the anatomic position, so we may speak of the "electrocardiographic position" of the heart. For instance, the mean electrical axis of a horizontal heart may be directed toward the left shoulder. This obviously does not imply that the long axis of the heart is rotated until the apex lies above the base of the heart (see Fig. 8–21B).

Analysis of the electrical position of the heart has been extended in recent years to include rotation around three axes: the anteroposterior, the transverse and the longitudinal (see Fig. 8–21B). In view of the transitional stages of rotation around any or all of three axes, the heart can occupy innumerable electrical positions. Examples of electrocardiographic patterns in normal hearts oriented vertically or horizontally are presented (Figs. 8–23 and 8–24).

EFFECTS OF HEART ORIENTATION ON UNIPOLAR LIMB LEADS

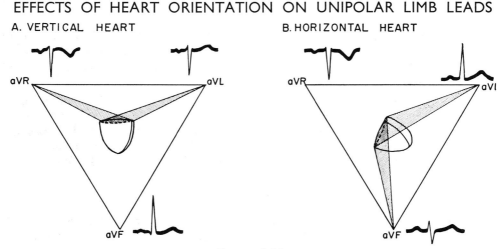

FIGURE 8-23

A, When the heart is oriented vertically, the QRS complexes are similar in leads aV_R and aV_L.

B, In the horizontal heart, aV_R and aV_L are essentially mirror images, a phenomenon which suggests that the wave of excitation actually progresses from right to left. This is confirmed by the diphasic QRS in aV_F. The designation aV_R or aV_F refers to a technical shortcut in recording which approximates the configuration of complexes obtained from unipolar limb leads (V_R or V_F).

HEART ORIENTATION ON ROUTINE E.C.G. LEADS

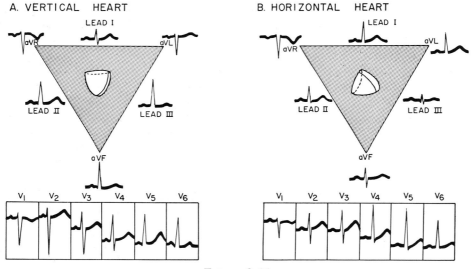

FIGURE 8-24

*A,*When the heart is oriented vertically within the thorax, the potentials viewed from the right and left shoulders are similar, so the patterns obtained from aV_R and aV_L are also similar. The QRS in lead I has low potentials and is diphasic, since it represents the difference between aV_R and aV_L (see Fig. 8–19). The transitional zone between V_3 and V_4 indicates a slight shift of the interventricular septum toward the right. The intrinsicoid deflections are within normal limits throughout, indicating that these changes are not due to ventricular conduction disturbances or hypertrophy.

B, The horizontal heart has a small diphasic lead III which may be slurred or notched. The augmented extremity leads are similar to those illustrated in Figure 8–23 and the V leads show a transitional zone at about V_3, which indicates a counterclockwise rotation of the ventricles around their longitudinal axis (Fig. 8–21*B*).

ELECTROCARDIOGRAPHIC SIGNS OF CHAMBER ENLARGEMENT

For many years, routine electro-cardiographic interpretation was based almost exclusively on the standard limb leads. Ventricular pre-ponderance or hypertrophy was recognized by those changes in QRS con-figuration which cause the mean elec-trical axis to deviate beyond the range of normal (see Fig. 8–21). The basis for these changes in QRS configuration could be convincingly rationalized in accordance with accepted electrocar-diographic theory. More recently, the widespread utilization of unipolar precordial and limb leads has greatly broadened the scope of electrocardio-graphic interpretation to include more complete information concerning the orientation of the heart, the intrinsi-coid deflection and changes in the S-T, T complex. The criteria for predomi-nant hypertrophy of each ventricle have become diversified, more empiri-cal and more controversial.

LEFT VENTRICULAR HYPERTROPHY

Selecting a "typical" series of electrocardiograms to illustrate left ventricular hypertrophy is extremely difficult because such diverse records are obtained from patients with ap-parently similar degrees of ventricular enlargement. Signs of left ventricular hypertrophy appear in the example presented in Figure 8–25. This is a rather extreme case, chosen to show clues which may be useful in recog-nizing the condition.

In Figure 8–25 the R wave is tall in lead I and very small in lead III. The very deep S_{III}, combined with a tall R_I, is responsible for the deviation of the mean electrical axis to the left

beyond the normal range. The QRS interval is less than 0.10 second, so the altered QRS configuration is presum-ably due to hypertrophy rather than to a ventricular conduction disturbance (see below). The augmented extremity leads (aV_R, aV_L and aV_F) indicate that the electrocardiographic position of the heart is horizontal. In the precor-dial leads, R waves predominate in V_2 through V_6, so the transitional zone has shifted strongly toward the right. In this example, the horizontal position of the ventricles is accompanied by marked counterclockwise rotation around the longitudinal axis. The T waves are inverted in leads I, aV_L, V_4, V_5 and V_6; this situation is fre-quently described as a ventricular "strain pattern."

EXPLANATIONS FOR THE ELECTROCARDIOGRAPHIC SIGNS OF VENTRICULAR ENLARGEMENT

The electrocardiographic signs of ventricular enlargement could be caused by: (a) rotation of the heart around its longitudinal axis (see be-low), (b) a thicker ventricular wall or (c) delayed conduction within the myocardium (e.g., ventricular conduc-tion disturbances). Distinguishing between these explanations is difficult. Indeed, each of them has been in-voked to explain the signs of ventricu-lar hypertrophy.

Although ventricular preponder-ance is one of the most common elec-trocardiographic interpretations, the criteria used by various authorities are remarkably diverse. Dimond[19] quoted the answers given by eight authorities in response to the simple question "What are the electrocardiographic evidences of left ventricular hyper-trophy?" No two answers were alike, and the divergence of opinion was extreme. It is very important to recog-

LEFT VENTRICULAR HYPERTROPHY OF HORIZONTAL HEART

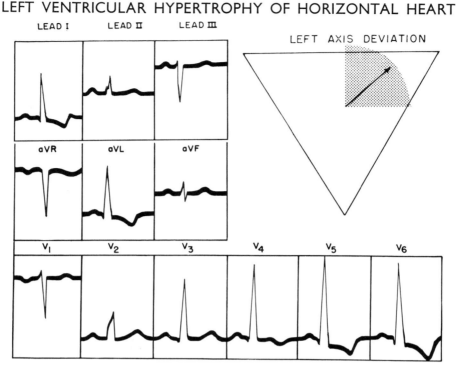

FIGURE 8–25

Electrocardiographic signs of left ventricular hypertrophy in this patient with a horizontal heart consist of a tall R_I, small R_{III} and deep S_{III}. These changes in the standard limb leads produce deviation of the mean electrical axis to the left beyond the normal range. The presence of a horizontal heart is affirmed by the tall R wave in aV_L and the diphasic deflection in aV_F (see also Fig. 8–24). The R wave predominates in V_2 through V_6, indicating that the transitional zone has been shifted to the right. The intrinsicoid deflection (peak of R) occurs more than 0.05 second after the beginning of the Q in $V_{5,6}$. Inversion of T waves and depression of the S-T segment (strain patterns) occur in leads I, aV_L, $V_{4,5,6}$. (From a record obtained through the courtesy of Dr. Samuel Aronson.)

nize that interpreting configurational changes in deflections remains a highly subjective process which depends in large measure on the experience and attitudes of the individual.

ELECTROCARDIOGRAPHIC SIGNS OF ABNORMAL VENTRICULAR CONDUCTION

Whenever a portion of the specialized conduction system in the ventricles is nonfunctional, the excitatory process must traverse the slowly conducting myocardial fibers. Thus,

excitation is delayed in the myocarddium served by the affected portion of the conduction system. If excitation of a sufficient mass of myocardium is delayed, the QRS interval is prolonged and the configuration of the QRS complexes is altered.

INTRAVENTRICULAR BLOCK

Grossly prolonged and distorted QRS complexes are generally attributed to a block in the main branches of the bundle of His (right and left bundle branches). Interference with

INTRAVENTRICULAR CONDUCTION DISTURBANCES

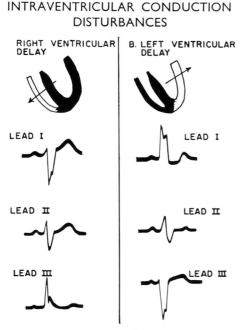

FIGURE 8–26

A, A ventricular conduction disturbance which delays the arrival of the wave of excitation to the right ventricle produces prolongation of the ventricular depolarization and wide QRS complexes, an example of which is shown. The mean electrical axis deviates to the right, beyond the normal limits in this case (arrow). The T waves tend to deflect in a direction opposite to the direction of the mean QRS deflection. This type of conduction disturbance is generally called right bundle branch block.

B, Delayed conduction to the left ventricular myocardium produces abnormal electrocardiographic patterns in the standard limb leads with the deformed portion of QRS predominantly upward in lead I and downward in lead III. The mean electrical axis tends to deviate to the left. However, the mean electrical axis is usually not equivalent to the resultant of the instantaneous electrical axis when severe conduction disturbances are present.

conduction along the right bundle branch would delay the arrival of excitation in the right ventricular wall (Fig. 8–26*A*). In this case, the following sequence is postulated: (*a*) atrial excitation beginning at the sino-atrial node follows a normal course, so the P wave and P-R interval are essentially normal; (*b*) excitation of the left side

of the septum and the left ventricular wall proceeds at normal speed; (*c*) the right ventricular wall is invaded after considerable delay by a wave of excitation along the slowly conducting myocardial fibers or by way of Purkinje bundles excited below the region of the block. Although the proximal portions of the bundle branches are generally indicated as the site of blocked conduction, a widespread interference with conduction in the peripheral distribution of the Purkinje fibers (e.g., at the junction of the Purkinje fibers with the myocardium) could have similar functional and electrocardiographic effects. The major deflections are delayed, slurred and deformed. When the right ventricular wall is depolarized late, the mean electrical axis tends to be directed from the center of the chamber toward the right ventricle (right axis deviation). The prolonged and slurred deflections are directed downward in lead I and upward in lead III. Repolarization begins in the regions activated first and tends to follow the same general course as the depolarization. Thus, the T wave is deflected in a direction opposite from that of the most prolonged QRS wave. The segment between the QRS and T waves is usually displaced from the baseline. There is no period when the ventricles are completely depolarized, and there is no isoelectric S-T segment.

Conversely, in left bundle branch block, conduction to the left ventricular wall may be delayed while the endocardial surface of the right ventricular cavity is excited promptly (Fig. 8–26*B*). Under these conditions, waves of excitation spread more or less simultaneously through the free wall of the right ventricle and through the interventricular septum. By the time a wave of excitation reaches the left ventricular wall, depolarization of the right ventricle and the septum is largely complete. Thus, the final deflection of the QRS is prolonged, slurred and deformed because it results from retarded activation of the left ventricular wall, unopposed by activity in the remainder of the heart (Fig. 8–26B). The prolonged QRS wave is generally downward in lead III and upward in lead I, and the T waves deflect in the opposite direction.

Clearly, alterations in the rate and sequence of excitation and repolarization can produce an unlimited variety of wave forms on the electrocardiographic records. All degrees of intraventricular conduction disturbance from simple slurring and notching of QRS deflections to grossly deformed and prolonged QRS complexes are encountered during routine electrocardiographic interpretation. As the correlation between pathologic lesions in the vicinity of the bundle branches and the electrocardiographic signs has been controversial, the rather complicated classification of such conduction disturbances has questionable value. For these reasons, it may be preferable to lump all the ventricular conduction disturbances into the single classification, intraventricular block. A notation of right or left ventricular delay may be warranted when electrocardiographic signs are clear (Fig. 8–26).

THE MEAN ELECTRICAL AXIS WITH ABNORMAL VENTRICULAR CONDUCTION

When the waves of excitation pursue abnormal courses through ventricular myocardium, the instantaneous and mean electrical axes generally deviate from their normal orientations. The mean electrical axis, determined in the routine manner

(Fig. 8–21), approximates the resultant of the instantaneous vectors only *so long as the height of the individual deflections is proportional to the area under them.* If each deflection of the QRS complexes conformed to an isosceles triangle subtending the same apical angle, the height of the deflection would be proportional to its duration and would therefore be proportional to the area under the deflection. When a deflection is markedly prolonged, its height is not related to the area under the deflections and the mean electrical axis, and the instantaneous vectors usually point in entirely different directions.

PREMATURE VENTRICULAR CONTRACTIONS

Ventricular excitation follows an abnormal course and sequence when a premature contraction is initiated at some ectopic focus in the ventricular myocardium. Distorted QRS complexes of widely varying form are produced by this mechanism. Premature ventricular contractions generally begin, without a P wave, very shortly after the T wave of a preceding normal cycle. The QRS-T pattern varies with the origin and course of the wave of excitation.

The patterns inscribed during normal cycles are very reproducible, while the premature ventricular contractions vary widely. The general direction taken by the wave of excitation as projected on the frontal plane is indicated by the electrical axis or vectorcardiogram. Considerable discrepancy between the mean electrical axis and the resultant of the instantaneous vectors occurs with premature ventricular contractions just as with ventricular conduction disturbances.

ABNORMALITIES OF VENTRICULAR REPOLARIZATION (S-T, T)

In contrast to the process of excitation, which is rapidly distributed by a specialized conduction system, the sequence of repolarization depends only on the duration of the depolarized state in the various myocardial fibers. The duration of the excited state is varied by temperature, pressure, electrolyte concentration (e.g., potassium, calcium) and other factors such as administration of various drugs or the oxygen supply, as they affect the "physiologic" condition of the myocardium. For this reason, the T wave has the most labile configuration of all the major deflections. Since the repolarization process occurs during the inscription of both the S-T segment and T wave, changes in the T waves are often but not always associated with changes in the duration of the S-T segment. It is not considered appropriate to embark upon a comprehensive discussion of the many factors which can affect repolarization. Certain causes of altered S-T, T complexes are mentioned because they pertain to subjects covered in other chapters.

ABNORMAL SEQUENCE OF REPOLARIZATION

As indicated in the preceding section, ventricular conduction disturbances delay excitation of certain regions of the heart walls and correspondingly retard completion of repolarization in those areas. The abnormal sequence of excitation is reflected in an abnormal sequence of repolarization which changes the configuration of the S-T, T complex. Generally, the S-T, T complex and the main (prolonged) QRS deflection deviate in opposite directions. This signifies that in abnormal cycles the process of repolarization follows the sequence of excitation more nearly than it does in normal cycles. Thus, the changes in S-T, T complex coincident with an abnormal course of ventricular excitation result from an abnormal sequence of repolarization.

ABNORMAL DEGREES OF POLARIZATION

Changes in the functional state of the myocardial fibers can change the extent of polarization. For example, whenever the S-T segment and the T-Q segment are isoelectric, the ventricular myocardium is uniformly depolarized during systole and uniformly polarized during diastole (Fig. 8–27A). If, during diastole, the depolarized state persisted in a region of myocardium sufficiently large to affect external electrodes, a potential difference would exist which would depress the T-Q interval below the S-T segment (Fig. 8–27B). If the same region remained partially polarized during both systole and diastole, precisely the same electrocardiographic pattern would be produced with the S-T segment elevated and the T-Q segment depressed (Fig. 8–27C). Finally, if the same area remained polarized throughout the cycle, a potential difference during electrical systole would elevate the S-T segment (Fig. 8–27D). Whenever a region of myocardium retains the same degree of polarization through a cardiac cycle, identical patterns can be produced by any one of the three mechanisms illustrated in Figure 8–27. The only difference between the three patterns lies in the level of a "zero" potential, which cannot be distinguished on electrocardiographic records.

ABNORMALITIES IN THE EXTENT OF POLARIZATION AND REPOLARIZATION

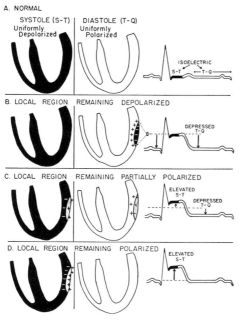

FIGURE 8–27

A, When the ventricular myocardium is uniformly polarized or depolarized, no potentials can be recorded by an external electrode. For this reason, the S-T and T-Q intervals are normally isoelectric.

B, If a local region in the left ventricle remained depolarized during diastole, a potential difference would exist between the polarized and depolarized regions. The junction between these two zones could be represented by a charged membrane with the negative charges facing the exploring electrode as indicated above. At this electrode, a negative potential would produce a downward deflection during diastole (T-Q interval) but not during systole. Thus, the T-Q segment would be displaced downward in relation to the S-T segment. If the local region became partially polarized, the T-Q segment would again be displaced but not quite so far.

C, If a region remained partially polarized to the same extent during both systole and diastole, the S-T segment would be somewhat elevated and the T-Q interval would be similarly depressed, producing a picture very similar to that indicated in *B,* above.

D, If a local region remained polarized through the cycle, the S-T segment would be elevated in relation to the T-Q segment. If the exploring electrode were placed on the opposite side of the heart, the S-T and T-Q segments would be displaced in the opposite direction. (Adapted from Kossmann.[22])

ABNORMAL RATES OF REPOLARIZATION

Although the myocardium might ultimately reach uniform polarization and depolarization, acceleration or retardation of these processes can affect the levels of the S-T and T-Q segments. For example, if a region of the myocardium remained depolarized for an abnormally long time, potential differences similar to those illustrated in Figure 8–27*B* would become manifest during the latter part of the S-T segment. The S-T segment would ascend and terminate in a tall T wave. This mechanism actually operates in causing the abnormal S-T and T complex associated with severe ventricular conduction disturbances in which delayed depolarization produces delayed repolarization. In contrast, therapeutic doses of digitalis accelerate the process of repolarization. If the rate of repolarization is not uniform throughout the ventricular myocardium, the S-T segment is displaced and the T wave is altered. Changes in the concentration of certain electrolytes in and about the myocardial cells also affect the repolarization process. For example, if the concentration of calcium in the blood is abnormally low, the process of repolarization is prolonged, which is evidenced by prolongation of electrical systole (Q-T interval). High blood calcium levels have the opposite effect. Hypopotassemia also changes the duration of the Q-T interval and alters the S-T, T complex.

Direct information concerning the rate and sequence of repolarization is scarce. Not even the rate and sequence of repolarization of normal ventricles have been described, to say nothing of the changes which result from disease. For this reason, the interpretation of the configurational changes in the S-T complex is almost completely empirical.

RECOGNIZING CHANGES IN THE MYOCARDIUM

ACUTE CORONARY OCCLUSION

Acute coronary obstruction produces characteristic changes in electrocardiograms; some of these changes are rarely observed during spontaneous attacks in patients but may be reproduced in experimental animals.

Bayley, LaDue and York[20] temporarily obstructed the anterior descending branch of the left coronary artery in dogs and recorded the following sequence of events with exploring electrodes on the surface of hearts (Fig. 8–28). Within 3 or 4 seconds after occlusion, the T waves, which had been positive, became sharply inverted, reaching maximal inversion in about 20 to 25 seconds. Thereafter the inverted T deflections diminished in amplitude as the S-T segment became elevated and rounded with the convexity upwards. The dia-stolic baseline (T-Q) was deflected in the opposite direction. After 3 to 5 minutes striking displacement of the S-T junction and upward peaking of T waves developed. When the occlusion was released after 2 to 5 minutes, S-T deviation and the large T waves vanished within 5 to 7 seconds, indicating that the procedure did no permanent damage to the myocardium. These striking electrocardiographic changes result from a functional change in the state of the affected myocardium rather than from demonstrable pathologic changes. The changes in the S-T segment and T waves develop very rapidly and are easily demonstrable by experiments like those illustrated in Figure 8–28 because the electrode is placed directly on the site of myocardial ischemia. They mimic the sequence of electrocardiographic alterations which develop over a much longer period of time following occlusion of coronary arteries in man.

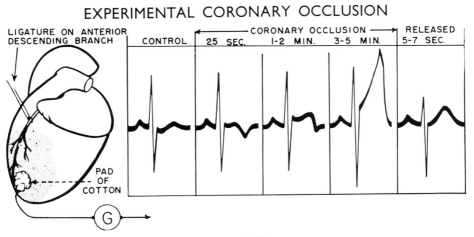

EXPERIMENTAL CORONARY OCCLUSION

FIGURE 8–28

Experimental coronary obstruction rapidly produces dramatic changes in electrocardiograms recorded from cotton electrodes positioned over the ischemic area. The initial change is a marked inversion of the T wave (at about 25 seconds), followed by elevation of the S-T segment in about 1.5 minutes. After 3 to 5 minutes, the S-T segment and T waves are both displaced upward. These changes largely disappear in 5 to 7 seconds after release of the ligature.

MYOCARDIAL INFARCTION

The evolution of the electrocardiographic patterns during myocardial infarction is illustrated in Figure 8–29. Since the electrocardiographic patterns change progressively following an attack, it is important to obtain serial electrocardiograms at intervals dictated by the patient's progress.

PHASE I

If the infarcted region includes the epicardial surface, ischemia of the affected myocardium apparently alters the process of repolarization. The T waves in various leads become either sharply inverted or very tall and peaked, depending upon the orientation of the electrodes in relation to the infarct. The patterns depicted in Figure 8–29 represent records obtained from a unipolar electrode facing the infarcted region. The changes in T waves are so transient that they are rarely recorded clinically. This initial phase of the sequence was first discovered following experimentally induced infarction in dogs (Fig. 8–28). Frequently, the rate of repolarization is sufficiently changed locally so that the S-T segment also is displaced, generally in the same direction as the T wave (see Fig. 8–28). The changes in the S-T segment and T wave deflection in any particular lead depend upon the size, location and orientation of the affected area in relation to the particular electrodes involved.

PHASE II

As ischemia continues, the rate of repolarization becomes progressively slower. This causes the T wave to reverse in direction. At the same time, the extent of polarization or depolarization diminishes, which causes displacement of the S-T segment, because the latter is a combined effect of an altered rate of repolarization (primary T wave changes) and changes in the extent of depolarization or repolarization (see the S-T segment shifts in Fig. 8–29). These two effects have different time courses, and are generally attributed to two different degrees of myocardial dysfunction. Probably the blood supply to the tissue at the periphery of the infarcted area is only slightly diminished because collateral channels of capillary size extend into this area from the normal tissue. Deeper within the infarct, a greater degree of myocardial ischemia would be expected as the distance from normal vessels increases. There is probably a gradient in the degree of ischemia from the normal tissue toward the central portion of the infarct where the myocardium will ultimately die and be replaced by connective tissue. However, for the sake of convenience, this ill defined shell of damaged myocardium is divided into two zones: (a) a zone of ischemia, which lies near the normal tissue and is believed to be responsible for the primary T wave changes, and (b) a zone of injury with an abnormal extent of polarization or depolarization producing S-T segment deviations (see Fig. 8–29).

PHASE III

Eventually, the myocardium near the center of the infarct becomes mechanically and electrically inactive. The spread of excitation does not invade the inactive myocardial tissue, which does not contribute to the QRS complex. Electrodes facing the infarct register a prominent negative deflection because the waves of excitation spreading through distal regions of

ELECTROCARDIOGRAPHY OF MYOCARDIAL INFARCTION

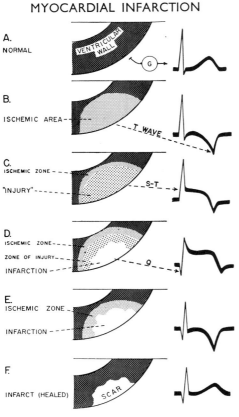

FIGURE 8–29

The sequence of electrocardiographic patterns recorded from unipolar electrodes over the site of a developing infarct is presented as reconstructed by Bayley.[23]

A, A normal electrocardiographic pattern recorded from a precordial electrode is illustrated for comparison.

B, Immediately after occlusion of a coronary artery, the myocardium served by the vessel becomes ischemic. A change in the rate of repolarization in the area produces a strongly inverted T wave (see also Fig. 8–28).

C, Within a short time myocardial hypoxia interferes with the repolarization process to the point that the affected myocardium fails to polarize to the normal extent. Incomplete repolarization produces an "injury" current by the mechanism illustrated in Figure 8–27. The S-T segment assumes a different level than the T-Q segment; this is generally described as a displacement of the S-T segment.

D, Within the center of the ischemic region, some of the myocardium dies and fails to contribute to the potentials during either systole or diastole. Under these conditions. a Q wave appears because the proximal tissue fails to

the heart are moving away from the electrode. This negative potential appears early in the process of excitation and produces prominent Q waves in records from particular leads. Pardee[24] noted early that Q waves with an amplitude greater than 25 per cent of the R wave occurred in lead III records taken from a substantial proportion of patients with clinical or pathologic evidence of myocardial infarction. The Q waves become deeper as more and more myocardium in the center of the infarct dies. At the same time, the myocardium which has been "injured" either dies or recovers as collateral circulation is augmented, so the S-T segment deviation tends to dwindle as the Q wave becomes more pronounced. The T wave remains inverted, indicating continued ischemia in the fringe around the dead myocardium.

PHASE IV

Over a period of months, the ischemic myocardium either fully recovers or dies. The inverted T waves may become upright, leaving Q waves as the sole remaining sign of the previous infarction.

If this sequence of electrocardiographic patterns appeared consistently in all patients with myocardial infarction, diagnosis would be very simple. Actually, these changes occur in only

balance the potentials in more distant regions where the wave of excitation is moving away from the electrode.

E, The myocardium in the zone of injury either dies or is incorporated in the ischemic zone, so the "injury" current disappears and the S-T segment returns to the baseline. The ischemic zone persists, as indicated by the sharply inverted T wave.

F, In a healed infarct, the ischemic zone is supplied by collateral vessels and returns to normal. The only residual sign is the Q wave, which is attributed to the presence of electrically inactive scar tissue.

about two-thirds of patients. In the remainder, the typical patterns tend to be masked by such preexisting conditions as bundle branch block, ventricular pacemaker, left heart strain or previous infarction. A very wide variety of electrocardiographic changes is encountered owing to differences in the extent and location of the infarcted region. An intramural infarct produces no change in electrocardiograms for the same reason that a uniformly polarized cell produces no external potential. At the same time, a number of other conditions may be associated with electrocardiographic patterns which closely resemble those characteristic of infarction. For example, right and left ventricular hypertrophy and strain may produce QRS-T patterns which can easily be confused with those of myocardial infarction. The reasons for the similar patterns resulting from different functional states are obvious, since the electrocardiographic patterns change only because the course, rate and extent of polarization and depolarization are affected.

In spite of its recognized limitations, electrocardiographic interpretation is a valuable adjunct in the diagnosis of myocardial infarction. By utilizing the various standard electrode positions one can determine the location and extent of most myocardial infarctions. Sample electrocardiograms from two common types of infarction are illustrated schematically in Figure 8–30. An infarct on the anterolateral surface of the heart results from occlusion of the anterior descending branch of the left coronary artery. A prominent Q wave develops in lead I, the S-T segment is elevated and the T wave is deeply inverted. A unipolar precordial electrode placed over the affected region produces a similar pattern, illustrated in Figure 8–29D. As the infarct heals, the S-T segment

returns to the baseline, leaving a prominent Q wave and an inverted T wave in lead I. This produces the well known Q_1T_1 pattern of anterior (or anterolateral) infarction.

Conversely, an infarct on the posterior or diaphragmatic aspect of the

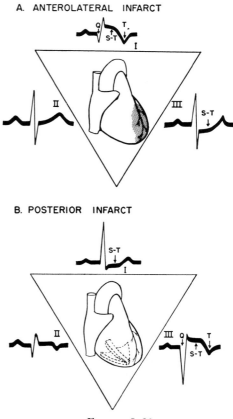

A. ANTEROLATERAL INFARCT

B. POSTERIOR INFARCT

FIGURE 8–30

A, An anterolateral infarct produced by occlusion of the anterior descending branch of the left coronary artery produces a fairly characteristic pattern. In lead I, a prominent Q wave appears with elevation of the S-T segment and inversion of the T wave. This pattern resembles that presented in Figure 8–29D. During recovery, the S-T segment returns to the baseline, leaving a Q wave and an inverted T wave in lead I (the Q_1T_1 pattern). In lead III the S-T segment is depressed and the T wave is upright, so the pattern reverts to normal more quickly in lead III than in lead I.

B, A posterior infarct produces a prominent Q wave in lead III with an elevated S-T segment and an inverted T wave. During recovery, this infarct produces the Q_3T_3 pattern.

heart usually results from occlusion of a posterior descending branch. In this case, the Q wave appears in lead III, where the S-T segment is elevated and the T wave inverted. As the infarct heals, a Q_3T_3 pattern develops. Infarction in different regions of the heart changes the patterns in the various leads. Additional details can be obtained from standard texts on electrocardiographic interpretation.[19, 21]

SUMMARY

The fundamental difficulty in electrocardiographic interpretation stems from the fact that the changes in configuration of the complexes are rather nonspecific and limited in number. For example, the QRS and T waves can have major deflections upright, downward or deformed. The S-T segment can be isoelectric, elevated, depressed or curved. Since a vast number of disease states may directly or indirectly affect the electrocardiographic complexes, certain electrocardiographic patterns must be common to many different pathologic conditions. The theoretical approach which has been followed in this chapter emphasizes the fact that interpreting changes in the configuration of individual waves and complexes frequently involves recognizing rather subtle differences which have been discovered empirically. Contrary to the usual discussion of electrocardiography, the points of similarity between complexes and mechanisms have been emphasized rather than the differences which can be demonstrated by selected examples. This attitude is not intended to depreciate or cast doubt upon electrocardiographic interpretation, but to help place it in a proper perspective. Although certain characteristic differences can be de-scribed to distinguish the patterns produced by ventricular conduction disturbances, ventricular hypertrophy and strain, myocardial infarction, and myocarditis, the basic similarities in the patterns must not be overlooked. In less extreme examples, the differences may be difficult to distinguish, particularly when more than one of these conditions is present in one patient. While a truly remarkable amount of important information can be gleaned from a routine electrocardiographic examination by a competent cardiologist, his interpretation must always be viewed in relation to all other sources of information concerning the patient under consideration. By correlating the electrocardiographic patterns with other signs and symptoms, a large number of disease states can be excluded from the differential diagnosis and a specific diagnosis often can be made. Serial electrocardiograms taken at appropriate intervals and accompanied by parallel clinical studies during the progress of a disease state will frequently establish a diagnosis when the cardiac status is in doubt at the initial examination.

Since electrocardiographic interpretation has been approached on a theoretical basis, the empirical approach has been neglected. To illustrate the kinds of patterns commonly encountered in electrocardiographic interpretation, a few examples have been presented. However, for a comprehensive discussion of electrocardiographic interpretation, the reader is referred to standard texts on the subject.

REFERENCES

1. WOODBURY, L. A., WOODBURY, J. W., and HECHT, H. H. Membrane resting and action potentials of single cardiac muscle fibers. *Circulation*, 1:264–266, 1950.

2. DRAPER, M. H., and WEIDMANN, S. Cardiac resting and action potentials recorded with an intercellular electrode. *J. Physiol.*, 115:74–94, 1951.

3. HODGKIN, A. L., and HUXLEY, A. F. Currents carried by sodium and potassium ions through the membrane of the giant axon of Loligo. *J. Physiol.*, 116:449–472, 1952.

4. HECHT, H. H. Some observations and theories concerning the electrical behavior of heart muscle. *Am. J. Med.*, 30:720–746, 1961.

5. MANNING, G. W., and AHUJA, S. P. *Electrical Activity of the Heart.* A Symposium sponsored by the Ontario Heart Assn. Springfield, Illinois, Charles C Thomas, 1969.

6. AMURA, Y. Relationship between transmembrane action potentials of single cardiac cells and their corresponding surface electrograms in vivo and in vitro and related electromechanical phenomena. *Trans. N. Y. Acad. Sci.*, 32:874–910, 1970.

7. WOODBURY, J. W., and CRILL, W. E. On the problem of impulse conduction in the atrium in nervous inhibitions. *Proc. of an International Symposium.* Oxford, Pergamon Press, 1961.

8. SANO, T., and YAMAGISHI, S. Spread of excitation from the sinus node. *Circ. Res.*, 16:423–430, 1965.

9. IRISAWA, H., and NINOMIYA, I. Repolarization phase at various sites of the right atrium. *Circ. Res.*, 19:96–103, 1966.

10. ZIMMERMAN, H. A., BERSANO, E., and DICOSKY, C. *The Auricular Electrocardiogram.* Springfield, Illinois, Charles C Thomas, 1968.

11. DURRER, D., ROOS, J. P., and BULLER, J. The spread of excitation in canine and human heart. *Electrophysiology of the Heart*, Proc. of a meeting held October 11–13, 1963 in Milan. Oxford, Pergamon Press, 1964.

12. TRAUTWEIN, W., AND KASSEBAUM, D. G. On the mechanism of spontaneous impulse generation in the pacemaker of the heart. *J. Gen. Physiol.*, 45:317–330, 1961.

13. PATTEN, B. M., and KRAMER, T. C. The initiation of contraction in the embryonic chick heart. *Amer. J. Anat.*, 53:349–375, 1933.

14. HOFF, H. E., and NAHUM, L. H. The supernormal period in the mammalian ventricle. *Amer. J. Physiol.*, 124:591–595, 1938.

15. ROSENBLUETH, A., and RAMOS, J. G. Studies on flutter and fibrillation, II. The influence of artificial obstacles on experimental auricular flutter. *Amer. Heart J.*, 33:677–684, 1947.

16. SCHERF, D., and SCHOTT, A. *Extrasystoles and Allied Arrhythmias.* New York, Grune & Stratton, 1953, 531 pp.

17. WILSON, F. N., JOHNSTON, F. D., MacLEOD, A. G., and BARKER, P. S. Electrocardiograms that represent the potential variations of a single electrode. *Amer. Heart J.* 27:19–85, 1944.

18. DOLGIN, M., GRAU, S., and KATZ, L. N. Experimental studies on the validity of the central terminal of Wilson as an indifferent reference point. *Amer. Heart J.* 37:868–880, 1949.

19. DIAMOND, E. G., *Electrocardiography.* St. Louis, C. V. Mosby Co., 1954.

20. BAYLEY, R. H., LaDUE, J. S., and YORK, D. J. Electrocardiographic changes (local ventricular ischemia and injury) produced in the dog by temporary occlusion of a coronary artery, showing a new stage in the evolution of myocardial infarction. *Amer. Heart J.* 27:164–169, 1944.

21. LAMB, L. E., *Electrocardiography and Vectorcardiography: Instrumentation Fundamentals and Clinical Applications.* Philadelphia, W. B. Saunders, 1965.

22. KOSSMANN, C. E. The electrocardiographic effects of myocardial and pericardial injury. Chap. 11 in *Disorders of the Circulatory System*, R. L. Craig, ed. New York. The Macmillan Co., 1952.

23. BAYLEY, R. H. On certain applications of modern electrocardiograph theory to the interpretation of electrocardiograms which indicate myocardial disease. *Amer. Heart J.*, 26:769–831, 1943.

24. PARDEE, H. E. B. The significance of an electrocardiogram with a large Q in lead 3. *Arch. Intern. Med.* 46:470–481, 1930.

INDEX

Numbers in *italics* refer to illustrations; (t) refers to tables.

291